Respiratory Medicine

Series Editor:
Sharon I.S. Rounds

For further volumes:
http://www.springer.com/series/7665

Linda Chlan · Marshall I. Hertz
Editors

Integrative Therapies in Lung Health and Sleep

Humana Press

Editors
Linda Chlan
School of Nursing
University of Minnesota
Minneapolis, MN 55455, USA
chlan001@umn.edu

Marshall I. Hertz
Department of Pulmonary, Allergy,
Critical Care, and Sleep Medicine
University of Minnesota
Minneapolis, MN 55455, USA
hertz001@umn.edu

ISBN 978-1-62703-912-3 ISBN 978-1-61779-579-4 (eBook)
DOI 10.1007/978-1-61779-579-4
Springer New York Dordrecht Heidelberg London

Printed on acid-free paper

Humana Press is part of Springer Science+Business Media (www.springer.com)

Foreword

In Pursuit of Well-Being

A question I often get from colleagues in medicine and nursing is some variation of "Why are people so interested in complementary or integrative therapies?" The question is sometimes posed in the context of a conversation around whether we should be teaching health professional students about these therapies, whether there is enough evidence to support their use in clinical settings, or whether they should be reimbursed or integrated into a comprehensive program of care.

While evidence shows that the largest group of people who use integrative therapies are people with chronic conditions who are seeking symptom relief, conversations with patients and clinicians have convinced me that stories and studies together paint a clearer picture.

Many years ago, a woman in her mid-thirties with advanced breast cancer came to see me explicitly to talk about her experiences in the healthcare system. She was a mother of two young children, unable to work or even care for her kids given the symptoms related to both her disease and treatment. She was grateful for the access she had to conventional cancer care—and she wisely recognized that she needed it all—chemotherapy, radiation, and surgery. The story she wanted me to understand was how much her life was improved when she began to access integrative therapies. Acupuncture helped her manage nausea; meditation and yoga put her mind at ease and reduced her anxiety and helped her sleep better. Paying attention to her diet gave her more energy. Recognizing the value of both biomedical and integrative approaches, she remarked that biomedicine helped cure her cancer while integrative therapies saved her life.

Maggie, like many of our patients, was seeking well-being in the midst of a complicated medical regimen that was focused on her medical diagnosis. Well-being encompasses not only physical health but also psychological, emotional, and spiritual health. For Maggie, being able to be an active participant in making decisions about her care contributed to her well-being. Choosing which mind/body therapy she would try, seeing a health coach, and trying acupuncture made her feel in control of a situation that seemed hopeless and beyond control. And these approaches also helped her attain better symptom management and improved her quality of life.

Well-being is not a particularly new concept. In 1946, the World Health Organization defined health as a state of complete physical, mental, and social well-being and not merely the absence of disease or infirmity. Over 30 years ago Aaron Antonovsky, a professor of sociology, coined the term *salutogenesis* to describe an approach to care that focuses on factors that support human health and well-being rather than on factors that cause disease. In many respects, the emerging field of integrative medicine or health is ideally suited to study the art and science of well-being.

Patients diagnosed with chronic lung disease, experiencing critical illness, or a sleep disorder face a myriad of complex symptoms and often an unfavorable or uncertain prognosis. I applaud Doctors Chlan and Hertz for recognizing both the challenges and opportunities we face in providing comprehensive, whole person care to this patient population. This text will heighten awareness of integrative therapies and provide an objective analysis of the evidence to support their use. The field is in its infancy and we are only beginning to see studies that are rigorously designed and that point toward understanding the mechanism of action. As with biomedicine, evidence-informed practice is important and that includes a careful examination of all kinds of evidence including studies of clinical effectiveness, randomized controlled clinical trials, qualitative studies, clinician judgment and experience, and patient preference.

Does well-being really matter? Our patients tell us definitively that it does. Even when they are struggling or suffering with a chronic or life-threatening illness, having their anxiety or depression eased, having less pain, or being able to sleep enables them to live whatever life they have more fully. As clinicians and scientists, this doesn't mean that we uncritically assume that anything and everything is safe, nor does it mean that we dismiss out of hand therapies that we are unfamiliar with. I hope that this book inspires you to become more informed, that you will seek opportunities to build strong interdisciplinary teams that include clinicians who provide integrative therapies, and that you will contribute to the important mission of generating research to rigorously evaluate all therapies, biomedical and integrative. And, I hope that it sparks a curiosity so that you will ask your patients about what they are doing to improve their well-being in the midst of their disease or health challenge.

Minneapolis, MN, USA Mary Jo Kreitzer, PhD, RN, FAAN

Preface

Complementary and Alternative Medicine (CAM) includes a group of diverse medical and healthcare systems, practices, and products that are generally not considered to be part of conventional medicine [1]. One method to organize these numerous and diverse group of practices, systems, and products is into four domains: Mind–body practices, Biologically based practices, Manipulative- and body-based practices, and Energy medicine. Whole Medical Systems, which cut across all of the domains, include homeopathic medicine, naturopathic medicine, Ayurveda, and Traditional Chinese Medicine. Some persons and cultures exclusively use Whole Medical Systems rather than allopathic or Western medicine for their health care.

The use of CAM therapies among adults in the United States is common and shows no sign of decreasing. According to a recent report from the National Health Interview Survey [2], over 35% of adults use some form of CAM treatment, modality, or practice. Adults with one or more chronic health conditions, including asthma and emphysema, are the most likely to use CAM modalities [3]. Many reasons are provided by patients for their use of CAM, including personal philosophy, need for greater control in healthcare decisions, and general dissatisfaction with conventional treatments. Today's consumers and their family members advocate that CAM therapies be continued and/or included in the plan of care for acutely ill patients. Thus, it is incumbent upon healthcare providers to be knowledgeable about the broad field of CAM, including those providers working with persons who experience acute or chronic lung disorders and sleep issues. Equally important is for healthcare providers to be knowledgeable in the evaluation of specific CAM therapies and how to advise patients on their use or nonuse, including potential dangerous interactions of herbal supplements with prescribed medications. Likewise, persons with chronic, debilitating lung diseases may be desperate for any treatment or modality that promises to palliate shortness of breath and other symptoms. There are, however, 'sham' modalities that should not be used, as they may be totally worthless and may even be dangerous if used by certain patients. Healthcare providers need to be informed regarding all therapies in which their patients may engage, including all CAM practices, which could positively or adversely affect the plan of care.

The purposes of this text are to provide clinicians caring for patients with acute or chronic lung disorders and sleep conditions with: (1) an overview of integrative therapies and their scientific bases; and (2) information and suggestions for evaluating the implementation of integrative therapies into practice. The term "Integrative" was chosen in order to focus the scope of this textbook on those CAM treatments, modalities, and practices that are combined with conventional medical treatment and for which there is some evidence of safety and efficacy. Whole Medical Systems, with a specific focus on Traditional Chinese Medicine (TCM), are addressed in a separate chapter.

This text is not intended to be an exhaustive review of integrative therapies, nor is it intended to include all pulmonary and sleep disorders. Each of the chapters that address a specific health condition or illness provides a brief overview of its incidence, clinical features, and challenges associated with clinical management. Each of the chapters addresses the current state of the science in the four organizing CAM domains, as reported in available literature including any benefits, risks, or safety considerations.

Unique aspects of this text are the chapters related to evaluation of integrative therapies evidence; ground-breaking animal model research with herbal preparations focused on the serious problem of sepsis in the ICU; guidance for counseling patients with chronic lung illness who may be desperate for a cure; and palliative and end-of-life care for chronic lung conditions.

Our hope is that clinicians in various healthcare settings will find the information contained in this text beneficial to their practice and the patients for whom they provide care.

Minneapolis, MN, USA

Linda Chlan
Marshall I. Hertz

References

1. NCCAM Fact Sheet. www.nccam.nih.gov. Accessed June 2010.
2. U.S. Department of Health and Human Services, Centers for Disease Control and Prevention, National Center for Health Statistics. Complementary and alternative medicine use among adults and children: United States, 2007. National Health Statistics Reports 12; December 10;2008.
3. Saydah S, Eberhardt M. Use of complementary and alternative medicine use among adults with chronic diseases: United States 2002. J Altern Complement Med. 2006; 12: 805–12.

Acknowledgments

We would like to take this opportunity to thank all of our chapter authors for their contributions to this text. Their content expertise was invaluable. We appreciate their commitment to the care and outcomes for patients with lung disorders, experiencing the challenges of critical illness, or sleep disorders.

We would also like to extend our gratitude to Barbara Lopez-Lucio, our Springer Developmental Editor. Barbara was tenacious in keeping us all on track to meet our publication deadline while ensuring the best quality text possible. Thank you, Barbara. We could not have done all the work without your assistance.

Contents

Contributors

Scott C. Bell, MBBS, MD, FRACP Department of Thoracic Medicine, The Prince Charles Hospital, Brisbane, QLD, Australia

Linda Berg-Cross, PhD, ABPP, CBSM Department of Psychology, Howard University, Washington, DC, USA

Yongjun Bian, MD, PhD Guang An Men Hospital, China Academy of Chinese Medical Science, Beijing, China

Malcolm N. Blumenthal, MD Department of Medicine, Pediatrics and Laboratory Medicine, University of Minnesota, Minneapolis, MN, USA

Claire A. Butler, MB, BCh, BAO, MRCP Department of Thoracic Medicine, The Prince Charles Hospital, Brisbane, QLD, Australia

Margaret-Ann Carno, PhD, MBA, CPNP, DABSM, FNAP School of Nursing, University of Rochester, Rochester, NY, USA

Jessie Casida, PhD College of Nursing, Wayne State University, Detroit, MI, USA

Hunter C. Champion, MD, PhD, FAHA Division of Pulmonary, Allergy and Critical Care Medicine, Dorothy P. and Richard P. Simmons Center for Interstitial Lung Disease, University of Pittsburgh, Pittsburgh, PA, USA

Annette DeVito Dabbs, PhD, RN, FAAN School of Nursing, University of Pittsburgh, Pittsburgh, PA, USA

DorAnne M. Donesky, PhD, RN Department of Physiological Nursing, University of California, San Francisco, CA, USA

Yvette Erasmus, MEd Department of Clinical Psychology, American School of Professional Psychology, Twin Cities, Eagan, MN, USA

Lauren M. Fine, MD Department of Pulmonary, Allergy and Critical Care, University of Minnesota, Minneapolis, MN, USA

Kevin F. Gibson, MD Department of Pulmonary, Allergy and Critical Care Medicine, Dorothy P. and Richard P. Simmons Center for Interstitial Lung Disease, University of Pittsburgh, Pittsburgh, PA, USA

Sandra W. Gordon-Kolb, MD, MMM Department of Palliative Medicine, Fairview Health Services, Minneapolis, MN, USA

Margo A. Halm, RN, PhD, ACNS-BC Department of Nursing Administration, Salem Hospital, Salem, OR, USA

Kate M. Hathaway, PhD, LP Center for Spirituality and Healing, University of Minnesota, Minneapolis, MN, USA

Department of Clinical Psychology, American School of Professional Psychology, Twin Cities, Eagan, MN, USA

Julie K. Katseres, DNP, MSN, BSN, Diploma Department of Hospice and Palliative Care, Minneapolis VA Health Care System, Minneapolis, MN, USA

Mary Jo Kreitzer, PhD, RN, FAAN School of Nursing, Center for Spirituality and Healing, University of Minnesota, Minneapolis, MN, USA

Guangxi Li, MD Mayo Clinic, Rochester, MN, USA

Guoqin Li, MD Guang An Men Hospital, China Academy of Chinese Medical Science, Beijing, China

Kathleen Oare Lindell, PhD, RN Department of Pulmonary, Allergy and Critical Care Medicine, Dorothy P. and Richard P. Simmons Center for Interstitial Lung Disease, University of Pittsburg, Pittsburgh, PA, USA

Kathryn L. Miele, MA Department of Emergency Medicine, North Shore University Hospital, Manhasset, NY, USA

LuAnn Nowak, PhD College of Nursing, Wayne State University, Detroit, MI, USA

Andrew E. Sama, MD Department of Emergency Medicine, North Shore University Hospital, Manhasset, NY, USA

Kathleen F. Sarmiento, MD, MPH Division of Pulmonary and Critical Care Medicine, University of Maryland School of Medicine, Baltimore, MD, USA

Alice C. Shapiro, PhD, RD, LN Department of Oncology Research, Park Nicollet Health Services, St. Louis Park, MN, USA

Mi-Kyung Song, PhD, RN School of Nursing, University of North Carolina at Chapel Hill, Chapel Hill, NC, USA

Karen K. Swenson, PhD Department of Oncology Research, Park Nicollet Health Services, St. Louis Park, MN, USA

Sheila D. Switzer, BSN University of Pittsburgh School of Nursing, Camp Hill, PA, USA

Yi Tian, MD, MSc Guang An Men Hospital, China Academy of Chinese Medical Science, Beijing, China

Mary Fran Tracy, PhD, RN University of Minnesota Medical Center, Minneapolis, MN, USA

Amy T. Wang, MD Mayo Clinic, Rochester, MN, USA

Fang Wang, MD, PhD Department of Pulmonary Medicine, Guang An Men Hospital, China Academy of Chinese Medical Science, Beijing, China

Haichao Wang, PhD Department of Emergency Medicine, North Shore University Hospital, Manhasset, NY, USA

Jie Wang, MD, PhD Guang An Men Hospital, China Academy of Chinese Medical Science, Beijing, China

Lei Wang, MD, PhD Guang An Men Hospital, China Academy of Chinese Medical Science, Beijing, China

Shihan Wang, MD, PhD Guang An Men Hospital, China Academy of Chinese Medical Science, Beijing, China

Mary F. Ward, MS, RN Department of Emergency Medicine, North Shore University Hospital, Manhasset, NY, USA

Shu Zhu, MD, PhD Department of Emergency Medicine, North Shore University Hospital, Manhasset, NY, USA

Part I
General

Chapter 1
Overview of Integrative Therapies and Healing Practices

Mary Jo Kreitzer

Abstract Growth in the use of integrative therapies has been stimulated by consumer interest in a more comprehensive, holistic approach to care that includes both conventional medical practices and complementary or integrative therapies. Increased utilization has also been fueled by the growing evidence base that has documented safety and efficacy for many of these unconventional practices. Increasingly, health professional students are exposed to integrative therapies within their curriculum and within clinical sites where they practice. Students, faculty teaching in health professional schools, and practitioners recognize the importance of educating students about integrative health and offering services that provide patients choice and the opportunity to integrate the best of conventional and CAM approaches. The policy issues surrounding integrative health/medicine are complex and include education and workforce development, care delivery, and economics and financing issues. For patients facing chronic health issues such as pulmonary disease and sleep disorders, integrative health approaches may offer improved symptom management and quality of life.

Keywords Integrative health • Integrative medicine • Complementary and alternative medicine • CAM utilization

According to the National Health Interview Survey (NHIS) conducted in 2007, approximately 38% of adults in the United States and close to 12% of children aged 17 and under use some form of complementary and alternative medicine (CAM) [1]. The survey, developed by the National Center for Complementary and

M.J. Kreitzer, PhD, RN, FAAN (✉)
School of Nursing, Center for Spirituality and Healing, University of Minnesota, Minneapolis, MN 55455, USA
e-mail: Kreit003@umn.edu

L. Chlan and M.I. Hertz (eds.), *Integrative Therapies in Lung Health and Sleep*, Respiratory Medicine 4, DOI 10.1007/978-1-61779-579-4_1,

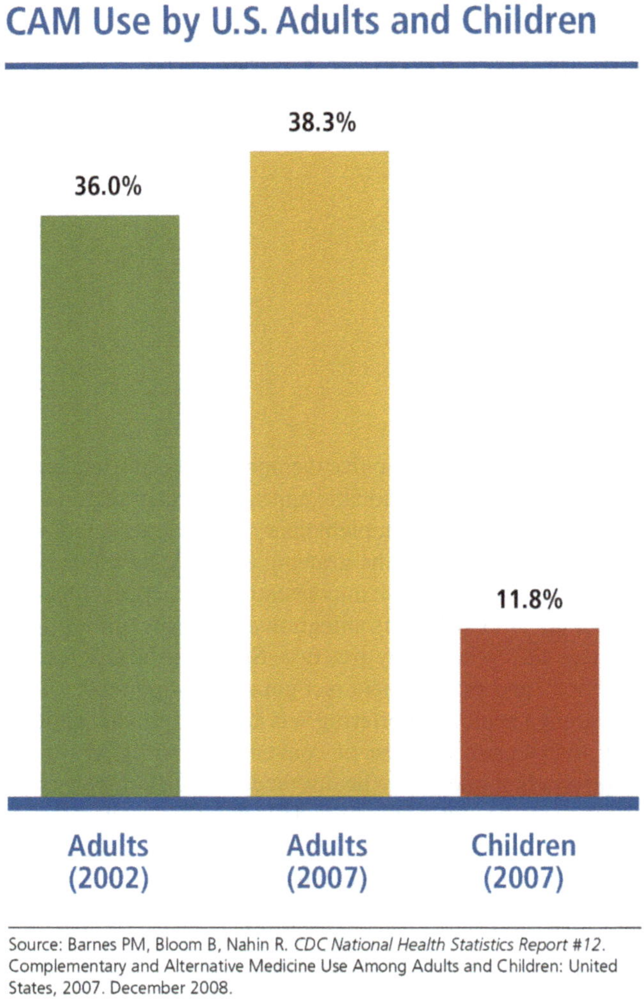

Fig. 1.1 CAM use in US adults and children. Percentage of US adults in 2002 vs. 2007 and children in 2007 who used complementary and alternative medicine (CAM) in the past 12 months. The figures show that CAM use among adults has remained relatively steady from 2002 to 2007. From National Center for Complementary and Alternative Medicine, NIH, DHHS

Alternative Medicine (NCCAM), part of the National Institutes of Health (NIH) and the National Center for Health Statistics (NCHS), a part of the Centers for Disease Control and Prevention (CDC), included questions on 36 types of CAM therapies commonly used in the United States and represents the most comprehensive survey to date on the utilization of CAM in the United States. As noted in Fig. 1.1, CAM use by adults remained relatively stable between 2002 and 2007.

CAM is defined by NCCAM as a group of diverse medical and healthcare systems, practices, and products not generally considered to be part of conventional medicine, though NCCAM acknowledges that the boundaries between CAM and conventional medicine are not absolute and that specific CAM practices may, over time, become widely accepted [2]. The term "complementary medicine" refers to the use of CAM together with conventional medicine while the phrase "alternative medicine" implies that CAM is used in lieu of conventional medicine. Over the past 5 years, integrative health, integrative therapies, and integrative medicine have emerged as descriptions of an approach to care that combines both conventional and CAM treatments that are safe and effective.

The purpose of this chapter is provide an overview of the diverse field commonly called alternative, complementary, or integrative health/medicine and to highlight broad issues related to education, practice, regulation, and policy.

Taxonomy of CAM

While the field of CAM is very diverse and is estimated to include over 1,800 different therapies/modalities, NCCAM has informally organized CAM practices into the following categories: mind–body medicine, natural products, manipulative and body-based practices, and a category—other CAM practices—that includes energy healing such as Reiki and healing touch and whole medical systems such as traditional Chinese and Ayurvedic medicine. The NCCAM categories have changed over time and are considered by many practitioners in the field to be fairly arbitrary and not particularly descriptive. The "other" category is extremely diverse and as large as the other three categories combined.

Mind–Body Medicine

Mind–body practices include meditation, yoga, tai chi, guided imagery, clinical hypnosis, biofeedback, deep breathing exercises, progressive relaxation, and creative arts therapies such as music, dance, and art therapy. Mind–body approaches are designed to enhance the mind's capacity to affect bodily function and symptoms and are based on the science of psychoneuroimmunology, a field of study that focuses on how the mind and emotions are connected to the autonomic nervous, endocrine, and immune systems.

Natural Products

The natural products category includes herbal or botanical medicine including aromatherapy, vitamins, dietary supplements, and the use of probiotics. Probiotics are live organisms, usually bacteria, that are similar to microorganisms found in the human digestive tract and that may have beneficial effects. An example of a commonly used probiotic is yogurt, which contains lactobacillus.

Manipulative and Body-Based Practices

Manipulative and body-based practices focus on the structures and systems of the body including the bones, joints, soft tissues, and circulatory and lymphatic systems. Massage, lymphatic drainage, cranial–sacral therapy, and spinal manipulation are examples of commonly used therapies.

Other CAM Practices

Just as allopathic medicine is a complete system of care based on a particular set of theories and practices, there are other whole medical systems that have evolved over time in different cultures and are considered to fall within CAM. Examples of whole medical systems include Ayurvedic (east Indian) medicine, traditional Chinese medicine, Tibetan medicine, and Native American medicine. Naturopathy and homeopathy are also examples of whole medical systems.

NCCAM also recognizes other CAM practices including movement therapies such as the Feldenkrais method and Pilates, energy therapies such as healing touch and Reiki, and the practice of indigenous/traditional healers. The NCCAM website includes detailed descriptions of each of the therapies and systems of healing identified above [3].

Patterns of CAM Utilization

Among adults in the United States, the most commonly used CAM therapies include natural products, deep breathing exercises, meditation, chiropractic or osteopathic manipulation, and yoga [1] (Fig. 1.2). Among natural products, the most commonly used substances were fish oil/omega 3, glucosamine, echinacea, flaxseed oil or pills, and ginseng. Therapies with the most significant increase in use between 2002 and 2007 were deep breathing (11.6–12.7%), meditation (7.6–9.4%), massage (5.0–8.3%), and yoga (5.1–6.1%).

The demographic pattern of use reported in the NHIS survey has remained consistent between 2002 and 2007. The highest users of CAM are women (42.8%, compared to men 33.5%), with more education (masters, doctorate, or professional degree 55.4%), and higher incomes. Multiple studies have confirmed that the highest users of CAM are people with chronic illnesses including asthma [4], cancer [5], and musculoskeletal pain [6]. These findings are consistent with the belief that users of CAM are seeking symptom relief and often use CAM in conjunction with conventional approaches. In a study of oncology patients, Lafferty et al. [7] found that pain was the most common presenting complaint to CAM providers and that CAM was being used to augment proven treatments rather than to replace them.

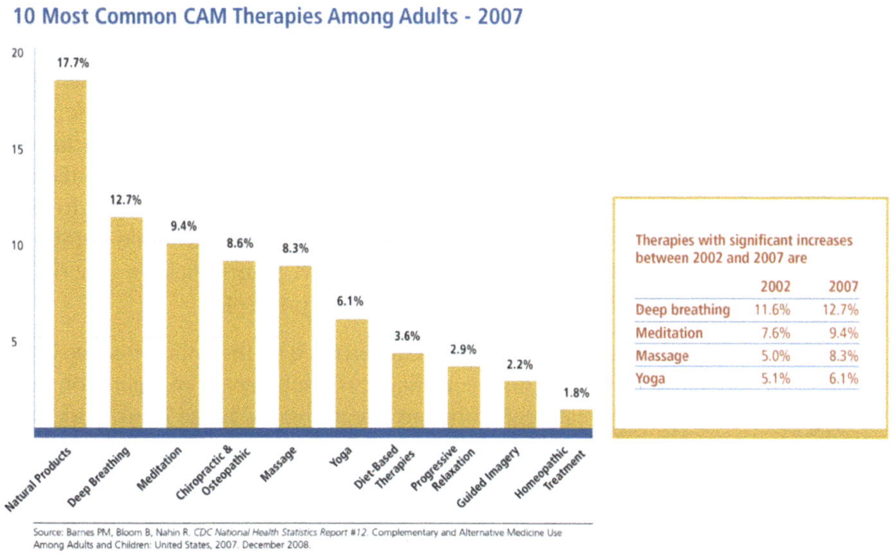

Fig. 1.2 Ten most common CAM therapies among adults—2007. Percentage of adults in 2007 who used the ten most common complementary and alternative medicine (CAM) therapies. The most commonly used CAM therapy among adults in 2007 was nonvitamin, nonmineral natural products. *Box* shows therapies with significant increases in use between 2002 and 2007: deep breathing, meditation, massage, and yoga. From National Center for Complementary and Alternative Medicine, NIH, DHHS

While some CAM is offered to patients at no additional charge in inpatient care settings or is covered by third party reimbursement, the majority of CAM charges are paid out of pocket. The 2007 NHIS survey [8] found that 83 million adults spent $33.9 billion out of pocket on visits to CAM practitioners and on purchases of CAM products, classes, and materials. This represents 11.2% of total out-of-pocket expenditures on health care in the United States. Of the $33.9 billion spent, $22 billion or 64.9% were self-care costs including CAM products, classes, and materials and $11.9 billion (35.1%) were practitioner costs.

Philosophic Beliefs Underlying Integrative Health and Integrative Medicine

While the terms alternative, complementary, and integrative medicine are often used interchangeably, they do reflect very different philosophical perspectives. As the name implies, alternative medical practices are used in place of standard medical treatments. In the treatment of chronic pain, acupuncture has been found to be a safe and effective alternative that may be used in lieu of pharmacological management. In contrast, there are no alternative treatments that have been found effective for curing cancer. The phrase complementary medicine suggests that CAM modalities are used to complement standard medical treatments. While there are many occasions when CAM and conventional therapy are complementary to each other, the term implies that CAM is secondary. Patients who are anxious or experiencing chronic stress may elect to use approaches such as meditation or yoga that in fact may become their primary mode of treatment. The phrase integrative medicine, coined by the physician Andrew Weil, refers to a comprehensive approach to care that engages the patient's body, mind, and spirit. Integrative medicine combines standard medical treatment with evidence-based CAM approaches. In describing integrative medicine, Weil [9] identified the following principles:

- Natural healing power—Integrative medicine is based on the notion that the body has an innate capacity for healing, self-diagnosis, self-repair, regeneration, and adaptation. The goal of treatment within an integrative medicine framework is to support, facilitate, and augment that innate capacity.
- Whole person care—Integrative medicine embraces the understanding that the body, mind, and spirit are inextricably linked and that all of these dimensions are relevant to health and the effective treatment of disease.
- Importance of lifestyle—Lifestyle choices that people make may have a larger impact on their overall health than their genetic predisposition.
- Health-care provider–patient relationship—Therapeutic relationships contribute to health and healing and are critical for patients and providers.

While these principles are beginning to shape and inform the practice of medicine and many other disciplines, these ideas have always been considered to be the essence of nursing. Florence Nightingale wrote in the 1860s that the role of the nurse was to put the patient in the best possible condition so that nature could act and self-healing occur. Ms. Nightingale stressed the importance of fresh air, natural light, touch, music, spirituality, presence, and caring [10]. Nursing theories have long embraced concepts of self-care [11], health as expanding consciousness [12], adaptation [13], transpersonal caring [14], unitary human beings [15], and human becoming [16]. Given the focus of nursing on human health, human potential, and health promotion, as well as management of illness and disease, the profession more often uses the phrase integrative health or holistic health to reflect the concepts more recently defined by Dr. Weil as integrative medicine.

NIH National Center for Complementary and Alternative Medicine

In large part in response to consumer demand, the US Congress passed legislation in 1991 to establish an office within NIH to study unconventional medical practices. In 1993, the Office of Alternative Medicine (OAM) was created within NIH with the directive that they were to facilitate the study and evaluation of complementary and alternative medical practices and to disseminate the resulting information to the public. Legislation passed by Congress in 1998 elevated the OAM to the NCCAM. The mission of NCCAM [17] is to:

- Explore complementary and alternative healing practices in the context of rigorous science.
- Train CAM researchers.
- Disseminate authoritative information to the public and professionals.
- NCCAM currently has a staff of approximately 65 FTE (full-time equivalent) and an annual budget (FY10) of $128.8 million.

A considerable amount of CAM research is funded by other federal agencies. For example, in FY 2008, the National Cancer Institute (NCI) supported $121.5 million in CAM-related research [18]. This represented over 444 projects in the form of grants, cooperative agreements, supplements, or contracts. Within NCI and other NIH institutes, CAM research is integrated throughout various intramural and extramural program areas.

While the majority of NCCAM funding has been directed to research, two requests for proposals (RFAs), described below, have focused on education of health professionals.

Health Professional Education and Attitudes of Health Professionals

As consumer interest and evidence supporting the safety and efficacy of integrative therapies continue to grow, academic institutions that prepare health professionals have begun to incorporate content on integrative therapies into their curricula. Over a period of 7 years beginning in 2000, NCCAM funded 15 institutions to develop curricula under a program announcement called the "Complementary and Alternative Medicine (CAM) Education Project Grant." Twelve grants went to medical schools, one grant to a nursing school, one grant to the American Medical Student Association, and one grant to an institution (University of Minnesota) that launched a curriculum project focused on three schools—nursing, medicine, and pharmacy. The immediate goal of the program was to encourage and support the incorporation of CAM information into medical, dental, nursing, and allied health professional school curricula into residency programs and into continuing education courses. The longer term goal of this initiative was to accelerate the integration of CAM and conventional medicine [19].

In 1999, eight institutions formed the Consortium of Academic Health Centers for Integrative Medicine (CAHCIM). These academic health centers each had medical schools with formally established integrative medicine programs. Between 1999 and 2010, the consortium experienced exponential growth and now includes 46 highly esteemed medical schools in the United States and Canada [20]. Within nursing, accreditation standards of undergraduate- and graduate-level programs reflect a focus on person-centered, holistic care and the incorporation of integrative therapies; several programs offer specialization in integrative or holistic health. Examples of graduate programs offering specialization include:

- The University of Minnesota School of Nursing offers a doctorate of nursing practice (DNP) in integrative health and healing [21].
- The University of Portland offers a DNP with a family nurse practitioner and integrative health specialization [22].
- New York University offers a holistic nurse practitioner master's degree [23].

Academic institutions that prepare CAM practitioners such as chiropractors, massage therapists, naturopathic physicians, and traditional Chinese medicine practitioners are also modifying curricula to better prepare students to work within integrative health-care settings. NCCAM offered a grant program to CAM institutions to enhance the quality and quantity of research content in curricula [24]. Supported by this initiative, CAM schools are making a concerted effort to teach students principles of evidence-informed practice. One of the grantees, Northwestern Health Sciences University, is integrating evidence-informed practice into three programs: chiropractic, massage, and acupuncture/Oriental medicine. The long-term objective of Northwestern's initiative is to facilitate the practice of evidence-based health care among CAM practitioners [25]. As further evidence of the maturing of the field, a new organization was formed in 2004, the Academic Consortium for Complementary and Alternative Health Care (ACCAHC). The mission of ACCAHC is to create and sustain a network of national CAM educational organizations and agencies to promote mutual understanding, collaborative activities, and interdisciplinary health-care education. Members include councils of colleges and schools, accrediting agencies, and certification and testing organizations associated with the five distinctly licensed complementary health-care professions which have a federally recognized accrediting agency: acupuncture and Oriental medicine, chiropractic, direct entry midwifery, massage therapy, and naturopathic medicine [26].

As evidence regarding the safety and efficacy of integrative approaches has increased, attitudes among health professionals have also evolved. In a study of attitudes toward CAM among medical, nursing, and pharmacy faculty and students, Kreitzer et al. [27] found that more than 90% of faculty and students believe that clinical care should integrate the best of conventional and CAM practices and that health professionals should be prepared to advise patients about commonly used CAM therapies; 88% of faculty and 84% of students indicated that CAM should be included in their school's curriculum. While there were similarities among the three faculty groups, the nursing faculty expressed the greatest interest in practicing CAM. Kurtz et al. [28] conducted a study of primary care physicians' attitudes and practices regarding CAM. Physicians were most likely to either use or refer patients for CAM for chronic problems (82%), failure of traditional modes of therapy (71.9%), psychiatric disorders (53.2%), and behavioral problems (50.8%). The most common modes of therapy referred to were massage therapy, acupuncture, self-help groups, biofeedback, and relaxation therapy. Female physicians were more likely to talk with their patients about CAM or refer them for CAM. Younger doctors were more likely to use CAM for themselves or their family. Family physicians and general internists were more likely to discuss CAM with their patients than were pediatricians. In a survey of clinical nurse specialists at the Mayo Clinic, Rochester, MN, 57% reported that CAM therapies were highly beneficial to patients while 43% indicated that CAM therapies had some benefit. Therapies believed to be most beneficial to patients were massage, meditation, music, and guided imagery [29].

Health Policy and Integrative Health/Medicine

In February 2009, the US Senate Committee on Health, Education, Labor, and Pensions held two hearings on integrative health as the early conversation on health-care reform began in Washington. The titles of the hearings reflect the interest at a federal level in what is now commonly called integrative health—Integrative Health: Pathway to Health Reform and Integrative Health: Pathway to a Healthier Nation [30]. The hearings included evidence on consumer demand for expanded health-care options and on clinical outcomes of integrated care.

The same week as these two senate hearings, the Institute of Medicine (IOM) and the Bravewell Collaborative convened a summit to explore the science and practice of integrative medicine and examine ways that integrative approaches might shift the orientation of our health-care system from the current sporadic, reactive, and physician-centric approach to one that fosters an emphasis on health, wellness, early intervention for disease, and patient empowerment. The proceedings of the summit *Integrative Medicine and the Health of the Public* describe a vision for integrative health and medicine and information on models of care, the science of integrative medicine, workforce and education issues, economics, and policy implications [31].

Prior to 2009, there were two other national policy initiatives on CAM: the White House Commission on Complementary and Alternative Medicine Policy (WHCCAMP) [32] and the IOM CAM Study Committee [33]. President William J. Clinton issued an executive order (Executive Order No. 13147) in March 2000 that established the WHCCAMP. The primary task of the commission was to provide the Secretary of Health and Human Services (HHS) with legislative and administrative recommendations for "ensuring that public policy maximizes the potential benefits of CAM therapies to consumers" [32]. The 20-member commission focused on the following four areas:

- Education and training of health-care practitioners
- Coordination of research to increase knowledge about CAM products
- Provision of reliable and useful information on CAM to health professionals
- Provision of guidance on the appropriate access to and delivery of CAM

The 29 recommendations addressed CAM information development and dissemination, access and delivery of safe and effective CAM services, coverage and reimbursement, use of CAM to promote wellness and health, the importance of incorporating CAM information in the education of health professionals, and the need for coordinated federal efforts. The final recommendation was that the president, Secretary of HHS, or Congress create an office to coordinate federal CAM activities and to facilitate the integration into the nation's health-care system of those complementary and alternative health-care practices and products determined to be safe and effective. With a change in administration at the executive level and within Congress, there was not a clear mandate for implementing the White House Commission recommendations, although a number of them were acted on incrementally within various public and private organizations and bodies at federal and state levels. For example, accreditation bodies such as the American Association of Colleges of Nursing incorporated content on integrative therapies within documents that detail accreditation requirements. Some states have continued to expand their regulation of CAM providers, and hospitals and health systems have continued to increase their offerings of integrative services to the public. NCCAM has continued to receive increases in funding, though modest in the last 5 years.

In 2002, 16 NIH institutes, centers, and offices and the Agency for Healthcare Research and Quality (AHRQ) asked the IOM to convene a study committee to explore scientific, policy, and practice questions that arise from the significant and increasing use of CAM therapies by the American public. The report [33] emphasized that decisions about the use of specific CAM therapies should primarily depend on whether or not they have been shown to be safe and effective; it concluded that the goal should be the provision of comprehensive health care that:

- Is based on the best scientific evidence available regarding benefits and harm
- Encourages patients to share in decision-making about therapeutic options
- Promotes choices in care that include CAM therapies when appropriate

The committee also cited the need for tools such as guidelines that would aid conventional practitioners' decision-making about offering or recommending CAM, where patients might be referred, and what organizational structures are most appropriate for the delivery of integrated care. In recommending the development of such tools, the committee noted that the goal is to provide comprehensive care that is safe, effective, interdisciplinary, and collaborative. Recommendations were identified that would strengthen the Dietary Supplement Health and Education Act of 1994, expand research funding, promote teaching CAM content in health profession schools, and expand the number of providers able to work in integrated care.

Summary

The growth of integrative therapies had been stimulated by consumer interest in a more comprehensive, holistic approach to care that includes both conventional medical practices and complementary or integrative therapies. Increased utilization has also been fueled by the growing evidence base that has documented safety and efficacy for many of these unconventional practices. Recognizing the importance of these modalities and integrative models of care, NIH established an institute, the NCCAM, which is focused on generating and disseminating the science underlying CAM.

Increasingly, health professional students are exposed to integrative therapies within their curriculum and within clinical sites where they practice. Students, faculty teaching in health professional schools, and practitioners recognize the importance of educating students about integrative health and offering services that provide patients choice and the opportunity to integrate the best of conventional and CAM approaches.

The policy issues surrounding integrative health/medicine are complex and include education and workforce development, care delivery, and economics and financing issues. For patients facing chronic health issues such as pulmonary disease and sleep disorders, integrative health approaches may offer improved symptom management and quality of life.

References

1. Barnes PM, Bloom B, Nahin R. CDC National Health Statistics Report #12. Complementary and alternative medicine use among adults and children: United States, 2008
2. http://nccam.nih.gov/health/whatiscam/. Accessed Jan 19, 2011.
3. http://nccam.nih.gov/health/atoz.htm. Accessed Jan 19, 2011
4. Joubert A, Kidd-Taylor A, Christopher G, Nanda J, Warren R, Lindong I, Bronner Y. Complementary and alternative medical practice: self-care preferred vs. practitioner-based care among patients with asthma. J Natl Med Assoc. 2010;102(7):562–9.
5. Vapiwaia R, Mick R, Hampshire M, Metz J. Patient initiation of complementary and alternative medical therapies (CAM) during conventional cancer treatment. J Clin Oncol. 2005;23(16s):8131.
6. Artus M, Croft A, Lewis M. The use of CAM and conventional treatments among primary care consulters with chronic musculoskeletal pain. BMC Fam Pract. 2007;8:(26). doi:10.1186/1471-2296-8-26.
7. Laffery WE, Bellas A, Corage A, Tyree PT, Standish L, Patterson R. The use of complementary and alternative medical providers by insured cancer patients in Washington State. Cancer. 2004;100(7):1522–30.
8. Nahin R. Barnes PM, Stussman BJ, Bloom B. Costs of complementary and alternative medicine (CAM) and frequency of visits to CAM practitioners: United States; 2007.
9. Weil A. Why integrative oncology? In: Abrams D, Weil A, editors. Integrative oncology. New York, NY: Oxford University Press; 2009. p. 3–14.
10. Nightingale F. Notes on Nursing. London: Harrison; 1860.
11. Orem D. Nursing: Concepts of Practice (5th ed). St. Louis: Mosby; 1995.
12. Newman M. Health as Expanding Consciousness. 2nd ed. New York, NY: National League for Nursing; 1994.
13. Roy C, Andrews H. The Roy Adaptation Model. 2nd ed. Stamford, CT: Appleton & Lange; 1999.
14. Watson J. Human Science and Human Care. New York, NY: National League for Nursing; 1988.
15. Rogers M. The Theoretical Basis for Nursing. Philadelphia: FA Davis; 1970.
16. Parse R. Human becoming: parse's theory of nursing. Nurs Sci Q. 1992;2:35–42.
17. http://nccam.nih.gov/about/ataglance/. Accessed Jan 22, 2011.

18. http://www.cancer.gov/cam/research_portfolio.html. Access Jan 19, 2011.
19. http://nccam.nih.gov/grants/types/r25/. Accessed Jan 20, 2011.
20. http://www.imconsortium.org/home.html. Accessed Jan 20, 2011.
21. http://www.nursing.umn.edu/DNP/Specialties/IntegrativeHealthandHealing/home.html. Accessed Jan 30, 2011.
22. http://nursing.up.edu/default.aspx?cid=8002&pid=207. Accessed Jan 20, 2011.
23. http://www.nyu.edu/nursing/academicprograms/masters/programs/holistic.html. Accessed Jan 20, 2011.
24. http://grants.nih.gov/grants/guide/pa-files/PAR-08-095.html. Accessed Jan 20, 2011
25. http://www.nwhealth.edu/research/WHCCS/projects/nccamed.html. Accessed Jan 30, 2011.
26. http://www.accahc.org/. Accessed Jan 30, 2011
27. Kreitzer MJ, Mitten D, Shandeling J. Attitudes toward CAM among medical, nursing, and pharmacy faculty and students: a comparative analysis. Altern Therap Health Med. 2002: 8(6):44–7, 50–53.
28. Kurtz M, Nolan R, Rittinger W. Primary care physicians' attitudes and practices regarding complementary and alternative medicine. J Am Osteopath Assoc. 2003;103(12):597–602.
29. Cutshall S, Derscheid D, Miers A, et al. Knowledge, attitudes and use of complementary and alternative therapies among clinical nurse specialists in an academic health center. Clin Nurse Spec. 2010;24(3):125–31.
30. U.S. Senate Committee on Health, Education, Labor and Pensions. (2009). Hearings and executive sessions. http://help.senate.gov/Hearings.html. Accessed January 11, 2010.
31. Institute of Medicine. Integrative medicine and the health of the public. Washington, DC: National Academies; 2009.
32. White House Commission on Complementary and Alternative Medicine Policy. (2002). Final report. www.whccamp.hhs.gov/finalreport.html. Accessed Jan 11, 2010.
33. Institute of Medicine. Complementary and alternative medicine in the United States. Washington, DC: National Academies; 2005.

Chapter 2
Evaluation of Integrative Therapies for Research and Practice

Margo A. Halm and Julie K. Katseres

Abstract This chapter provides an overview of evaluating integrative therapies from both a scientific, empirical standpoint, as well as from a practical clinical perspective. The challenges of evaluating integrative therapies are outlined, including prevailing research paradigms and the nature of integrative therapies themselves and the conditions they are often used to ameliorate. Major steps to achieving evidence-based integrative therapy practice are highlighted: (1) formulating an answerable question, (2) conducting an efficient literature search, (3) critically appraising the evidence, (4) applying results in healthcare decisions, and (5) evaluating outcomes. Within these steps, considerations for appraising explanatory, pragmatic, and qualitative trials are discussed. Similarly, readers are enlightened on patient, practitioner, and institutional factors to consider in the application of integrative therapies to practice in order to achieve good clinical care for patients.

Keywords Integrative therapies • Biological vs. clinical plausibility • Inquiry paradigms • Randomized controlled trials (explanatory vs. pragmatic) • Evidence hierarchy • Personal readiness (patient, practitioner) • Institutional philosophy • Feasibility

An integrative therapy is one that is used instead of ("alternative") or in addition to ("complementary") the conventionally accepted therapy for a condition and for which there is safety and effectiveness; it refers to a holistic approach to health, not

M.A. Halm, RN, PhD, ACNS-BC (✉)
Department of Nursing Administration, Salem Hospital, 890 Oak Street SE, Salem, OR 97301, USA
e-mail: margo.halm@salemhospital.org

J.K. Katseres, DNP, MSN, BSN, Diploma
Department of Hospice and Palliative Care, Minneapolis VA Health Care System, One Veterans Drive, Minneapolis, MN 55417, USA

L. Chlan and M.I. Hertz (eds.), *Integrative Therapies in Lung Health and Sleep*, Respiratory Medicine 4, DOI 10.1007/978-1-61779-579-4_2,

only physical but also mind and spirit [1, 2]. Over 200 modalities constitute integrative therapies. The original five domains defined by the National Center for Complementary and Alternative Medicine (NCCAM) have recently been modified to four domains: natural products, mind–body medicine, manipulative and body-based practices, and "other integrative practices."

Natural products refer to the use of botanicals (herbal and spices), vitamins (high dose), minerals, and other natural products such as probiotics [1]. The 2007 National Health Interview Survey indicated the use of fish oil was reported as the greatest used natural product in U.S. adults. Mind–body therapies as defined by NCCAM promote the mind's capacity to have an impact on the functioning of the body and health; however, Snyder and Lindquist [2] suggest a holistic view to include the impact on spirit and vice versa, the body's ability to impact the mind and spirit. Such therapies include yoga, meditation, prayer, music therapy, humor, acupuncture, deep breathing exercises, guided imagery, hypnotherapy, animal-assisted therapy, qigong, and tai chi. Manipulative and body-based practices focus on the structure and systems of the body including bones, joints, tissues, circulation, and lymphatics. Two main categories are spinal manipulation used by chiropractors, osteopaths, and physical therapists, and massage. The last category defined by NCCAM, "other practices," includes a variety of therapies such as movement therapies (Pilates, Rolfing), energy therapies (Reiki, healing touch, magnet, and light), traditional healers, and whole medical systems (Ayurvedic, traditional Chinese medicine, homeopathy, naturopathy). The purpose of this chapter is to provide a framework for the clinician to evaluate integrative therapy studies and consider their application to one's practice. Content will be addressed in the area of describing the nature and challenges in conducting integrative therapy research, exploring the utilization of evidence-based practice (EBP) as a model for critically appraising integrative therapy studies, and factors to consider when recommending implementation of integrative therapies in practice.

Shaping whether an idea, therapy, or practice will be actively utilized depends on its plausibility. Plausibility is a formula for determining whether therapies are accepted as conventional. Biological plausibility implies there may be a cause and effect or mechanism of action between a biological factor and a specific disease or adverse event. Whereas, clinical plausibility demonstrates efficacy and is established through epidemiological studies, case reports, and well-designed clinical trials. Therapies become standards of care depending on demonstrated clinical efficacy through well-designed clinical studies or because its biological rationale is in sync with the scientific biomedical framework. However, the more biologically implausible a therapy appears, the greater demand put forth for clinical plausibility by the greater scientific community [3]. In some respects, this requirement may be viewed as a double standard as the Institute of Medicine (IOM) report [4] discusses how, prior to our current EBP environment, many therapies that are now conventional were used before research demonstrated efficacy or effectiveness.

Challenges of Integrative Therapy Research

Nature of Conditions and Symptoms

Many of the symptoms and ailments integrative therapies are pursued for have variable natural histories or unpredictable course, lack definitive cures, and include nonspecific, multifactorial conditions such as insomnia, anxiety, and pain that are highly subjective or complex chronic conditions such as fibromyalgia [4, 5]. Integrative therapies may be practiced as adjuvant therapy to other aggressive conventional therapies such as concurrent chemotherapy and radiation in the treatment of cancer. Health promotion activities may also include integrative therapies, and while one is not focused on treating a specific disease or cluster of symptoms, the goals of one or more therapies may be targeted toward enhancing overall sense of holistic well-being or prevention of illness.

Nature of Integrative Therapies

Research on integrative therapies is not only challenging because of the types of conditions and symptoms they are used to ameliorate but also due to the nature of the therapies themselves. Topping the list is the fact that integrative therapies are frequently complex interventions. Many integrative therapies incorporate multiple modalities simultaneously (e.g., relaxation and guided imagery, use of essential oils with massage), making it difficult to tease out the effects of a given therapy. Integrative therapies also usually place strong emphasis on the patient-provider relationship and so the impact of the healer on the therapeutic outcome must be considered when assessing overall therapy effect. To complicate matters more, many integrative therapies are not standardized. Rather, these modalities are delivered in a flexible manner so they can be individualized to meet the patient's specific and changing needs [2, 6, 7]. As a result, trial recruitment and randomization may prove challenging if patients have strong preferences for one integrative modality over another. Adherence to randomization may be threatened if patients do not stay true to their therapy assignment and either stop, change, or add other modalities to their daily repertoire [5–7].

The integrative therapy field has been plagued by a lack of Phase I and Phase II trials that establish the optimal dose (i.e., how much, how often, how long) for full clinical value. As a result, Phase III trials may inappropriately reject an integrative therapy as ineffective in relation to a control group and/or comparison therapy simply because the optimal dose was not previously established [5]. Additional design challenges include identifying appropriate placebos to account for the nonspecific effects of therapies, as well as reasonable treatments for comparison groups. As a result, integrative therapies may be difficult, if not sometimes impossible, to double-blind either because the practitioner is providing a procedure-based intervention (e.g., biofeedback or acupuncture), or active participation is required due to the modality's nature (e.g., tai chi, qigong, yoga, meditation) [6, 7]. When blinding to reduce expectation effects is not possible, the selection of outcome measures is particularly important. Both subjective and outcome measures are critical to limit this validity threat [5].

Nature of Inquiry Paradigms

The scientific community has long upheld the double-blind randomized controlled trial (RCT) as the gold standard for evaluating allopathic and integrated therapies. This perspective can be located within the positivist paradigm that has dominated the physical and social sciences for over 400 years. Positivism aims to objectively explain, control, and predict phenomenon, asserting that hypotheses can be empirically tested and therefore verified as truth at a high level of probability if the design has strong controls for reliability and internal validity [8]. Many argue that this reductionist approach ignores the holistic orientation of integrative therapies and strips the research of the context that is imperative to understand an individual's experience with a particular therapy [6, 7]. While the postpositivism paradigm holds many of the same basic beliefs around inquiry as positivism, its methodology may incorporate qualitative methods. Pure qualitative methodology aligns itself with the constructivism or critical theory paradigm, emphasizing the dialectical or hermeneutical approach to understand phenomenon from the perspective of multiple realities [8]. Indeed, qualitative research provides a lens for which to understand human experience. This research paradigm has a unique ability to provide insight into the meaning, beliefs, expectations, and perceptions of the impact integrative therapies may have on clinical conditions and symptoms or a patient's overall sense of holistic well-being.

Given the evolution of scientific paradigms, coupled with the many challenges related to symptoms/conditions and integrative therapies, a variety of methodologies may be appropriate to evaluate integrative therapies. As Lindquist and Snyder [2] point out, RCTs are not the only type of design that builds knowledge about a therapy. Indeed, the IOM Committee on the Use of Complementary and Alternative Medicine [4] outlined the following recommendations for study designs that can provide essential information about the effectiveness of integrative therapies:

- *Observational and cohort*—Evaluations of patients receiving specified treatments
- *Case control*—Retrospective evaluations of patients with good or bad outcomes to find aspects of treatment associated with outcome profiles
- *Preference*—Comparisons of outcomes of patients who chose a particular treatment with those who were randomly assigned to it
- *Therapy bundle*—Evaluations of the effectiveness of a whole package of care
- *Placebo effect*—Evaluations that account for placebo effects as a part of the therapy's main mechanism of action (and not extraneous effects)

- *Attribute-treatment interactions*—Evaluations that account for differences in effectiveness outcomes within and among studies of varying design

As a thorough review of study designs is outside the scope of this chapter, readers are referred to the IOM report *Complementary and Alternative Medicine in the United States* [4] and other classic research texts for further information. The following section will focus on evaluating RCTs and qualitative studies in establishing the efficacy, effectiveness, acceptability, and feasibility of integrative therapies for clinical practice. But before critical appraisal is discussed, practitioners must first consider the comprehensive steps involved in achieving evidence-based decisions. The model of EBP outlined below begins in the process of clinical inquiry to clearly identify the question(s) about the integrative therapy that are of primary significance. By articulating what aspect of the therapy one is most interested in, a focused and efficient search for the literature best able to answer that question can unfold.

Achieving Evidence-Based Practice

EBP is a model for clinical decision-making that encompasses five classic phases. These phases include formulating answerable questions, conducting efficient literature searches, critically appraising the evidence, applying the results in healthcare decisions, and evaluating outcomes.

Formulate Answerable Question

The first phase of EBP begins in clinical inquiry. The PICOT and PS methods for framing clinical questions are helpful to narrow your topic to an answerable inquiry. PICOT is often used with more quantitative-oriented questions where "P" stands for problem or patient population, "I" for the intervention, "C" for the comparison, "O" for the outcome, and "T" for timing (when applicable). An example might be: What is the effect of music therapy on anxiety of mechanically ventilated patients during weaning trials as compared to anxiolytic medications? PS questions explore the patient's experience which lends itself to qualitatively oriented research. Again, "P" stands for problem or patient population but "S" refers to the situation. An example PS question could be: What is the lived experience of patients with asthma that regularly practices mindfulness-based stress reduction?

Clinical questions may be further classified into categories. These categories include issues related to (1) etiology (cause of conditions/diseases), (2) diagnosis (sensitivity/specificity of a test), (3) prognosis (clinical course or natural progression of conditions/diseases), (4) treatment (effect of integrative therapy on particular symptom or outcome of interest), (5) cost (economics associated with an integrative therapy), or (6) meaning (experience with particular integrative therapy).

Generally speaking, the PICOT format lends itself well to etiology, diagnosis, prognosis, treatment, and cost inquiries, while meaning questions lend themselves more to the PS format.

Conduct Efficient Literature Search

Once the PICOT or PS question is sufficiently stated, the next step in EBP is to conduct an efficient literature search. The hierarchy of preprocessed evidence [9] is especially useful for the busy provider to find answers to questions about the application of integrative therapies to clinical practice. Starting at the top of the pyramid are clinical practice guidelines. Evidence-based clinical practice guidelines may be found in a multitude of professional journals or professional organization websites. One popular resource is the National Guidelines Clearinghouse (www.guidelines.gov). Systematic reviews lie in the middle of the hierarchy. The Cochrane Library is a ready source of systematic reviews and contains an entire section targeted to integrative therapies (www.cochrane.org). The Database on Abstracts of Reviews of Effects (DARE) is another repository of systematic reviews on the effects of health care that have been critically analyzed according to a high standard of criteria (www.crd.york.ac.uk/crdweb). When clinical practice guidelines or systematic reviews are not available on the topic, then individual databases such as Pub Med should be searched to locate individual studies on the integrative therapy of interest.

Critically Appraise the Evidence

After the databases have been searched, the next phase turns to critically appraising available literature. This process is first applied to each individual piece of literature (clinical practice guideline, systematic review, or single study). A wide variety of critical appraisal tools are available for evaluating guidelines, systematic reviews, or single studies including the Appraisal of Guidelines Research and Evaluation (AGREE) available at www.agreecollaboration.org or CASP tools available at www.gla.ac.uk/departments/generalpracticeprimarycare/ebp/checklists. Additional tools for evaluating single studies based on research design are discussed below.

Explanatory Trials

RCTs (or meta-analyses of multiple RCTs) are the preferred study design to appraise when addressing questions about an integrative therapy [4]. Such trials are focused on establishing whether the intervention works as intended and identifying risk and benefits and who benefits from the therapy [10]. RCTs can be classified as *explanatory* or *pragmatic*. Explanatory RCTs test the efficacy of an integrative therapy in relation to clinically meaningful endpoints (i.e., morbidity/ mortality, symptom relief, functional ability, health-related quality of life). Most suitable with acute conditions, these trials test standardized intervention protocols with highly selected participants under tightly controlled conditions [11–13]. Explanatory studies tend to be *superiority* trials and are interested in showing one therapy is better than standard treatment. However, such trials are feasible only when it is possible to double-blind and evaluate the efficacy of the intervention against a placebo [14]. Some integrative therapies have the potential to be blinded to both the practitioner and patient, such as herbs, essential oils, or even intercessory prayer. For instance, an explanatory trial could be designed to test the efficacy of an herbal supplement in reducing insomnia, compared to an inert placebo substance.

Explanatory trials are strengthened with the addition of subjective measures. Subjective measures add another dimension to RCTs that cannot be obtained through the objective measurement of variables alone. Subjective measures often move beyond assessment of physical endpoints and include holistic concepts such as meaning and purpose, spirituality, or wholeness [6, 7, 15]. Even so, subjective measures can be significantly affected by context, contrast, or expectation effects. These effects can be minimized by features built into the design such as assessment of a subjective outcome on two scales to establish convergent validity. Contrast effects can be minimized by carefully selecting patients with similar characteristics in terms of severity of symptoms or conditions at the time of treatment [4], while expectation effects can be reduced by blinding methods.

The critical appraisal process for explanatory trials involves assessing internal validity, including the appropriateness of data analysis, and external validity (Table 2.1) [11–14, 16, 17]. In explanatory designs, internal validity is of prime importance since they test therapies under ideal experimental conditions. External validity is a measure of the applicability of the findings to the larger intended target population. Because explanatory trials test interventions under highly controlled conditions, findings generally lack external validity and thus, have lower relevance and impact on practice.

Pragmatic Trials

In contrast, pragmatic RCTs are designed to compare therapy effectiveness in the routine care setting with a wider population. These trials provide practitioners freedom to treat patients as they do in normal everyday practice by using individual approaches. Consequently, these trials are helpful to make decisions between two interventions and thus, inform decisions about practice [13]. More suitable with chronic conditions, pragmatic trials are used to evaluate complex integrative therapy interventions or to compare the overall effectiveness of a package of care with another treatment (and not a placebo as with explanatory trials). However, these trials cannot evaluate the contributions of subcomponents of the package of care, nor can they assess the contribution of the therapeutic relationship to the overall

Table 2.1 Critical appraisal criteria for explanatory and pragmatic trials on integrative therapies [11–14, 16, 17]

	Criteria	Yes	No	Unsure
INTERNAL VALIDITY	**Appropriateness of Design**	Yes	No	Unsure
	RESEARCH QUESTIONS: • Are research questions clearly stated? *SAMPLE*: • Is population clearly specified with inclusion/exclusion criteria? *Pragmatic Trials*: Wide inclusion/exclusion criteria used? • Is sample sufficiently powered for primary outcome? *OUTCOME MEASUREMENT*: • Are primary and secondary outcomes clinically meaningful? Do they match research question(s)? *Pragmatic Trials*: Is there depth of clinically meaningful outcomes (e.g., QOL, pain, mood/coping, patient satisfaction)? • Are outcomes of reasonable follow-up to assess benefits & harms? Are responses for treatment success or failure defined? • Do outcome measures have sound psychometric properties? *LEVEL OF SIGNIFICANCE*: • Is the alpha level specified a priori?			
	Validity of Results	Yes	No	Unsure
	SELECTION BIAS: • Are patients randomly assigned to groups? Was randomization list concealed and maintained? *Pragmatic Trials*: If partial randomization done, were patients asked if they had a preference & if so assigned to this treatment, with remaining patients randomized to all treatment options? *PERFORMANCE BIAS*: • Are double-blinding methods achieved? *Pragmatic Trials*: When blinding not possible, was outcome assessment done by third party (i.e., not a therapist?) ▪ Is a reasonable intervention and comparison tested? *Pragmatic Trials*: -Was 2nd treatment a fair comparison with similar chances of response (i.e., as similar to integrative therapy as possible)? -Were following factors standardized for the two treatments: ☐ Duration, frequency & number of sessions ☐ Physical environment where treatment administered ☐ Amount/content of conversation ☐ Credibility of treatment to patient and therapist - Was more than one therapist used? Did they treat similar numbers in each arm to control for therapist variability? • Is there fidelity to research protocol for all groups (i.e., groups were treated equally aside from experimental treatment)? *Pragmatic Trial*: Did treatment protocol specify what variability was allowed (open vs. tightly standardized)? *ASSESSMENT BIAS*: • Are assessors blinded? • Is intention-to-treat analysis performed? *ATTRITION BIAS*: • Is there zero or minimal missing data (<5–10%) unless thorough intention-to-treat analysis is done?			
	Appropriateness of Statistical Analysis	Yes	No	Unsure
	• Are statistical tests appropriate to research questions? • Were clinical & psychological variables assessed at baseline between groups? (e.g., mood/coping style, locus of control) • Are all randomized patients accounted for? Analyzed in groups as randomized? • Is a reasonable method for imputing missing values used? • Are problems with selective outcome reporting observed?			
EXTERNAL VALIDITY	**Applicability of Findings**	Yes	No	Unsure
	EFFECT SIZE: • Is treatment effect large enough to be clinically beneficial? Is effect precise (are confidence intervals presented)? • Is risk or harm associated with the treatment minimal? *GENERALIZABILITY*: • Were groups similar at start of trial? • Is there great likelihood that the results would apply to the wider population based on size of target population, inclusion/exclusion criteria, and baseline characteristics?			

benefit of the therapy. Therefore, the specific effects of the therapy cannot be isolated from their nonspecific or contextual effects (as is generally the case with explanatory trials) [2, 7, 13, 14]. As a result, pragmatic trials can be classified as either *superiority* (one intervention is better than another in some significant way) or *noninferiority* (new intervention is as good as, or no worse than, the comparison therapy) depending on the study's goal [18].

A number of design differences are evident with pragmatic designs. Typically, a variety of treatment settings are utilized and the therapy is administered by the same type of clinician who provides the treatment in nonstudy settings. Larger sample sizes are necessary since recruitment is derived from a wider population leading to more heterogeneity. Since patient preference may limit recruitment or randomization, preference trials can allocate patients to a preferred modality followed by randomization of remaining patients to all treatment options, thereby limiting this threat to validity. Additionally, it is often not possible to blind interventions to the patient or therapist; for example, a researcher may desire to test the effectiveness of qigong, an integrative therapy that requires active participation, and thus patient blinding is not possible. Like in real life, patients enrolled in these trials may be allowed to change treatments, and as a result, there is considerable risk that the treatment effect will be diluted. However, if patients are compared in the groups to which they were randomized with an intention-to-treat model, the integrity of the trial is not jeopardized. Outcome assessment generally should not only be relevant to everyday life such as functional ability or quality of life (QOL) but also span a wider spectrum such as changes in attitude, behavior, or outlook. Longer follow-up is typically needed due to the greater variability between patients that may dilute the treatment effect, as well as to show how treatment benefits are sustained. Furthermore, some therapeutic changes associated with integrative therapies take place over a considerable period of time along the natural trajectory of chronic symptoms and conditions [14, 19].

The critical appraisal process for pragmatic trials also involves assessing internal validity, including the appropriateness of data analysis, and external validity. Similar critical appraisal criteria apply with pragmatic trials. However, since the aim of these trials is to establish treatment effectiveness, then some RCT features create problems in generalizing findings to routine care settings. As indicated on Table 2.1, a few design deviations may apply. Therefore, while internal validity tends to be lower, pragmatic trials afford greater external validity with high relevance and impact on practice [14].

Qualitative Trials

Qualitative trials are increasingly being used to evaluate integrative as well as allopathic therapies. Qualitative research is the appropriate method when the primary interest relates to understanding the meaning, beliefs, and expectations of a patient's experience with an integrative therapy for a condition or symptom within a particular context. By using these methods, researchers learn about patients' experiences with particular integrative therapies, including any physical, emotional, or spiritual changes they attribute to the therapy [7, 15, 20, 21]. For example, qualitative trials may explore patients' perceptions about the impact of a therapy such as meditation on overall well-being and health-related QOL or guided imagery on frequency of insomnia and sleep quality. For these reasons, qualitative research is case-oriented as opposed to variable-oriented quantitative research [7].

Additionally, qualitative methods may be useful to determine holistic changes perceived to be relevant to patients. In fact, the most important change experienced may not be relevant to the primary aim of the study at all. If these changes are ignored and not explored, researchers may lose insight into useful data that may help to understand the effects of integrative therapies and their mechanisms of action [21]. Verhoef et al. [7] argues that just as RCTs can generate statistically significant effects without any clinical significance, it is also possible to have non-statistically significant results with meaningful implications for individual patients. Consequently, if an intervention shows no effect on the outcomes of interest, these results cannot inform whether some specific individuals benefited from the intervention or if the therapy worked in other desirable ways than expected. As a result, qualitative changes may serve an important role in identifying relevant outcomes for further hypothesis testing.

Another purpose of qualitative methods is to gain knowledge about how integrative therapies, practices, and protocols play out realistically in a patient's life. By collecting data on the natural context in which patients act, researchers can get a better picture of the influence of that context on the patient's actions in relation to the integrative therapy [7, 15]. This ability to evaluate the impact of context may be especially relevant for those integrative therapies that require active participation such as guided imagery, meditation, or tai chi. Thus, qualitative trials can be especially useful in evaluating the acceptability and feasibility of integrative interventions for patients with various symptoms and from different populations. By exploring why participants continue or withdraw from treatment, researchers can evaluate recruitment and retention strategies that may be feasible to keep patients who might benefit most from particular integrative therapies. Thus, qualitative methods may be especially helpful in teasing out variables in the natural context that may be related to various levels of satisfaction with particular integrative therapies [21].

Critical appraisal of qualitative research also involves evaluating internal and external validity, although different terms are applicable because of the fundamental differences in these research methods (Table 2.2) [22–25]. Qualitative research draws on interview and observation methods to collect subjective data to describe phenomenon as they occur in the natural setting (as opposed to the use of strict control of variables with explanatory or pragmatic studies). Thus, the analysis of qualitative data differs substantially from traditional statistical analysis. By immersing themselves in the data, researchers use content analysis to derive common themes and patterns of the phenomenon of interest.

Accordingly, critical appraisal of qualitative research is centered on establishing the *trustworthiness* of the data. Trustworthiness of the data reflects both internal and external validity. The internal validity for qualitative research includes the following: (1) appropriateness of the design (i.e., congruency of the design and method with the research question, sampling strategies to identify key informants, verifiable data collection methods, content analysis); (2) *reflexivity* or *signposting*, accounting for what is going on while researching; (3) *dependability* or *auditability*, reporting all decisions involved in the analysis and transformation of qualitative data; (4) *credibility*, providing vividness and faithfulness in the description of the phenomenon; and (5) *confirmability*, adequately addressing issues of dependability, credibility, and transferability. The trustworthiness of qualitative data also has implications for external validity; this concept is known as *transferability*. Transferability demonstrates the applicability of findings to similar contexts, as opposed to generalizability which is the focus of external validity with quantitative research [22–25]. Unlike generalizability, transferability is the responsibility of the reader to consider comparable contexts where the findings might be worth further exploration.

Table 2.2 Critical appraisal criteria for qualitative studies on integrative therapies [22–25]

INTERNAL VALIDITY	**Appropriateness of Design**	Yes	No	Unsure
	DESIGN CONGRUENCY: • Are research questions clearly stated? Do research questions fit the analytic methods used? • Is there sufficient congruence between description of the research process and qualitative methodology used? *SAMPLING STRATEGY*: • Is the strategy for sampling both patients and settings adequately described? Is it clear why they were chosen? • Are most productive informants & relevant settings used? • Are characteristics of the informants described? *DATA COLLECTION METHODS*: • Are methods described in enough detail? • Are methods reliable and independently verifiable (e.g., audio/videotape, field notes)? • Were observations taken over a range of circumstances (e.g., at different times of day or days or week)? *DATA ANALYSIS*: • How were themes derived from the data? • Did more than one researcher perform analysis? What method was used to resolve discrepancies in interpretation? Were discrepancies fully addressed?			
	Reflexivity (Signposting)	Yes	No	Unsure
	• Is the manner in which the researcher locates himself/herself within the research process explicit (*if applicable*)? • Does the researcher account for his/her background, philosophical perspective, biases, and potential patient's reactions to their role and status? *Check all that are applicable:* ☐ Age ☐ Race & ethnicity ☐ Sexual orientation ☐ Gender ☐ Appearance ☐ Political affiliation ☐ Authority ☐ Professional role ☐ Marital/parental/elder status • Are strategies used by researcher to reflect upon his/her interactions and participation in the research process? ☐ Journal ☐ Field notes			
	Dependability (Auditability)	Yes	No	Unsure
	• Is there evidence that processes, procedures & decisions of the researcher are logical and consistent (audit trail)?			
	Credibility	Yes	No	Unsure

(continued)

Table 2.2 (continued)

	• Which strategies were used to achieve trustworthy findings? ☐ Journaling of process ☐ Multiple data sources ☐ Peer debriefing (validation by colleagues engaged with research issue) ☐ Negative case analysis ☐ Prolonged engagement in field ☐ Member checking (patient response to analysis)			
	Confirmability	Yes	No	Unsure
	• Is there sufficient evidence that findings, conclusion and recommendations are supported by the data, as evidenced by: ☐ Direct quotations from informants to amplify themes • Is there sufficient evidence of internal agreement between the data and the researcher's interpretations? ☐ Plausible and coherent explanations ☐ Exploration of alternative explanations for results			
EXTERNAL VALIDITY	**Transferability**	Yes	No	Unsure
	• Is there sufficient evidence that the findings may be applicable to other contexts or settings, as evidenced by: ☐ Similarity of patients to contexts of interest ☐ Thick description ☐ Validation by colleagues			

Evidence Grading Systems

After all individual studies, systematic reviews, and clinical practice guidelines have been appraised, the next step is to collectively evaluate them against a selected evidence hierarchy system. An example is the grading system developed by the U.S. Preventive Services Task Force (Table 2.3) [26]. This grading system evaluates the quality of the evidence by assigning hierarchical ranking to study designs. This hierarchy of evidence is then used to assess the strength of the recommendations for or against the intervention based on the balance of benefits and harms from the available evidence. Similarly, the hierarchy from the National Health Service Center for Evidence-Based Medicine focuses on the design, number of studies, and consistency of results. In this hierarchy, evidence is assigned the following weight, from highest to lowest: (1) combined results of several RCTs (meta-analyses), (2) results of a single well-designed RCT, (3) combined results of observational studies or non-RCT designs, and (4) case series or anecdotal reports and professional consensus [4]. In treatment effectiveness research, it has also been argued that the results of a

Table 2.3 Clinical evidence rating system of U.S. Preventive Services Task Force [26]

Quality of evidence	
I	Evidence from at least one properly designed randomized controlled trial
II-1	Evidence obtained from well-designed controlled trials without randomization
II-2	Evidence from well-designed cohort or case-control studies, preferably from more than one center or research group
II-3	Evidence from multiple time series with or without the intervention
	Important results in uncontrolled experiments (such as introduction of penicillin treatment in 1940s) could be considered as this type of evidence
III	Opinions of respected authorities, based on clinical experience; descriptive studies; or reports of expert committees
Strength of recommendations	
A	Good evidence to support intervention (benefits substantially outweigh harms)
B	Fair evidence to support intervention (benefits outweigh harms)
C	Insufficient evidence to recommend for or against intervention (lack of evidence on clinical outcomes), but recommendation might be made on other grounds
D	Fair evidence against intervention (ineffective or harms outweigh potential benefits)
E	Good evidence against intervention (ineffective or harms outweigh potential benefits)

Table 2.4 Hierarchy of evidence: ranking of research evidence evaluating healthcare interventions

	Effectiveness	Appropriateness	Feasibility
Excellent	• Systematic review • Multicenter studies	• Systematic review • Multicenter studies	• Systematic review • Multicenter studies
Good	• RCT • Observational studies	• RCT • Observational studies • Interpretive studies	• RCT • Observational studies • Interpretive studies
Fair	• Uncontrolled trials with dramatic results • Before and after studies • Nonrandomized controlled trials	• Descriptive studies • Focus groups	• Descriptive studies • Action research • Before and after studies • Focus groups
Poor	• Descriptive studies • Case studies • Expert opinion • Studies of poor methodological quality	• Expert opinion • Case studies • Studies of poor methodological quality	• Expert opinion • Case studies • Studies of poor methodological quality

From Evan [10]; used with permission

single well-designed outcomes study should be considered as compelling as those of a single well-controlled RCT [4, 19].

Evan [10] advocates that a limitation of current evidence hierarchies is the sole focus on effectiveness, while more robust evaluation of healthcare interventions should include other crucial considerations, namely, appropriateness and feasibility (Table 2.4). These distinctions are significant since the value of a healthcare intervention—no matter how effective—will remain uncertain if it is unacceptable to the patient or cannot be implemented adequately. Thus, if the evidence hierarchy focuses solely on effectiveness, valid evidence related to the appropriateness or feasibility of an intervention may be appraised at a lower level.

Apply Results in Healthcare Decisions and Evaluate Outcome

Widespread use of the internet makes ascertaining information on integrative therapies easy; however, determining the value and relevance of the information for use in clinical practice can be challenging and daunting in a busy, time-constrained practice. Multiple studies indicate self-use of integrative therapies by healthcare professionals influences both knowledge of and recommending/referring for use of integrative therapies [4, 27–29]. There is a growing body of scientific literature on integrative therapies, and developing a procedure for accessing and evaluating studies as noted earlier in this chapter may be helpful in advising patients. Indeed, the remaining two phases of EBP involve applying the results of the evidence about an integrative therapy to individual patients in clinical practice and then evaluating the outcome. Understanding patient, institutional, and practitioner factors are essential for successful application to practice.

Patient Factors

While one in three Americans reports the use of integrative therapies [1], the majority of them do not disclose use to their physician despite being seen during the times of integrative therapy use [30]. Reasons for not disclosing varied from "It wasn't important for the doctor to know," "The doctor never asked," to "The doctor would not understand." A recent publication by the IOM [4] recommends shared decision-making between patients and providers regarding treatments, which includes both conventional and integrative therapies. Integrative healthcare interventions should address not only absence of disease and quality of life measures but include levels of wellness too [31].

Determining whether a particular integrative therapy has documented benefit in targeted outcomes for a clinical condition or group of symptoms requires one to obtain credible information and analyze whether or not the results apply to a specific patient or group of patients, how great the benefit of therapy might be, and to what extent the findings are transferable to other clinical settings. The clinical risk and therapeutic posture [4] is one framework for advising patients about the use of integrative therapies:

- *Option A*—Supports both safety and efficacy: *Recommend and monitor* (examples: meditation, yoga, folic acid in pregnancy)
- *Option B*—Supports safety, however, inconclusive evidence regarding efficacy: Tolerate, provide caution, and closely monitor effectiveness (example: healing energy therapies such as Reiki)

- *Option C*—Supports efficacy but inconclusive evidence regarding safety: Consider tolerating, providing caution, and closely monitoring safety (example: ingestion of herbal products like garlic during concomitant aspirin or antiplatelet therapy)
- *Option D*—Indicates serious risk or inefficacy: *Avoid and actively discourage* (example: use of herbal products such as Echinacea that influence the immune system in transplant patients)

As one of the three primary components of EBP [32], patient preferences are a staunch consideration in recommending treatment options. Would your patients' values and preferences be satisfied by the intervention offered? Are you able to facilitate frank discussions on the known risks, benefits, and alternatives in language understood by your patient? Are resources, both products and experienced practitioners, for integrative therapies available to your patient population? While some HMOs and insurance companies have covered some integrative therapies such as chiropractic care, most are paid for out of pocket with recent estimates at $27 billion [4]. As important as it is to follow up regarding any treatments recommended or prescribed, it is especially prudent to follow up on effectiveness and satisfaction of integrative therapies [33, 34].

Institutional Factors

While integrative therapies are becoming mainstream, the acclimatization into healthcare institutions varies widely depending on institutional philosophy regarding health and well-being, financial sustainability, and readiness for integrative therapy of interest both internally (staff resources, provider perceptions) and externally (economic and social trends, patient interest). Some institutions implement the use of integrative therapies system-wide (Woodwinds Hospital, Woodbury, MN), while others begin in one particular area with the vision of implementing incrementally (Palliative Integrated Care Unit, Minneapolis VA). Additionally, issues of liability, professional licensure or certification, and ongoing education competencies must also be addressed [4].

One may begin by checking specific state requirements for licenses of practitioners providing a particular integrative therapy. Acupuncture.com is an example of a website that provides links to each state's laws regarding acupuncture. Some states also provide avenues like the following website (http://www.docboard.org/mn/df/mndf.htm) to assist in searching for a licensed professional practitioner such as an acupuncturist or naturopathic doctor in a targeted area. Accessing information on integrative therapies utilizing certification as its educational documentation source can be more challenging, although some states have web sources providing this information (http://www.iowaholisticresources.com/id42.html). Unfortunately, "word of mouth" tends to be a highly practiced avenue in locating reliable, certified practitioners of integrative therapies in one's community or local region.

Practitioner Factors

Institutional practitioners including nurses, providers (MD, physician assistant, advanced practice nurse), and other healthcare practitioners (physical therapists, occupational therapists, pharmacists) are likely to have some awareness of at least one integrative therapy; however, acceptability and personal readiness of a given practice may be met with resistance. Implementing integrative therapies may pose a feasibility issue, for example, expecting nursing staff in a chemotherapy infusion unit to begin utilizing essential oils in the management of treatment-related nausea without the availability of education, equipment, and support is likely to produce frustration and poor execution. A different example about feasibility might entail a practitioner who may have both a professional license (MD) and a certification in an integrative therapy (acupuncture) and, thus, be able to apply knowledge from both licenses/certifications in their hired position. For instance, at the Minneapolis VAMC, a physical medicine and rehabilitation physician was hired who also had certification and licensure in acupuncture. As a result, this physician is able to provide acupuncture in an outpatient clinic one day a week. Unfortunately, this situation is not a sustainable avenue in providing acupuncture long term, nor is it accessible to inpatient veterans.

Identifying credible community practitioners may be problematic in some areas. However, once a decision has been made to pursue a specific integrative therapy (e.g., Reiki, massage, acupuncture), assisting patients in locating a practitioner with acceptable expertise should be a priority [4]. Exploration should include ascertaining licensure, certifications, experience, scope of practice, and any history of malpractice or professional discipline [4]. It would be prudent to develop a collegial relationship with any integrative therapy practitioner where shared patients may be treated as the practitioner relationship may influence outcomes which may or may not be measureable [6, 34, 35].

References

1. National Center for Complementary and Alternative Medicine. What is complementary and alternative medicine. 2010. http://nccam.nih.gov/health/whatiscam/. Accessed October 16, 2010.
2. Lindquist R, Snyder M, Song Y. Perspectives on future research and practice. In: Snyder M, Lindquist R, editors. Complementary/alternative therapies nursing. 6th ed. New York: Springer; 2010. p. 485–98.
3. Hoffer J. Complementary or alternative medicine: the need for plausibility. JAMC. 2003; 168(2):180–2.
4. Institute of Medicine. Complementary and alternative medicine in the United States. Washington: National Academy Press; 2005.
5. Nahin R, Berman J, Stoney C, et al. Approaches to clinical trials of complementary and alternative medicine. In: Vogel J, Krucoff M, editors. Integrative cardiology: complementary and alternative medicine for the heart. New York: McGraw Hill; 2005. p. 63–86.
6. Carter B. Methodological issues and complementary therapies: researching intangibles? Complement Ther Nurs Midwifery. 2003;9:133–9.

7. Verhoef M, Casebeer, Hilsden R. Assessing efficacy of complementary medicine: Adding qualitative research methods to the 'gold standard'. Alternative Compl Med. 2002;8(3): 275–81.
8. Guba E, Lincoln Y. Competing paradigms in qualitative research. In: Denzin D, Lincoln Y, editors. The landscape of qualitative research: theories and issues. London: Sage; 1998. p. 195–220.
9. Haynes R. Of studies, syntheses, synopses, summaries, and systems: the "5S" evolution of information services for evidence-based healthcare decisions. Evid Based Nurs. 2007;10:6–7.
10. Evan D. Hierarchy of evidence: a framework for ranking evidence evaluating healthcare interventions. J Clin Nurs. 2003;12:77–84.
11. Critical appraisal checklist. 2010. www.delfini.org. Accessed November 19, 2010.
12. Walker L, Anderson J. Testing complementary and alternative therapies within a research protocol. Eur J Cancer. 1999;35(11):1614–8.
13. Zwarenstein M, Treweek S, Gagnier J, et al. for CONSORT and Practihc groups. Improving the reporting of pragmatic trials: an extension of the CONSORT statement. BMJ. 2008; 337:1–8.
14. MacPherson H. Pragmatic clinical trials. Complement Ther Med. 2004;12:136–40.
15. Schumacher K, Koresawa S, West C, et al. Qualitative research contribution to a randomized clinical trial. Res Nurs Health. 2005;28:268–80.
16. Evidence-based practice checklists. 2010. www.gla.ac.uk/departments/generalpracticeprimarycare/ebp/checklists/#d.en.19536. Accessed November 19, 2010.
17. Schulz K, Altman D, Moher D; for CONSORT group. CONSORT 2010 statement: updated guidelines for reporting parallel group randomized trials. Ann Intern Med. 2010;152(11):1–8.
18. Piaggio G, Elbourne D, Altman D, et al.; for CONSORT group. Reporting of noninferiority and equivalence randomized trials: An extension of the CONSORT statement. JAMA. 2006;295(10):1152–60.
19. Institute of Medicine. Gulf war veterans: treating symptoms and syndromes. Washington: National Academy Press; 2001.
20. Paterson C, Britten N. Acupuncture for people with chronic illness: combining qualitative and quantitative outcome assessment. J Altern Complement Med. 2003;9(5):671–81.
21. Vuckovic N. Integrating qualitative methods in randomized controlled trials: the experience of the Oregon center for complementary and alternative medicine. J Altern Complement Med. 2002;8(3):225–7.
22. Bailey P. Assuring quality in narrative analysis. West J Nurs Res. 1995;18(2):186–94.
23. Burns N. Standards for qualitative research. Nurs Sci Q. 1989;2(1):44–52.
24. Koch T, Harrington A. Reconceptualizing rigour: the case for reflexivity. J Adv Nurs. 1998;28(4):882–90.
25. Sandelowski M. Rigor or rigor mortis: the problem of rigor in qualitative research revisited. Adv Nurs Sci. 1993;16(2):1–8.
26. U.S. Preventive Service Task Force Hierarchy of Research Design and Quality Rating Criteria. 2010. www.ncbi.nlm.nih.gov. Accessed November 5, 2010.
27. Cutshall S, Derscheid D, Miers A, et al. Knowledge, attitudes, and use of complementary and alternative therapies among clinical nurse specialists in an academic medical center. Clin Nurse Spec. 2010;24(3):125–31.
28. Polich G, Dole C, Kaptchuk T. The need to act a little more "scientific": biomedical researchers investigating complementary and alternative medicine. Sociol Health Illn. 2010;32(1): 106–22.
29. Tracy M, Lindquist R, Savik K, et al. Use of complementary and alternative therapies: a national survey of critical care nurses. Am J Crit Care. 2005;14(5):404–14.
30. Eisenberg D, Davis R, Ettner S, et al. Trends in alternative medicine use in the United States, 1990–1997: results of a follow-up national survey. JAMA. 1998;280(18):1569–75.
31. Verhoef M, Mulkins A, Boon H. Integrative health care: how can we determine whether patients benefit? J Altern Complement Med. 2005;11(Supp 1):S57–65.
32. Sackett D, Rosenberg W, Gray J, et al. Evidence-based medicine: what it is and what it isn't. BMJ. 1996;312:71–2.

33. Mason S, Tovey P, Long A. Evaluating complementary medicine: methodological challenges of randomized controlled trials. Br Med J. 2002;325:832–4.
34. Long A, Mercer G, Hughes K. Developing a tool to measure holistic practice: a missing dimension in outcomes measurement within complementary therapies. Complement Ther Med. 2000;8:26–31.
35. Brown C. Methodological problems of clinical research into spiritual healing: the healer's perspective. J Altern Complement Med. 2000;6(2):275–81.

Part II
Integrative Therapies in Chronic Pulmonary Conditions

Chapter 3
Integrative Therapies for People with Asthma

Lauren M. Fine and Malcolm N. Blumenthal

Abstract Asthma is a complex disease with many phenotypes. Its definition and treatment by a number of cultures around the world may play a role in the efficacy of such treatments. Western medicine defines asthma based on inflammation, obstruction, and mucus production which are reversible with treatment. A number of studies focusing on natural products, mind–body medicine, manipulative therapy, and others have not been able to reproducibly demonstrate efficacy in treating asthma. This may be due to a number of factors including methodology, study design, and—most importantly—the definition of asthma used for each study. The Western definition of asthma may differ greatly from the definition used by those cultures which originally created the therapies used in studies of complementary and alternative medicine (CAM). Because of this difference, the outcome of the studies may not be an accurate reflection of the ability of these therapies to treat the disease process they were originally designed to treat. Future studies in CAM will likely need to address these differences.

Keywords Asthma • Complementary and alternative medicine • Natural products • Herbal medicine • Mind–body medicine

L.M. Fine, MD (✉)
Department of Pulmonary, Allergy and Critical Care, University of Minnesota,
420 Delaware Street SE, MMC 276, Minneapolis, MN 55455, USA
e-mail: laurenmfine@gmail.com

M.N. Blumenthal, MD
Department of Medicine, Pediatrics and Laboratory Medicine, University of Minnesota,
420 Deleware Street SE, Minneapolis, MN 55440, USA

L. Chlan and M.I. Hertz (eds.), *Integrative Therapies in Lung Health and Sleep*,
Respiratory Medicine 4, DOI 10.1007/978-1-61779-579-4_3,

Introduction

Asthma is a chronic airways disease that affects both children and adults worldwide. Airways inflammation, increased mucus production, and bronchospasm result in variable degrees of airflow obstruction which present clinically as breathlessness, cough, and wheeze. However, the frequency and severity of these symptoms vary from person to person [1]. Asthma differs from chronic obstructive lung disease (COPD) in that in asthma the airflow obstruction is reversible with the administration of bronchodilators, and the obstruction can be induced by challenge with a bronchoconstricting chemical such as methacholine or histamine. Additionally, inflammation in asthma may involve airway eosinophilia which often results from an imbalance toward Th2 lymphocytes.

We performed a literature search for English-language articles and reports on the use of various alternative and integrative therapies for the treatment and prevention of asthma. Over 250 articles and references were found, most of which were directly used in the composition of this chapter. This chapter does not encompass all therapies that might be used in integrative medicine although it does address many of the most common. As we will discuss, most articles published in English used a Western definition of asthma. Therefore, conclusions drawn regarding the efficacy of treatment interventions are based on the use of the Western definition of asthma, rather than the definition of asthma used by the group or culture that originally created each treatment or intervention. The difference in definition of asthma may be one of the many reasons that otherwise similar studies yield inconsistent results. Asthma is a complex disease which involves a multitude of different factors. In addition, it is well-documented that behavior and environmental exposures, and possibly epigenetics, impact the clinical course of asthma. Therefore, environmental factors and their impact on genes and phenotype should be considered when comparing studies using Western vs. Eastern medicine.

Traditional Chinese Medicine (TCM) and traditional Western medicine are similar in that both believe that one symptom, such as wheezing, can be explained by a number of different etiologies or disease diagnoses. For example, in traditional Western medicine, airway obstruction leading to wheeze is explained as being secondary to disease in the lungs, heart (congestive heart failure [CHF]), liver (carcinoid), or immune system activation (eosinophilia). In TCM, airway obstruction is attributed to dysfunction of any of the organ systems listed above, as well as the kidney, spleen, or the central nervous system (CNS) [2]. However, the diagnosis of asthma, as defined in Western medicine, is not existent in TCM. This is because in TCM a group of symptoms do not define a diagnosis. Each patient's illness has a particular set of symptoms that the physician must analyze in order to determine the stage, location, and balance of Qi (energy) in the particular disease. Because symptoms may vary from person to person and disease is treated based on symptoms, the treatment for what may be considered the same disease by standards and definitions in Western medicine may vary from person to person in TCM. Treatment of airway disease in TCM is individualized for each person and focuses on correcting the imbalance in Qi, which is considered the source of the constellation of symptoms in each patient. In contrast, in Western medicine, treatment of the Western diagnosis of asthma is focused on managing airways inflammation and obstruction. This is generally done with a limited number of medications that are prescribed for the vast majority of patients, such as beta-agonists and corticosteroids. TCM focuses on the mind–body-spirit connection and energy balances, in particular two opposite but balancing forces called yin and yang. TCM therapies include acupuncture, herbal therapies, meditation, and other mind–body practices. We refer the reader to Chap. 15 for more background on TCM treatment and history.

Economic and Noneconomic Costs of Asthma

The burden of asthma manifests in both morbidity and cost of disease management. As many as 34 million Americans have been diagnosed with asthma during their lifetime and 300 million worldwide suffer from it, with half of them suffering at least one exacerbation in the preceding year [3–5]. Asthma affects almost 10% of pediatric patients, and is the most common chronic disease in children [6]. The cost of asthma includes not only direct healthcare costs but also those related to missed days of work and school, as more than 20 million days of both school and work are missed each year due to asthma [4]. Healthcare costs children with asthma are 92% greater than in those without asthma. In adults, the healthcare cost is 66% greater for those who have asthma. Asthma costs an individual more than $2,000 a year and total direct annual expenditure for asthma, not including indirect costs, has been estimated at $37.17 billion [3]. In 1997, the out-of-pocket expenditure for all alternative medicine practitioners, not including self-administered therapies, approached $12.2 billion, nearly one-third of the expenditure for traditional asthma therapies as listed above [7]. The cost of CAM in comparison to traditional medicine has been examined in a Swiss population, where CAM services were paid by insurance. Those with access to free CAM services under their insurance were compared to those who did not have these services covered by their insurance. While the cost of traditional medicine therapies did not go up, the cost of CAM therapies did rise, although only 6% of those with access to CAM used it [8]. In Israel, where all have basic insurance by law, 94% of citizens purchase supplementary insurance which includes CAM coverage. In this population of asthmatic children, more than one in seven were treated for asthma with CAM [9]. In China, the trend has been toward greater use of Western medicine, with a resulting decline in the use of TCM. This is most pronounced in urban areas of China although the trend has also been noted in rural communities [10].

Overview of Integrative Therapy Use in Asthmatics: Who Uses It and Why?

The use of complementary, alternative, and integrative therapies in asthmatics is high. Up to 49% of those with asthma or allergic rhinitis report having used complementary therapies, with herbal therapies and breathing techniques being the most common [11, 12] Those who report use of complementary medicine tend to be more highly educated, are younger, suffer from chronic disease, and are concerned about risks of and dependency on traditional medications [9, 11, 13–16]. Most who use integrative therapies do so because they may provide symptom relief rather than because of dissatisfaction with conventional therapies. In support of this finding is the fact that most of those who use nonconventional therapies do so in addition to, not as a substitute for, traditional medicines. However, up to 26% use alternative therapies as their only form of treatment [11, 13, 15, 17]. Despite the apparently high rate of reported use of complementary therapies, up to 41% of those with asthma are unaware of complementary therapies and up to 33% are aware of them but have not considered their use. Interestingly, despite the concerns about risks with traditional medicines that sometimes lead to use of herbal therapies, many caregivers either were unsure about or did not think that herbal products interact with over-the-counter or prescription medications. The source of information regarding safety often comes primarily from friends and relatives, with less than half reporting or discussing use of herbal therapies with their child's primary physician [12, 15, 17, 18]. Additionally, the source of the actual herb varies from backyards to supermarkets to herbalists, herbal shops, and pharmacies [15].

It is difficult for the practitioner to educate patients on therapies for which there is little guidance from the literature or medical societies. The British Thoracic Society (BTS) attempted to provide such guidance in their 2003 and 2008 summary statements on CAM [19, 20]. The BTS recognized that, in general, there is a lack of evidence for CAM but that because these treatments may have some effect on disease, further studies need to be conducted. After examining acupuncture, air ionizers, breathing techniques, herbal and TCM, homeopathy, hypnosis and relaxation, massage and spinal manipulation, physical exercise training, and family therapy, the only treatment suggested by the BTS to have some therapeutic benefit was family therapy [20].

The National Institutes of Health (NIH) National Center For Complementary and Alternative Medicine (NCCAM) has categorized CAM into four categories: (1) natural products, including herbal medicines, vitamins, minerals, and other products sold over-the-counter as dietary supplements; (2) mind–body medicine, including meditation, yoga, and acupuncture; (3) manipulative and body-based practices, including massage and spinal manipulation; and (4) movement techniques, manipulation of energy such as through light or magnet therapy, and whole medical systems including Ayurvedic medicine, TCM, and homeopathy, among others [21]. The remainder of this chapter will review the literature on the use of selected areas in integrative medicine in each of these CAM categories.

Natural Products

Herbal and Supplemental Therapies

Herbal therapies are among the most common types of complementary medicine used by those with allergic diseases and asthma. Much of the basis for Japanese, Indian, and Latin American herbal medicine is influenced by Chinese medicine, but is also varied and individualized based on the philosophies and beliefs of the culture in which it is used [22]. Herbal remedies from plant sources from any location worldwide may include leaves, flowers, stems, roots, seeds, and berries in any number of forms including pills, powders, syrups, and teas taken internally as well as topical salves, ointments, and shampoos [16]. The Food and Drug Administration (FDA) Dietary Supplement Health and Education Act of 1994 defines dietary supplements as any of the following: a vitamin; a mineral; an herb or other botanical; an amino acid; a dietary substance for use by man to supplement the diet by increasing the total dietary intake; or a concentrate, metabolite, constituent, extract, or combination of any of the above ingredients [23]. However, despite the establishment of this definition, there is little regulation of herbal and supplementary therapies, allowing them to be marketed without the rigorous research performed on pharmaceutical medicines. The fact that many herbal and supplemental therapies are marketed and sold in pharmacies may confuse the consumer who may believe that they are tested and regulated by the FDA like other medications sold there. Adolescents and adults may therefore confuse over-the-counter and prescription medicines with alternative medicines, thinking that they are equally regulated and safe [24]. The lack of regulation of herbal remedies leads to questions about safety. Up to 20% of herbal remedies sold in the United States and over the Internet have been found to contain potentially intoxicating lead, mercury, and arsenic and medicines such as phenytoin, indomethacin, and corticosteroids, none of which are necessarily revealed openly to the consumer [25–27]. More dangerous is the risk of bronchospasm and allergic reactions ranging from dermatitis to anaphylaxis which have been reported with the use of various herbal preparations [28]. *Ephedra sinica,* also known as *ma huang,* first appeared in Chinese medicine over 2,500 years ago and was marketed in the United States in 1994 as a weight loss supplement. However, it was also used by asthmatics as an alternative treatment for asthma, many who were unlikely aware of the danger of combining it with albuterol [18]. In 2004, after a decade of reports of cardiovascular events and deaths linked to its use, *Ephedra* was withdrawn from the United States market [29–31].

In summary, there are countless herbal therapies used for various complaints. The few studies with a sufficiently strong design are not comparable enough to make a statement on the efficacy of herbal therapies in asthma. This is because of differences in definition of asthma, primary outcomes studied, and the fact that many herbs have been included in only one or two studies with strong design. A Cochrane review found only 27 studies that met their search criteria, excluding 225 because of inadequate study design [29]. The small number of studies, few of which are for the same herbal remedy, in addition to the lack of consistency in study design or primary outcome, makes it difficult to draw conclusions on the efficacy and safety of any particular herbal remedy. While studies using preparations of combinations of herbs appear to find some efficacy in the treatment of asthma, several concerns arise. First, the herbs are not standardized with regards to source, processing, and content. The formulation in which the herbal remedy is provided, for example, pill/capsule, powder, or other varies from one study to the next. None of the individual herbs have been studied sufficiently to determine their efficacy or safety when taken alone. When combined with other herbs, over-the-counter or prescription medications, there may both beneficial and harmful interactions, the mechanisms of which are not yet clear. Further studies of these remedies, both singly and in combination, are needed before one can conclude that they are a safe and efficacious treatment for asthma.

There are numerous studies on herbal preparations for the prevention and treatment of asthma. These have been thoroughly reviewed elsewhere and the reader is encouraged to refer to these reviews [22, 29, 32–34]. Table 3.1 summarizes the results of a 2008 Cochrane review [29]. Other notable herbs not reported on or included in the Cochrane review include Chamomile, *Nigella sativa, Cannabis sativa* (Marijuana), *Solanum xanthocarpum*, and *Solanum tribobatum*. Chamomile should be used cautiously in those with known allergy to the Compositae family of plants such as ragweed, chrysanthemum, and chamomile, as anaphylaxis to this supplement has been reported [16, 35]. *N. sativa* is an Arabian plant that has been shown to improve symptom severity and frequency in both adults and children with allergic rhinitis and allergic asthma and may reduce medication use and improve spirometry [36, 37]. Marijuana is thought to have bronchodilating properties due to the active component, delta-9-tetrahydrocannabinol. Studies on smoked marijuana for the treatment of asthma are poorly constructed, with few studies being double-blind and randomization methods which are poorly described. Significant bias was identified because of previous experience with smoking marijuana in study subjects. Common side effects were intoxication and tachycardia [38, 39]. The herbal remedies *S. xanthocarpum* and *S. tribobatum* have been studied as treatments for asthma, but poorly so. Few trials have used control groups and their methods have been criticized [32]. One trial showed a significant improvement in FEV1 but this improvement was still inferior to the use of conventional medicines [33]. The reported safety profile seems to be fairly benign with only one study reporting minor adverse events (dryness of mouth/throat and fever) [32] (in reference to its reference 42).

There are several studies examining combinations of herbs in the treatment of asthma. ASHMI is one such herbal combination made of three herbs (Ling-Zhi (*Ganoderma lucidum*), Ku-Shen (Radix *Sophora flavescentis*), and *Gan-Cao* (Radix *Glycyrrhiza uralensis*)) originally derived from a TCM 14-herb formula called MSSM-002. ASHMI may suppress the Th2 response, as it reduced IL-5 and IL-13 [40]. A randomized, placebo-controlled study showed that ASHMI used with prednisone placebo in those with moderate–severe persistent atopic asthma reduced symptom scores; rescued beta-agonist use; and improved FEV1, eosinophil counts, and IgE levels; however, these changes were not significantly different from the group treated instead with ASHMI placebo and prednisone. Reported side effects were weight gain and gastric discomfort [41]. The same group completed a phase I dose-escalation trial of ASHMI in 20 subjects, but this time the diagnosis of asthma was based on a previous physician diagnosis and was not confirmed with pulmonary function testing, making the results difficult to compare to the first trial [42].

STA-1 is a Chinese herbal preparation made up of Mai-Men-Dong-Tang (mMMDT) and Lui-Wei-Di-Huang-Wan (LWDHW) both of which were included in the Cochrane review (Table 3.1) [29, 43]. This preparation contains five herbs (*Ophiopogon*, American ginseng, *Pinellia*, raw Licorice, and Lantern tridax) and

Table 3.1 Summary of publications regarding the use of herbal remedies for asthma [29]

21 compounds or herbs studied				
5 TCM (Mai-Men-Dong-Tang, Liu-Wei_huang-Wan, Shen-Ling-Bia-Shu-San, Jai-Wei-Si-Jun-Zi-Tang)				
4 Indian (*Tylophora indica*, Devaduru compound, Pulmoflex, Herbal compound DCBT4567-Astha-15)				
1 Japanese (TJ-96 "saiboku-tu")				
11 Other (Ivy leaf extract, Gamma-linolenic acid-containing Borage oil, Ginkgolides or *Ginkgo* containing, 1.8-cineol (eucalyptol), Butterbur, Menthol vapor, Pycnogenol, Boswellic acids, Evening primrose oil, Propolis extract, Ginger)				
Study design	Study size	Age of participants	Inclusion criteria	Treatment duration
1 Quasi-randomized study	8–12 (2 studies)	Children (6 studies)	Reversibility (5 studies)	Mean 8.4 weeks
1 Randomized, single-blind placebo-controlled parallel study	15–30 (6 studies)	Adults (14 studies)	Met existing diagnostic criteria for asthma (11 studies)	Range
14 Randomized double-blind placebo-controlled parallel studies	31–99 (12 studies)	Adults and children (1 study)	Clinical diagnosis or history of asthma (10 studies)	3–7 days (8 studies)
10 Randomized, placebo-controlled crossover studies	100–200 (5 studies) Over 300 (1 study)	Unclear age range or not stated (6 studies)	No criteria stated (1 study)	2–16 weeks (17 studies) 4–12 months (3 studies)
Primary outcome measure FEV1, FEV1/FVC, PEFR, VC, FEF 25–75, maximum breathing capacity Other outcome measures Exacerbation rates, changes in medication use, symptom scores, subjective assessments		Adverse events *6 herbs/compounds with reported adverse events* Saiboku-tu—pneumonia and pneumonitis Tylophora—Giddiness, nausea, vomiting, abdominal pain, sore mouth Boswellic acids—Nausea, abdominal pain, hyperacidity Pycngenol—Gastrointestinal disturbance Eucalyptol—Heartburn and gastritis Menthol vapor—Upper airway discomfort No adverse events occurred: Ulmoflex, inkgolides, PDCT No adverse events reported: Evening primrose oil, Propolis, Butterbur, Ivy Leaf extract, Borage oil, Ginger		

has been shown to reduce levels of IL-4 after inhalational challenge and also to reduce airway inflammation [44, 45]. Ginseng, which is found in mMMDT, may reduce number of inflammatory cells and prevent airway remodeling [46]. In a double-blind, randomized, placebo-controlled trial in children with confirmed symptomatic atopic asthma, 4 months of mMMDT significantly improved FEV1 and symptom scores but had no effect on total IgE, dust mite-specific IgE, or IgG4 [45].

LWDHW is a combination of six herbs (*Rehmannia glutinosa*, *Cornus officinalis*, *Dioscorea opposite*, *Alisma orientalis*, *Paeonia suffruticosa*, and *Poria cocos*) and is available in pill or powder form, or may be made into a soup [47, 48]. Two components of the herbal combination, Cortex Moutan and Rhizoma Dioscoreae, may have antioxidant activity, although LWDHW has not been shown to share this property [47]. LWDHW has been shown to inhibit Th1 and Th2 cytokine gene expression from the activated peripheral blood mononuclear cells of asthmatics [48]. In animals, STA-1 lowered dust mite-specific IgE but not IgG levels. It was also shown to reduce airway hyperreactivity after allergen challenge as well as inflammation, based on reduced numbers of airway eosinophils and neutrophils after exposure to allergen [43]. In humans, STA-1 improved symptom scores and FEV1 and resulted in reduced steroid requirements and total and mite-specific IgE in atopic asthmatic adults and children [49].

Vitamins and Other Supplements

Airway inflammation is one of the major components of asthma pathophysiology. Asthmatics with severe persistent airway hyperresponsiveness have been found to have reduced blood levels of antioxidants such as beta-carotene, alpha-tocopherol, and total tocopherol [50]. Therefore, improved nutrition and intake of dietary antioxidants may be important in the prevention of inflammation in asthma and other inflammatory diseases. Various studies have suggested that diets rich in fruits, nuts, and vegetables containing high amounts antioxidants such as vitamins A, C, and E may have a protective effect in asthma [51–53]. Both adults and children consuming diets with higher amounts of antioxidant vitamins have improved lung function based on pulmonary function testing, as well as fewer reports of asthma [51, 52, 54]. Conversely, low serum vitamin A concentrations have been reported in children with asthma and low intake may correlate with reduced lung function in both healthy and asthmatic children [54–58]. Low vitamin C intake in both healthy and asthmatic children has been correlated with increased cough and wheeze as well as low FEV1 and FVC, and increased risk of asthma [54, 59, 60]. Vitamin C supplementation has been shown to attenuate exercise-induced bronchoconstriction, and postexercise eNO, improve symptom scores and pulmonary function and lower urinary and sputum leukotrienes and prostaglandins [61, 62].

A Cochrane review of vitamin C supplementation in asthmatics evaluated twelve studies ranging in size from 6 to 41 participants. All of the studies were reported to be randomized, but few reported the method of randomization, blinding, and allocation concealment and none reported methods for all three of these items. Overall, no studies found a significant difference in pre- or postexercise challenge FEV1 or FVC although one study did find that the percent drop in FEV1 after exercise was improved in the group given vitamin C. Based on the small trials, poor reporting, and variation in study design, there was insufficient evidence to recommend vitamin C in the treatment of asthma [63]. Vitamin E has also been examined as an antioxidant with possible disease-modifying ability in asthma, as it has been shown to protect against monocyte activation by LPS [64]. Low vitamin E intake may correlate with decreased lung function in children that does not appear to differ between healthy and asthmatic children [54]. The finding that vitamin E intake is positively associated with lower serum IgE levels and reduced risk of atopy suggests a role for vitamin E in protection against asthma [65]. However, a randomized placebo-controlled trial of vitamin E replacement in physician-diagnosed asthmatics on inhaled corticosteroids found no improvement in bronchial reactivity to methacholine, change in pulmonary function (FEV1, FVC, or peak expiratory flow rate), bronchodilator use, symptom scores, or serum IgE levels [66]. Other studies failed to consistently support a role for Vitamin E in protection from development of asthma, improvement in pulmonary function or sensitivity to methacholine [55, 64, 67]. The NIH sponsored NCCAM is currently investigating the safety of vitamin E in the form of gamma-tocopherol in asthmatics as well as the combination of vitamin E and C for the purpose of enhancing airway antioxidant levels in those with allergic asthma [68].

The antioxidant selenium has not been found to have a significant effect on pulmonary function, quality-of-life scores, bronchodilator use, or diagnosis of asthma [69, 70]. A recent Cochrane review found only one randomized double-blind, controlled trial that met their search criteria regarding the use of selenium to treat asthma [71]. Since that single study was published, another double-blind placebo-controlled study was carried out, but neither study found that selenium improved objective measures of lung function [69, 71]. Dietary magnesium has been repeatedly shown to reduce bronchial hyperresponsiveness to methacholine [69, 72–74] but has no apparent effect on airway inflammation based on eNO levels [74].

Vitamin D is a steroid hormone that can be activated by respiratory epithelium in situations such as viral infections [75]. The active form of vitamin D has been shown to modulate both the innate and adaptive immune system by increasing production of the cathelicidin antimicrobial peptide gene and inhibition of lymphocyte differentiation [76, 77]. Therefore, it may play a role in preventing the development of the atopic phenotype or of airway remodeling in sensitized asthmatics. Maternal intake of vitamin D, while it may reduce wheeze in infancy, does not appear to protect against other signs of inflammation and asthma including elevated FeNO, symptoms, allergic sensitization, and airflow obstruction on spirometry [65, 78]. Serum concentrations of 25-hydroxyvitamin D are positively correlated with FEV1 and negatively correlated with methacholine-induced airway hyperresponsiveness, which suggests a potential role for this vitamin in preventing or reversing airway obstruction [79, 80]. Deficiency of vitamin D in children may reduce FEV1 and increase exacerbations and the use of medications such as beta-agonists and inhaled corticosteroids [81, 82].

Coenzyme Q (ubiqinone) is an antioxidant that scavenges free oxygen radicals and therefore may be anti-inflammatory. While low plasma and whole blood concentrations have been reported in asthmatics as compared to controls, no well-designed studies have been able to confirm a positive effect on symptoms, medication use, or lung function in asthmatics [83, 84].

Eicosanoids are pro-inflammatory chemical messengers that are synthesized from three sources, including a polyunsaturated fatty acid called dihomo-gamma-linolenic acid, arachadonic acid, and eicosapentaenoic acid. The three eicosanoids important in asthmatic inflammation include prostaglandins, leukotrienes, and thromoboxanes which are produced when activated phospholipase A2 causes release of arachadonic acid from cell membranes [85]. Conjugated linoleic acid which is found in fish oil may compete with linoleic acid in cell membranes as a substrate from which to synthesize eicosanoids [85–87]. Animal studies have suggested that increased dietary linoleic acid or gamma-linolenic acid have immunomodulatory effects such as reduction in lymphocyte proliferation, NK cell activity, and expression of cell adhesion molecules [88–90]. One study suggests that in developed countries such as the United States, the United Kingdom, and Germany, a rise in consumption of linoleic acid in products containing polyunsaturated fat correlates to a rise in the incidence of asthma [52, 91] although others have not been able to confirm this association [67]. Diets low in n-3 fatty acids have been associated with increased chronic bronchitis symptoms, wheeze, and asthma [51]. Supplementation of conjugated linoleic acid has been shown to improve bronchial hyperresponsiveness to methacholine although it did not affect other measurable parameters in asthmatics including FEV1, beta-agonist use, quality-of-life scores, or levels of serum cytokines [87]. Additional reviews and individual studies were also unable to support the supplementation of fish oil or other unsaturated fatty acids for the prevention or treatment of asthma [60, 62, 67, 92–98].

Caffeine is a methylxanthine which is chemically related to a once-popular asthma medication, theophylline. The mechanism of action of methylxanthines, while still unclear, may be through inhibition of cAMP breakdown by phosphodiesterases, thereby having an effect on smooth muscle contraction [99, 100]. It may also be due to antagonistic action on adenosine receptors [100]. Caffeine has been shown to improve FEV1 in a dose–responsive manner in confirmed asthmatics, although studies disagree on whether it is as effective as equivalent doses of theophylline [101, 102]. Caffeine may also improve FEV1 and attenuate the drop in FEV1 seen in exercise-induced asthma and during dry gas hyperventilation [103–105]. A Cochrane review of the literature regarding caffeine in the treatment of asthma found that while caffeine may improve lung function, it does not improve asthma symptoms [99]. Studies do not agree on whether caffeine has an effect on FEV1 or PC20 during histamine bronchoprovocation studies, but this may be due to differences in the definition of asthma during subject recruitment as well as differing amounts of caffeine used in the studies [106, 107]. Caffeine and carbonated caffeinated drinks do not appear to have an effect on inflammation in asthmatics, based on FeNO levels [108, 109]. Common adverse effects of caffeine include shakiness, tremor, nervousness, and gastrointestinal upset [101, 102].

Mind–Body Medicine

The use of acupuncture in China dates back more than 5,000 years [2, 110]. However, it was not until 1971 that it became popular in the United States, after journalist James Reston, who traveled to China with President Richard Nixon, wrote of his experience [111, 112]. Acupuncture treatment is based on the flow of Qi energy, made up of Yin and Yang forces. This energy flows along pathways termed meridians that lie just beneath the skin and within blood vessels. The energy is manipulated by acupuncture to correct imbalances in disease [2, 110, 113]. As in traditional Western medicine, where several treatment forms may be used for the same disease, TCM uses acupuncture in conjunction with other forms of TCM to treat the diagnosed energy imbalances [2]. The most common rationale cited for acupuncture in clinical studies is that acupuncture stimulates release of neurochemicals [114]. Other proposed mechanisms of action include modulation of the autonomic nervous system and subsequent effects on smooth muscle [114]. There is suggestive evidence based on changes in levels of cytokines, neuropeptides, and nitric oxide levels, that acupuncture, by acting on nerve fibers, may have immune-modulating effects [110, 114–117].

Asthma is commonly treated by acupuncture in both China and the United States [118]. Acupuncture as a treatment for asthma has been systematically reviewed. There are few double-blind, randomized placebo-controlled trials with an n less than 50 [119–124]. Overall, there is no clear benefit of acupuncture as compared to sham acupuncture with regards to spirometric results, even after treatment periods as long as 1 year [117, 122, 124–130]. However, acupuncture may improve symptoms, based on questionnaires and quality-of-life scores [123, 124, 131]. Laser acupuncture is a painless method of acupuncture using the energy of a laser beam on acupuncture points as a surrogate for needle acupuncture that has only been evaluated in a limited number of studies [119–121, 132–134]. One small ($n=44$) double-blind, placebo-controlled study, looked at the effects of laser acupuncture on lung function and bronchial responsiveness in children and adolescents with exercise-induced asthma. It found that a single treatment did not provide any improvement in basal bronchomotor tone and additionally it did not provide protection against cold dry air hyperventilation-induced bronchoconstriction [120]. A randomized, double-blind, placebo-controlled study in asthmatic children attempted to treat both the intestines (with probiotics) and the lungs (with laser acupuncture therapy) as these organs are thought to be complementary, since the intestines are a Yang organ and the lungs a Yin organ. The study design was better than many, and employed spirometry to confirm asthma and maintained treatment for several months. The authors noted significant improvement in FEV1 in the treatment group and no adverse events, but the study lacked statistical power ($n=17$) and larger studies are needed before this form of treatment can be endorsed [119].

There are several methodological limitations related to the study of acupuncture in clinical trials; these relate primarily to methods used to blind the subjects. First, many double-blind, placebo-controlled trials using acupuncture use sham acupuncture as their control. Sham acupuncture uses nonspecific needling of areas of the body to mimic true acupuncture. There has been criticism of this technique, as some argue that nonspecific needling may have some of the effect that acupuncture does and therefore may provide a potential second treatment arm rather than a true placebo control arm [135]. In fact, some studies were later found to have used sham sites that were actually areas used to treat respiratory conditions and were therefore not truly sham acupuncture sites [135]. It is possible that sham acupuncture, like real acupuncture, modifies the autonomic nervous system and causes release of endorphins and substance P [2, 114, 136]. To date, no technique has been found which creates the same sensation as acupuncture without breaking the skin [2]. Second, the lack of a clear mechanism by which acupuncture affects the many organ systems in disease poses a problem because without a clear mechanism of action for a treatment, an appropriate placebo cannot be effectively chosen [114]. An additional major issue in trials is the lack of ability to blind all three involved individuals: the patient, the acupuncturist, and the evaluator. The acupuncturist must be aware they are inserting a needle into the skin [2]. This is as opposed to laser acupuncture where a light could be used as placebo since it could be made indistinguishable to the study provider. The patient can be blinded as long as they do not know information about point location and technique for acupuncture [2]. In April 1994, the FDA and the NIH Office of Alternative Medicine (NIH-OAM) conducted a workshop on acupuncture to reevaluate the status of acupuncture needles as investigational devices [137]. The issue of "proper" scientific methods in acupuncture research was brought up, and here as well it was noted that until sham acupuncture can be proven not to cause a significant effect beyond placebo, it should not be considered an appropriate control for scientific studies [137].

In 1998 the NIH published a consensus report on acupuncture, noting equivocal results and multiple methodological problems. Asthma was listed as one of many diseases for which there is insufficient evidence to support acupuncture as a solitary treatment, but it was noted that it may be effective in conjunction with other therapies in a comprehensive management program [138].

In 2003 the World Health Organization (WHO) also released a review of clinical trials using acupuncture, citing evidence for effectiveness of acupuncture for the treatment of 28 conditions based on clinical trials. Asthma was not among this group but was listed among 62 other conditions for which evidence is present, but the evidence was judged to be insufficient [111]. A 2009 Cochrane review on the use of acupuncture for chronic asthma cited insufficient evidence to make recommendations about the value of acupuncture as a treatment for asthma [139]. Major flaws in trials for acupuncture include small sample size, lack of appropriate placebo or other control, and lack of or poor definitions of asthma (including failure to confirm asthma by pulmonary function testing or failure to include pulmonary function testing as a measure of response to treatment), variations in acupuncture technique, continuation of other therapies in conjunction with acupuncture therapy, and lack of blinding. Another issue seen in trials is that many asthmatics cannot safely be taken off of their traditional medications such as corticosteroids and beta-agonists for prolonged periods of time. This means that results from trials using acupuncture may not see the full effects, as the study subject may not be given enough time off of their medication to be brought to baseline or the study duration was not long enough to see the full effects of acupuncture. Additionally, effects noted by the study may be in part because of effects of medications still in the subject's system or interactions of medications with acupuncture [2]. In general, the evidence for acupuncture for the treatment of asthma is tenuous. Even if the current evidence supported acupuncture, the lack of a clear definition of asthma or consistent study design, results cannot be compared. Therefore, no conclusion can be drawn regarding the effectiveness of acupuncture as a treatment for asthma.

Complications from acupuncture include those that are relatively benign, such as vasovagal episodes, pain, and bleeding; but also more serious complications such as acquisition of HIV or hepatitis B/C, hemothorax, pneumothorax, cardiac tamponade, visceral laceration, muscle hematomas, nerve compression due to hematomas, deep vein thrombosis, compartment syndrome, sepsis, CNS infections, endocarditis and deterioration of and even death from asthma [115, 140–150]. Additionally, in Japanese acupuncture, the needle may be cut and left in the body. There are reports of migration of needles to the spinal cord, upper urinary tract, nerves, and tendons which may cause secondary complications and pain [143]. One review found that at least half of all patients with acupuncture-induced pneumothorax were treated by acupuncturists who also had an MD degree [143]. An adjunctive therapy to acupuncture, termed moxibustion, has also resulted in adverse events. Moxibustion consists of burning cones filled with a dried herb (*Artemesia vulgaris*) directly on the acupuncture point until a blister forms, or to heat the needle to improve flow of Qi [2, 113, 140]. Several reports have been published of severe burns to the skin of patients undergoing this technique [140]. The National Certification Commission for Acupuncture and Oriental Medicine (NCCAOM) was established in 1982. It is a not-for-profit organization under which there are 19,000 diplomates practicing acupuncture, oriental medicine, Chinese herbology, and Asian bodywork therapy. It is the only nationally recognized certification and is required for state licensure in most states [151]. Safety precautions, particularly with regards to transmission of infectious diseases, have been established and published by the NCCAOM in their *Clean Needle Technique Manual*, which was reviewed by the Centers for Disease Control (CDC) [145, 152]. Every individual seeking national board certification must pass their Clean Needle Technique course [152].

Yoga, Breathing, and Relaxation Techniques

Based on the fact that asthma is a disorder of respiratory airflow, many have attempted to use breathing and relaxation techniques to improve asthma control. An Australian study found that after being taught how to use wind instruments and how to sing, indigenous children with asthma reported improved well-being and compliance with treatment [153]. After a 6-month period, breathing retraining taught by a physiotherapist appeared to have a significant effect on quality-of-life scores in asthmatics, as compared to nurse-directed asthma education, although the diagnosis of asthma was not confirmed by spirometry [154]. The same group carried out another study on breathing retraining in a prospective, parallel group, single-blind, randomized controlled trial, again looking at the difference in effect of breathing training and asthma education. In this study, spirometry and methacholine challenges were performed at baseline and 1 month, in addition to sputum cell count and differential and FeNO. Again, at 6 months the breathing retraining group had significantly improved quality-of-life scores in comparison to the asthma education group. Hyperresponsiveness to methacholine, FeNO and sputum cell counts and differential did not differ significantly between the two groups [155].

A Cochrane review on breathing retraining for patients with asthma found only seven studies that met their inclusion criteria. Even these did not consistently report data, preventing data from being compared from one study to the next. The authors concluded that due to the small number of studies, the low number of subjects in each study, and the variability in interventions used, "no reliable conclusions can be drawn as to the beneficial effects of breathing retraining in asthma" [156]. An earlier review of the literature which had very little overlap with the Cochrane studies found that breathing exercises in most studies did not significantly improve pulmonary function, symptom score, or medication use [157]. One pilot study successfully used breathing training with capnometry biofeedback and paced breathing assistance to reduce hyperventilation and raise pCO_2 levels in asthmatics. Subjects reported reduced symptoms but no change in FEV1 was appreciated [158].

Yoga, breathing, and relaxation techniques have been studied as potential interventions for asthma. A systematic review of relaxation therapies for asthma cited poor evidence for mental and muscular relaxation in the treatment of asthma, primarily because studies had significant methodological flaws [159]. Hypnosis, a treatment that may be categorized under relaxation techniques, has been studied for decades as a possible treatment for asthma. However, despite the existence of randomized, controlled trials, most are small and observed outcomes are not comparable, ranging from symptomatic improvement to spirometry results to airway hyperresponsiveness and even to the prevention of asthma. This variability makes it difficult to make a generalized statement on its efficacy [160].

Yoga, a practice of breathing and meditation in defined postures, has been studied in a double-blind randomized controlled trial in adults with confirmed asthma. Interestingly, both groups had significant improvement in post-bronchodilator FEV1, but there was no difference in quality of life, frequency of inhaler use, or pulmonary function [161]. Various types of yoga and breathing techniques such as Buyeyko breathing technique, Sahaja yoga, Hatha yoga, and Pranayama yoga have been studied in asthmatics [162–167]. Most of these studies, despite their generally small size, were randomized, double-blind, and placebo-controlled, although usual asthma therapy was not discontinued. Asthma diagnosis and response to therapy were confirmed with spirometry in most studies and some studies also evaluated for improvement in hyperresponsiveness to methacholine or histamine. In general, there was not consistent improvement in spirometry, quality-of-life measures, or steroid or beta-agonist requirements in these studies, although some showed reduced sensitivity to methacholine or histamine [162–164, 166]. Other studies failed to confirm asthma diagnosis or to measure FEV1, therefore making it difficult to objectively evaluate degree of improvement [165, 167]. More unusual techniques have been attempted, such as mouth taping at night to mimic the Buteyko yoga technique. Mouth taping forces one to inspire nasally, therefore warming and humidifying inspired air [168]. One small study on this technique ($n = 50$) did not show improvement in symptom scores or pulmonary function as determined by peak flow measurements [168]. Overall, adverse effects and events reported in studies on yoga and breathing techniques were either not reported or were mild, and included dyspnea and exacerbations of asthma [166, 168].

Manipulative and Body-Based Practices

Manual therapy includes chiropractic and osteopathic techniques, massage, and other physical maneuvers to improve expectoration of phlegm [169]. Chiropractic medicine is based on the concept that misaligned vertebrae negatively influence other systems and structures in the body, including the respiratory system. Spinal manipulations are thought to treat pulmonary disease by normalizing neurologic function, improving movement of the thoracic cage and even by improving pulmonary lymphatic flow [170–173]. Generally, studies on these approaches use randomization. However, sham spinal manipulation is used as placebo, which like acupuncture may be partially interventional rather than true placebo. The studies are generally methodologically poor as they often lack confirmation of asthma diagnosis and improvement of lung function with spirometry [170, 173, 174]. One methodologically adequate study in 80 children with asthma confirmed with spirometry found no improvement compared to placebo with regards to symptoms, quality of life, peak flow, or beta-agonist use [174]. In accord with these findings, a Cochrane review on manual therapy for the treatment of asthma concluded that more research is needed [169]. Adverse events reported in studies using chiropractic manipulation were generally mild but stroke has been reported [174–177].

Craniosacral fascial therapy is based on the concept that the brain and spinal cord exist in a normal balance and rhythm within the CSF, and that the brain "breathes" with the rest of the body in "cycles" as it expands and contracts. Because all tissues of the body are connected to one another, trauma to the fascia in one location can lead to abnormalities in another location, such as the respiratory system [178]. Craniosacral fascial therapy attempts to correct the abnormal cycle seen in disease states such as in asthma where the cycle length is thought to be abnormally short [178, 179]. However, the measurement of cycles in this technique is examiner dependent as the examiner does not use any objective measures or equipment to determine cycle length. Only two articles on the use of craniosacral therapy in the treatment of asthma were found in a literature search [178, 180]. One was a case report on the successful use of craniosacral fascial therapy to treat a young child with asthma and other was a relatively small ($n = 68$) randomized controlled trial on the use of acupuncture in conjunction with craniosacral therapy [178]. The latter trial, which confirmed asthma based on NHLBI criteria, symptoms, and pulmonary function testing, suggested that the combination of treatments resulted in an improved quality-of-life, but there was no clear improvement in objective measures such as pulmonary function [180]. There are no well-designed studies looking at craniosacral fascial therapy alone in the treatment of asthma. Although further studies are needed to determine its safety and effectiveness, the lack of objective diagnostic measures in this technique makes it unlikely to be properly and sufficiently studied or widely recommended.

Reflexology and massage therapy both use pressure to various parts of the body to relieve symptoms. Reflexology is the use of finger-pressure on the feet, back, and other parts of the body to treat disease states [181]. Few studies have been published on reflexology and massage for the treatment of asthma [181, 182]. Two small studies used spirometry to monitor for improvement, but there was either no improvement or improvement was only seen in certain age groups [181, 182]. The Alexander technique, a century-old method of "taught physical therapy," is based on correction of posture and realignment of the body so that it may relax and function more efficiently [183, 184]. While its most common use has been to improve coordination of the musculoskeletal system in the management of pain, it has been used by athletes, singers, dancers, and others to improve breathing and vocal production [183, 184]. This may be the basis on which it has been advocated as a treatment for asthma [183, 184]. Unfortunately, a systematic review concluded that more research is needed as it was unable to identify any controlled trials on this technique in the treatment of asthma [183].

Movement Techniques and Other Integrative Medicine Practices

As early as the 1960s, electro-aerosol therapy using ionized aerosols were being used to treat a number of respiratory diseases [185]. Negatively charged ions were thought to improve ciliary function and possibly even affect CNS function. Based on these theories, ionized water was used in the 1960s in aerosolized form for the treatment of bronchial asthma and bronchitis [185]. Several decades later the ability to ionize the air without using aerosolized water led several to question whether negatively ionized air could indirectly treat asthma by reducing allergens and irritants. Positively ionized air has been shown to have bronchoconstrictive effects in children with exercise-induced asthma [186]. Various studies, including a Cochrane review, have examined the effects of air ionizers on allergen levels, lung function, asthma symptoms, and bronchoprovocation sensitivity. Unfortunately these studies are small, have poor methodology (most use PEFR to monitor response, instead of spirometry), and report conflicting results, all of which makes even apparently significant results difficult to interpret or to apply clinically [186–191].

Homeopathy is an individualized treatment which is based on consumption of extremely dilute solutions (10^{-60}) of the substance, that in larger amounts, is felt to be causing the symptoms or disease to be treated [192, 193]. Studies do not consistently show a benefit of homeopathy in the treatment of allergic asthma [193–195]. One study was able to show that very dilute amounts of grass pollen (compared to placebo) was able to improve hay fever symptoms [196]. Two similar double-blind, randomized, placebo-controlled trials of homeopathic treatment in skin prick positive, dust mite-allergic asthmatics showed conflicting results. While homeopathy in one study resulted in improved spirometry, there was no improvement in symptoms. The other study found an improvement in symptoms but no improvement in spirometry [193, 195]. One study was able to show that successive dilutions of IgE antibodies generally resulted in decreasing basophil degranulation. However, some concentrations resulted in an increase in degranulation, a finding that was not explicable but was reproducible in several independent labs [197]. It has been proposed that these dilute concentrations may result in inhibition of IgE-mediated basophil degranulation, possibly through very dilute concentrations of histamine. These concentrations may also modulate the immune response through rearrangements in the variable region of the IgG molecule [197, 198]. These results suggest that the very dilute concentrations used in homeopathy may affect IgE and basophil degranulation differently than the concentration that causes symptoms. A recent Cochrane Database review on the use of homeopathy for the treatment of asthma concluded that more evidence is necessary before homeopathy can be recommended in the treatment of asthma [192].

Art therapy has been well studied as an intervention for children with cancer, cerebral palsy, and other chronic diseases but has not been well studied in children with respiratory disease [199–202]. In children with cystic fibrosis, art therapy has been used to better understand the role of spirituality and religion in coping with their illness [203]. Only one study has looked specifically at the role of art therapy in the management of asthma [204]. This randomized, placebo-controlled trial of 22 children with persistent asthma requiring daily treatment found that art therapy improved quality-of-life scores and reduced anxiety, with effects that lasted up to 6 months after completion of the therapy. There was no difference between placebo and treatment groups with regard to exacerbation rates. However, the authors correctly question whether combination of art therapy with traditional medical therapy might help the patient and family manage chronic diseases such as asthma and thereby improve control and reduce exacerbation rates [204]. In those with both confirmed asthma and panic disorder, teaching subjects how to differentiate the two diseases and use relaxation techniques was able to improve asthma symptom severity but not albuterol use during the treatment period. Pulmonary function did not improve significantly across all treatment groups examined [205].

Conclusion and Further Directions

Integrative medicine is becoming more popular in the treatment of chronic diseases such as asthma. Practitioners treating patients with asthma need to be aware of the variety of therapies available, the current body of evidence for their use in the treatment of asthma, and the risks and cost of using them, so that they may help educate their patients. As providers become more knowledgeable about these topics, patients may become more likely to reveal to their provider that they are using them. Many studies had positive outcomes, whether objective or based on symptom scores. We must ask why our patient is seeking care with integrative therapies. One might consider whether symptomatic improvement without improvement in an objective measure, (such as FEV1), is enough to validate the health risks and costs of each treatment.

Another issue that must be considered is that most studies we reviewed included subjects who were already on traditional asthma medications such as inhaled corticosteroids and beta-agonists. Studies that use patients who are on no medications or only on a rescue beta-agonist may be biased toward a different phenotype of asthma that may respond differently to treatment than those requiring inhaled or oral corticosteroids.

There is also a problem with the wide definition of asthma, as an inclusion criterion—which along with differences in treatment technique, duration, and study size and design factors such as randomization and use of placebo—likely contributes to the differences in outcome. Additionally, most of the studies reviewed used a Western definition of asthma, even if the definition was not clearly outlined in the article. Whether the outcome of these studies would have been different if one used the TCM or even another culture's definition of asthma is not known. It is possible that the outcomes of the studies are inconsistent not only because of differences in the Western definition of asthma used, but because none of the studies included those with definitions of asthma unique to the place of origin of the therapy being used. Once we are able to better define both the disease and the treatment, including the pathophysiologic response to treatment, we might be able to conduct properly powered and designed studies that will identify integrative therapies with reproducible effects. Until then, those who use integrative medicine should do so cautiously, keeping in mind the lack of strong evidence to support its benefit.

References

1. Centers for Disease Control and Prevention. 2007 National Health Interview Survey Data. Table 1–1, Lifetime asthma population estimates in thousands-by age, United States: National Health interview Survey 2007. Atlanta: Department of Health and Human Services, CDC [cited 2010 October 24]. http://www.cdc.gov/asthma/nhis/07/table1–1.htm.
2. Jobst KA. Acupuncture in asthma and pulmonary disease: an analysis of efficacy and safety. J Altern Complement Med. 1996;2(1):179–206.
3. Kamble S, Bharma M. Incremental direct expenditure of treating asthma in the united states. J Asthma. 2009;46(1):73–80.
4. CDC Asthma Statistics: Center For Disease Control. [cited 2009 November 29]. http://www.cdc.gov/nchs/data/hestat/asthma03–05/asthma03–05.htm.
5. WHO Asthma Statistics: World Health Organization [cited 2010 October 24]. http://www.who.int/mediacentre/factsheets/fs307/en/print.html.
6. WHO Chronic Respiratory Diseases. Asthma. World Health Orgainization [cited 2010 November 24]. http://www.who.int/respiratory/asthma/en/.

7. Eisenberg DM, Davis RB, Ettner SL, Appel S, Wilkey S, Van Rompay M, Kessler RC. Trends in alternative medicine use in the united states, 1990–1997: results of a follow-up national survey. JAMA. 1998;280(18):1569–75.
8. Sommer JH, Burgi M, Theiss R. A randomized experiment of the effects of including alternative medicine in the mandatory benefit package of health insurance funds in switzerland. Complement Ther Med. 1999;7(2):54–61.
9. Singer L, Karakis I, Ivri L, Gross M, Bolotin A, Gazala E. The characteristics of complementary and alternative medicine use by parents of asthmatic children in southern Israel. Acta Paediatr. 2007;96(11):1693–7.
10. Jin L. From mainstream to marginal? Trends in the use of Chinese medicine in china from 1991 to 2004. Soc Sci Med. 2010;71(6):1063–7.
11. Blanc PD, Trupin L, Earnest G, Katz PP, Yelin EH, Eisner MD. Alternative therapies among adults with a reported diagnosis of asthma or rhinosinusitis: data from a population-based survey. Chest. 2001;120(5):1461–7.
12. Ernst E. Complementary therapies for asthma: what patients use. J Asthma. 1998;35(8):667–71.
13. Astin JA. Why patients use alternative medicine: results of a national study. JAMA. 1998;279(19):1548–53.
14. Partridge MR, Dockrell M, Smith NM. The use of complementary medicines by those with asthma. Respir Med. 2003;97(4):436–8.
15. Clement YN, Williams AF, Aranda D, Chase R, Watson N, Mohammed R, Stubbs O, Williamson D. Medicinal herb use among asthmatic patients attending a specialty care facility in trinidad. BMC Complement Altern Med. 2005;5:3.
16. Woolf AD. Herbal remedies and children: do they work? Are they harmful? Pediatrics. 2003;112(1 Pt 2):240–6.
17. Shaw A, Noble A, Salisbury C, Sharp D, Thompson E, Peters TJ. Predictors of complementary therapy use among asthma patients: results of a primary care survey. Health Soc Care Community. 2008;16(2):155–64.
18. Lanski SL, Greenwald M, Perkins A, Simon HK. Herbal therapy use in a pediatric emergency department population: expect the unexpected. Pediatrics. 2003;111(5 Pt 1):981–5.
19. British Thoracic Society, Scottish Intercollegiate Guidelines Network. British guideline on the management of asthma. Thorax 2003;58 Suppl 1:i1–94.
20. British Guideline on the Management of Asthma: A National Clinical Guideline [cited 2010 November 30]. http://www.brit-thoracic.org.uk/clinical-information/asthma/asthma-guidelines.aspx.
21. What is CAM. [cited 2011 January 7]. http://nccam.nih.gov/health/whatiscam/#otherpractices.
22. Bielory L, Lupoli K. Herbal interventions in asthma and allergy. J Asthma. 1999;36(1):1–65.
23. Dietary Supplement Health and Education Act of 1994. Significant Amendments to the FD&C Act. [cited 2010 December 5]. http://www.fda.gov/RegulatoryInformation/Legislation/FederalFoodDrugandCosmeticActFDCAct/SignificantAmendmentstotheFDCAct/ucm148003.htm.
24. Klein JD, Wilson KM, Sesselberg TS, Gray NJ, Yussman S, West J. Adolescents' knowledge of and beliefs about herbs and dietary supplements: a qualitative study. J Adolesc Health. 2005;37(5):409.
25. Saper RB, Phillips RS, Sehgal A, Khouri N, Davis RB, Paquin J, Thuppil V, Kales SN. Lead, mercury, and arsenic in US- and Indian-manufactured ayurvedic medicines sold via the internet. JAMA. 2008;300(8):915–23.
26. Saper RB, Kales SN, Paquin J, Burns MJ, Eisenberg DM, Davis RB, Phillips RS. Heavy metal content of ayurvedic herbal medicine products. JAMA. 2004;292(23):2868–73.
27. Ernst E. Adulteration of Chinese herbal medicines with synthetic drugs: a systematic review. J Intern Med. 2002;252(2):107–13.
28. Ernst E. Harmless herbs? A review of the recent literature. Am J Med. 1998;104(2):170–8.
29. Arnold E, Clark CE, Lasserson TJ, Wu T. Herbal interventions for chronic asthma in adults and children. Cochrane Database Syst Rev. 2008;(1):CD005989.

30. FDA news release. FDA Acts to Remove Ephedra-Containing Dietary Supplements from the Market. [cited 2010 November 24]. http://www.fda.gov/NewsEvents/Newsroom/PressAnnouncements/2004/ucm108379.htm.
31. Haller CA, Benowitz NL. Adverse cardiovascular and central nervous system events associated with dietary supplements containing ephedra alkaloids. N Engl J Med. 2000;343(25):1833–8.
32. Singh BB, Khorsan R, Vinjamury SP, Der-Martirosian C, Kizhakkeveettil A, Anderson TM. Herbal treatments of asthma: a systematic review. J Asthma. 2007;44(9):685–98.
33. Huntley A, Ernst E. Herbal medicines for asthma: a systematic review. Thorax. 2000;55(11):925–9.
34. Li XM. Traditional chinese herbal remedies for asthma and food allergy. J Allergy Clin Immunol. 2007;120(1):25–31.
35. Benner MH, Lee HJ. Anaphylactic reaction to chamomile tea. J Allergy Clin Immunol. 1973;52(5):307–8.
36. Kalus U, Pruss A, Bystron J, Jurecka M, Smekalova A, Lichius JJ, Kiesewetter H. Effect of *Nigella sativa* (black seed) on subjective feeling in patients with allergic diseases. Phytother Res. 2003;17(10):1209–14.
37. Boskabady MH, Javan H, Sajady M, Rakhshandeh H. The possible prophylactic effect of *Nigella sativa* seed extract in asthmatic patients. Fundam Clin Pharmacol. 2007;21(5):559–66.
38. Tashkin DP, Shapiro BJ, Frank IM. Acute effects of smoked marijuana and oral delta9-tetrahydrocannabinol on specific airway conductance in asthmatic subjects. Am Rev Respir Dis. 1974;109(4):420–8.
39. Tashkin DP, Shapiro BJ, Lee YE, Harper CE. Effects of smoked marijuana in experimentally induced asthma. Am Rev Respir Dis. 1975;112(3):377–86.
40. Ko J, Busse PJ, Shek L, Noone SA, Sampson HA, Li XM. Effect of chinese herbal formulas on T-cell responses in patients with peanut allergy or asthma. J Allergy Clin Immunol. 2005;115:S34.
41. Wen MC, Wei CH, Hu ZQ, Srivastava K, Ko J, Xi ST, Mu DZ, Du JB, Li GH, Wallenstein S, Sampson H, Kattan M, Li XM. Efficacy and tolerability of anti-asthma herbal medicine intervention in adult patients with moderate-severe allergic asthma. J Allergy Clin Immunol. 2005;116(3):517–24.
42. Kelly-Pieper K, Patil SP, Busse P, Yang N, Sampson H, Li XM, Wisnivesky JP, Kattan M. Safety and tolerability of an antiasthma herbal formula (ASHMI) in adult subjects with asthma: a randomized, double-blinded, placebo-controlled, dose-escalation phase I study. J Altern Complement Med. 2009;15(7):735–43.
43. Chang TT, Huang CC, Hsu CH. Inhibition of mite-induced immunoglobulin E synthesis, airway inflammation, and hyperreactivity by herbal medicine STA-1. Immunopharmacol Immunotoxicol. 2006;28(4):683–95.
44. Hsu CH, Shyu YY, Li MH. The mechanisms of antiasthma formulas in traditional Chinese medicine in the treatment of allergen-induced airway inflammation. J Chin Med. 2000;11:111.
45. Hsu CH, Lu CM, Chang TT. Efficacy and safety of modified mai-men-dong-tang for treatment of allergic asthma. Pediatr Allergy Immunol. 2005;16(1):76–81.
46. Babayigit A, Olmez D, Karaman O, Bagriyanik HA, Yilmaz O, Kivcak B, Erbil G, Uzuner N. Ginseng ameliorates chronic histopathologic changes in a murine model of asthma. Allergy Asthma Proc. 2008;29(5):493–8.
47. Szeto YT, Lei PC, Ngai KL, Yiu AT, Chan CS, Kok EW, Leong CW. An in vitro study of the antioxidant activities and effect on human DNA of the Chinese herbal decoction 'liu wei di huang'. Int J Food Sci Nutr. 2009;60(8):662–7.
48. Shen JJ, Lin CJ, Huang JL, Hsieh KH, Kuo ML. The effect of liu-wei-di-huang wan on cytokine gene expression from human peripheral blood lymphocytes. Am J Chin Med. 2003;31(2):247–57.
49. Chang TT, Huang CC, Hsu CH. Clinical evaluation of the Chinese herbal medicine formula STA-1 in the treatment of allergic asthma. Phytother Res. 2006;20(5):342–7.
50. Wood LG, Gibson PG. Reduced circulating antioxidant defences are associated with airway hyper-responsiveness, poor control and severe disease pattern in asthma. Br J Nutr. 2010;103(5):735–41.

51. Burns JS, Dockery DW, Neas LM, Schwartz J, Coull BA, Raizenne M, Speizer FE. Low dietary nutrient intakes and respiratory health in adolescents. Chest. 2007;132(1):238–45.
52. Chatzi L, Apostolaki G, Bibakis I, Skypala I, Bibaki-Liakou V, Tzanakis N, Kogevinas M, Cullinan P. Protective effect of fruits, vegetables and the mediterranean diet on asthma and allergies among children in crete. Thorax. 2007;62(8):677–83.
53. Barros R, Moreira A, Fonseca J, de Oliveira JF, Delgado L, Castel-Branco MG, Haahtela T, Lopes C, Moreira P. Adherence to the mediterranean diet and fresh fruit intake are associated with improved asthma control. Allergy. 2008;63(7):917–23.
54. Gilliland FD, Berhane KT, Li YF, Gauderman WJ, McConnell R, Peters J. Children's lung function and antioxidant vitamin, fruit, juice, and vegetable intake. Am J Epidemiol. 2003;158(6):576–84.
55. Mizuno Y, Furusho T, Yoshida A, Nakamura H, Matsuura T, Eto Y. Serum vitamin A concentrations in asthmatic children in Japan. Pediatr Int. 2006;48(3):261–4.
56. Al Senaidy AM. Serum vitamin A and beta-carotene levels in children with asthma. J Asthma 2009;46(7):699–702.
57. Arora P, Kumar V, Batra S. Vitamin A status in children with asthma. Pediatr Allergy Immunol. 2002;13(3):223–6.
58. Zachman RD. Role of vitamin A in lung development. J Nutr. 1995;125(6 Suppl):1634S–8.
59. Omenaas E, Fluge O, Buist AS, Vollmer WM, Gulsvik A. Dietary vitamin C intake is inversely related to cough and wheeze in young smokers. Respir Med. 2003;97(2):134–42.
60. Huang SL, Pan WH. Dietary fats and asthma in teenagers: analyses of the first nutrition and health survey in Taiwan (NAHSIT). Clin Exp Allergy. 2001;31(12):1875–80.
61. Tecklenburg SL, Mickleborough TD, Fly AD, Bai Y, Stager JM. Ascorbic acid supplementation attenuates exercise-induced bronchoconstriction in patients with asthma. Respir Med. 2007;101(8):1770–8.
62. Al Biltagi M, Baset AA, Bassiouny M, Al Kasrawi M, Attia M. Omega-3 fatty acids, vitamin C and zinc supplementation in asthmatic children: a randomized self-controlled study. Acta Paediatr. 2009;98:737.
63. Kaur B, Rowe BH, Arnold E. Vitamin C supplementation for asthma. Cochrane Database Syst Rev. 2009;(1):CD000993.
64. Wiser J, Alexis NE, Jiang Q, Wu W, Robinette C, Roubey R, Peden DB. In vivo gamma-tocopherol supplementation decreases systemic oxidative stress and cytokine responses of human monocytes in normal and asthmatic subjects. Free Radic Biol Med. 2008; 45(1):40–9.
65. Fogarty A, Lewis S, Weiss S, Britton J. Dietary vitamin E, IgE concentrations, and atopy. Lancet. 2000;356(9241):1573–4.
66. Pearson PJ, Lewis SA, Britton J, Fogarty A. Vitamin E supplements in asthma: a parallel group randomised placebo controlled trial. Thorax. 2004;59(8):652–6.
67. Troisi RJ, Willett WC, Weiss ST, Trichopoulos D, Rosner B, Speizer FE. A prospective study of diet and adult-onset asthma. Am J Respir Crit Care Med. 1995;151(5):1401–8.
68. Antioxidant Supplements for Health: An Introduction [cited 2010 December 9]. http://nccam.nih.gov/health/antioxidants/introduction.htm.
69. Shaheen SO, Newson RB, Rayman MP, Wong AP, Tumilty MK, Phillips JM, Potts JF, Kelly FJ, White PT, Burney PG. Randomised, double blind, placebo-controlled trial of selenium supplementation in adult asthma. Thorax. 2007;62(6):483–90.
70. Burney P, Potts J, Makowska J, Kowalski M, Phillips J, Gnatiuc L, Shaheen S, Joos G, Van Cauwenberge P, van Zele T, Verbruggen K, van Durme Y, Derudder I, Wohrl S, Godnic-Cvar J, Salameh B, Skadhauge L, Thomsen G, Zuberbier T, Bergmann KC, Heinzerling L, Renz H, Al-Fakhri N, Kosche B, Hildenberg A, Papadopoulos NG, Xepapadaki P, Zannikos K, Gjomarkaj M, Bruno A, Pace E, Bonini S, Bresciani M, Gramiccioni C, Fokkens W, Weersink EJ, Carlsen KH, Bakkeheim E, Loureiro C, Villanueva CM, Sanjuas C, Zock JP, Lundback B, Janson C. A case–control study of the relation between plasma selenium and asthma in european populations: a GAL2EN project. Allergy. 2008;63(7):865–71.
71. Allam MF, Lucane RA. Selenium supplementation for asthma. Cochrane Database Syst Rev. 2004;(2):CD003538.

72. Soutar A, Seaton A, Brown K. Bronchial reactivity and dietary antioxidants. Thorax. 1997;52(2):166–70.
73. Britton J, Pavord I, Richards K, Wisniewski A, Knox A, Lewis S, Tattersfield A, Weiss S. Dietary magnesium, lung function, wheezing, and airway hyperreactivity in a random adult population sample. Lancet. 1994;344(8919):357–62.
74. Kazaks AG, Uriu-Adams JY, Albertson TE, Shenoy SF, Stern JS. Effect of oral magnesium supplementation on measures of airway resistance and subjective assessment of asthma control and quality of life in men and women with mild to moderate asthma: a randomized placebo controlled trial. J Asthma. 2010;47(1):83–92.
75. Hansdottir S, Monick MM, Hinde SL, Lovan N, Look DC, Hunninghake GW. Respiratory epithelial cells convert inactive vitamin D to its active form: potential effects on host defense. J Immunol. 2008;181(10):7090–9.
76. Pichler J, Gerstmayr M, Szepfalusi Z, Urbanek R, Peterlik M, Willheim M. 1 Alpha,25(OH)2D3 inhibits not only Th1 but also Th2 differentiation in human cord blood T cells. Pediatr Res. 2002;52(1):12–8.
77. Song Y, Qi H, Wu C. Effect of 1,25-(OH)2D3 (a vitamin D analogue) on passively sensitized human airway smooth muscle cells. Respirology. 2007;12(4):486–94.
78. Devereux G, Litonjua AA, Turner SW, Craig LC, McNeill G, Martindale S, Helms PJ, Seaton A, Weiss ST. Maternal vitamin D intake during pregnancy and early childhood wheezing. Am J Clin Nutr. 2007;85(3):853–9.
79. Black PN, Scragg R. Relationship between serum 25-hydroxyvitamin D and pulmonary function in the third national health and nutrition examination survey. Chest. 2005;128(6):3792–8.
80. Sutherland ER, Goleva E, Jackson LP, Stevens AD, Leung DY. Vitamin D levels, lung function, and steroid response in adult asthma. Am J Respir Crit Care Med. 2010;181(7):699–704.
81. Brehm JM, Schuemann B, Fuhlbrigge AL, Hollis BW, Strunk RC, Zeiger RS, et al.; Childhood Asthma Management Program Research Group. Serum vitamin D levels and severe asthma exacerbations in the childhood asthma management program study. J Allergy Clin Immunol. 2010;126(1):52-8.e5.
82. Searing DA, Zhang Y, Murphy JR, Hauk PJ, Goleva E, Leung DY. Decreased serum vitamin D levels in children with asthma are associated with increased corticosteroid use. J Allergy Clin Immunol. 2010;125(5):995–1000.
83. Gazdik F, Gvozdjakova A, Horvathova M, Weissova S, Kucharska J, Pijak MR, Gazdikova K. Levels of coenzyme Q10 in asthmatics. Bratisl Lek Listy. 2002;103(10):353–6.
84. Gvozdjakova A, Kucharska J, Bartkovjakova M, Gazdikova K, Gazdik FE. Coenzyme Q10 supplementation reduces corticosteroids dosage in patients with bronchial asthma. Biofactors. 2005;25(1–4):235–40.
85. Calder PC, Yaqoob P, Thies F, Wallace FA, Miles EA. Fatty acids and lymphocyte functions. Br J Nutr. 2002;87 Suppl 1:S31–48.
86. Calder PC. Effects of fatty acids and dietary lipids on cells of the immune system. Proc Nutr Soc. 1996;55(1B):127–50.
87. MacRedmond R, Singhera G, Attridge S, Bahzad M, Fava C, Lai Y, Hallstrand TS, Dorscheid DR. Conjugated linoleic acid improves airway hyper-reactivity in overweight mild asthmatics. Clin Exp Allergy. 2010;40(7):1071–8.
88. Sanderson P, Calder PC. Dietary fish oil diminishes lymphocyte adhesion to macrophage and endothelial cell monolayers. Immunology. 1998;94(1):79–87.
89. Yaqoob P, Newsholme EA, Calder PC. The effect of dietary lipid manipulation on rat lymphocyte subsets and proliferation. Immunology. 1994;82(4):603–10.
90. Yaqoob P, Newsholme EA, Calder PC. Inhibition of natural killer cell activity by dietary lipids. Immunol Lett. 1994;41(2–3):241–7.
91. Black PN, Sharpe S. Dietary fat and asthma: is there a connection? Eur Respir J. 1997;10(1):6–12.
92. Woods RK, Thien FC, Abramson MJ. Dietary marine fatty acids (fish oil) for asthma in adults and children. Cochrane Database Syst Rev. 2002;(3):CD001283.
93. Anandan C, Nurmatov U, Sheikh A. Omega 3 and 6 oils for primary prevention of allergic disease: systematic review and meta-analysis. Allergy. 2009;64(6):840–8.

94. Mickleborough TD, Lindley MR, Ionescu AA, Fly AD. Protective effect of fish oil supplementation on exercise-induced bronchoconstriction in asthma. Chest. 2006;129(1):39–49.
95. Peat JK, Mihrshahi S, Kemp AS, Marks GB, Tovey ER, Webb K, Mellis CM, Leeder SR. Three-year outcomes of dietary fatty acid modification and house dust mite reduction in the childhood asthma prevention study. J Allergy Clin Immunol. 2004;114(4):807–13.
96. Laerum BN, Wentzel-Larsen T, Gulsvik A, Omenaas E, Gislason T, Janson C, Svanes C. Relationship of fish and cod oil intake with adult asthma. Clin Exp Allergy. 2007;37(11): 1616–23.
97. Mihrshahi S, Peat JK, Webb K, Oddy W, Marks GB, Mellis CM, CAPS Team. Effect of omega-3 fatty acid concentrations in plasma on symptoms of asthma at 18 months of age. Pediatr Allergy Immunol. 2004;15(6):517–22.
98. Almqvist C, Garden F, Xuan W, Mihrshahi S, Leeder SR, Oddy W, Webb K, Marks GB. CAPS team. Omega-3 and omega-6 fatty acid exposure from early life does not affect atopy and asthma at age 5 years. J Allergy Clin Immunol. 2007;119(6):1438–44.
99. Welsh EJ, Bara A, Barley E, Cates CJ. Caffeine for asthma. Cochrane Database Syst Rev. 2010;(1):CD001112.
100. Daly JW. Caffeine analogs: biomedical impact. Cell Mol Life Sci. 2007;64(16):2153–69.
101. Gong H Jr, Simmons MS, Tashkin DP, Hui KK, Lee EY. Bronchodilator effects of caffeine in coffee. A dose–response study of asthmatic subjects. Chest. 1986; 89(3):335–42.
102. Becker AB, Simons KJ, Gillespie CA, Simons FE. The bronchodilator effects and pharmacokinetics of caffeine in asthma. N Engl J Med. 1984;310(12):743–6.
103. VanHaitsma TA, Mickleborough T, Stager JM, Koceja DM, Lindley MR, Chapman R. Comparative effects of caffeine and albuterol on the bronchoconstrictor response to exercise in asthmatic athletes. Int J Sports Med. 2010;31(4):231–6.
104. Kivity S, Ben Aharon Y, Man A, Topilsky M. The effect of caffeine on exercise-induced bronchoconstriction. Chest. 1990;97(5):1083–5.
105. Duffy P, Phillips YY. Caffeine consumption decreases the response to bronchoprovocation challenge with dry gas hyperventilation. Chest. 1991;99(6):1374–7.
106. Henderson JC, O'Connell F, Fuller RW. Decrease of histamine induced bronchoconstriction by caffeine in mild asthma. Thorax. 1993;48(8):824–6.
107. Colacone A, Bertolo L, Wolkove N, Cohen C, Kreisman H. Effect of caffeine on histamine bronchoprovocation in asthma. Thorax. 1990;45(8):630–2.
108. Taylor ES, Smith AD, Cowan JO, Herbison GP, Taylor DR. Effect of caffeine ingestion on exhaled nitric oxide measurements in patients with asthma. Am J Respir Crit Care Med. 2004;169(9):1019–21.
109. Turner SW, Craig LC, Harbour PJ, Forbes SH, Martindale S, McNeill G, Seaton A, Ayres JG, Devereux G, Helms PJ. Carbonated drink consumption and increased exhaled nitric oxide in atopic children. Eur Respir J. 2007;30(1):177–8.
110. Zijlstra FJ, Van den Bergde Lange I, Huygen FJ, Klein J. Anti-inflammatory actions of acupuncture. Mediators Inflamm. 2003;12(2):59–69.
111. Acupuncture: review and analysis of reports on controlled clinical trials. 2003 [cited 2011 March 2]. http://apps.who.int/medicinedocs/en/d/Js4926e/.
112. Consumer Reports. Acupuncture: what the experts think now. 1998(September):60–1.
113. Ceniceros S, Brown GR. Acupuncture: a review of its history, theories, and indications. South Med J. 1998;91(12):1121–5.
114. Moffet HH. How might acupuncture work? A systematic review of physiologic rationales from clinical trials. BMC Complement Altern Med. 2006;6:25.
115. Joos S, Schott C, Zou H, Daniel V, Martin E. Immunomodulatory effects of acupuncture in the treatment of allergic asthma: a randomized controlled study. J Altern Complement Med. 2000;6(6):519–25.
116. Kou W, Bell JD, Gareus I, Pacheco-Lopez G, Goebel MU, Spahn G, Stratmann M, Janssen OE, Schedlowski M, Dobos GJ. Repeated acupuncture treatment affects leukocyte circulation in healthy young male subjects: a randomized single-blind two-period crossover study. Brain Behav Immun. 2005;19(4):318–24.

117. Sternfeld M, Fink A, Bentwich Z, Eliraz A. The role of acupuncture in asthma: changes in airways dynamics and LTC4 induced LAI. Am J Chin Med. 1989;17(3–4):129–34.
118. Xu X. Acupuncture in an outpatient clinic in china: a comparison with the use of acupuncture in north America. South Med J. 2001;94(8):813–6.
119. Stockert K, Schneider B, Porenta G, Rath R, Nissel H, Eichler I. Laser acupuncture and probiotics in school age children with asthma: a randomized, placebo-controlled pilot study of therapy guided by principles of traditional Chinese medicine. Pediatr Allergy Immunol. 2007;18(2):160–6.
120. Gruber W, Eber E, Malle-Scheid D, Pfleger A, Weinhandl E, Dorfer L, Zach MS. Laser acupuncture in children and adolescents with exercise induced asthma. Thorax. 2002;57(3):222–5.
121. Morton AR, Fazio SM, Miller D. Efficacy of laser-acupuncture in the prevention of exercise-induced asthma. Ann Allergy. 1993;70(4):295–8.
122. Fung KP, Chow OK, So SY. Attenuation of exercise-induced asthma by acupuncture. Lancet. 1986;2(8521–22):1419–22.
123. Maa SH, Sun MF, Hsu KH, Hung TJ, Chen HC, Yu CT, Wang CH, Lin HC. Effect of acupuncture or acupressure on quality of life of patients with chronic obstructive asthma: a pilot study. J Altern Complement Med. 2003;9(5):659–70.
124. Choi JY, Jung HJ, Kim JI, Lee MS, Kang KW, Roh YL, Choi SM, Jung SK. A randomized pilot study of acupuncture as an adjunct therapy in adult asthmatic patients. J Asthma. 2010;47(7):774–80.
125. Shapira MY, Berkman N, Ben-David G, Avital A, Bardach E, Breuer R. Short-term acupuncture therapy is of no benefit in patients with moderate persistent asthma. Chest. 2002;121(5):1396–400.
126. Chu KA, Wu YC, Ting YM, Wang HC, Lu JY. Acupuncture therapy results in immediate bronchodilating effect in asthma patients. J Chin Med Assoc. 2007;70(7):265–8.
127. Medici TC, Grebski E, Wu J, Hinz G, Wuthrich B. Acupuncture and bronchial asthma: a long-term randomized study of the effects of real versus sham acupuncture compared to controls in patients with bronchial asthma. J Altern Complement Med. 2002;8(6):737–50; discussion 751–4.
128. Martin J, Donaldson AN, Villarroel R, Parmar MK, Ernst E, Higginson IJ. Efficacy of acupuncture in asthma: systematic review and meta-analysis of published data from 11 randomised controlled trials. Eur Respir J. 2002;20(4):846–52.
129. McCarney RW, Lasserson TJ, Linde K, Brinkhaus B. An overview of two cochrane systematic reviews of complementary treatments for chronic asthma: acupuncture and homeopathy. Respir Med. 2004;98(8):687–96.
130. Chu KA, Wu YC, Lin MH, Wang HC. Acupuncture resulting in immediate bronchodilating response in asthma patients. J Chin Med Assoc. 2005;68(12):591–4.
131. Zwolfer W, Keznickl-Hillebrand W, Spacek A, Cartellieri M, Grubhofer G. Beneficial effect of acupuncture on adult patients with asthma bronchiale. Am J Chin Med. 1993;21(2):113–7.
132. Nikitin AV, Esaulenko IE, Shatalova OL. Effectiveness of laser puncture in elderly patients with bronchial asthma accompanied by chronic rhinosinusitis. Adv Gerontol. 2008;21(3):424–6.
133. Nikitin AV, Esaulenko IE, Shatalova OL. Effectiveness of laser puncture in elderly patients with bronchial asthma. Vopr Kurortol Fizioter Lech Fiz Kult. 2008;(6):38–9.
134. Nedeljkovic M, Ljustina-Pribic R, Savic K. Innovative approach to laser acupuncture therapy of acute obstruction in asthmatic children. Med Pregl 2008;61(3–4):123–30.
135. Jobst KA. A critical analysis of acupuncture in pulmonary disease: efficacy and safety of the acupuncture needle. J Altern Complement Med. 1995;1(1):57–85.
136. Lewith GT, Kenyon JN. Physiological and psychological explanations for the mechanism of acupuncture as a treatment for chronic pain. Soc Sci Med. 1984;19(12):1367–78.
137. Eskinazi DP, Jobst KA. National institutes of health office of alternative medicine-food and drug administration workshop on acupuncture. J Altern Complement Med. 1996 Spring;2(1):3–6.
138. NIH consensus conference. Acupuncture. JAMA. 1998;280(17):1518–24.
139. McCarney RW, Brinkhaus B, Lasserson TJ, Linde K. Acupuncture for chronic asthma. Cochrane Database Syst Rev. 2004;(1):CD000008.

140. Carron H, Epstein BS, Grand B. Complications of acupuncture. JAMA. 1974;228(12): 1552–4.
141. Vittecoq D, Mettetal JF, Rouzioux C, Bach JF, Bouchon JP. Acute HIV infection after acupuncture treatments. N Engl J Med. 1989;320(4):250–1.
142. Kent GP, Brondum J, Keenlyside RA, LaFazia LM, Scott HD. A large outbreak of acupuncture-associated hepatitis B. Am J Epidemiol. 1988;127(3):591–8.
143. Norheim AJ. Adverse effects of acupuncture: a study of the literature for the years 1981–1994. J Altern Complement Med. 1996 Summer;2(2):291–7.
144. Birch S, Hesselink JK, Jonkman FA, Hekker TA, Bos A. Clinical research on acupuncture. part 1. What have reviews of the efficacy and safety of acupuncture told us so far? J Altern Complement Med. 2004;10(3):468–80.
145. Lao L. Safety issues in acupuncture. J Altern Complement Med. 1996 Spring;2(1):27–31.
146. Ogata M, Kitamura O, Kubo S, Nakasono I. An asthmatic death while under Chinese acupuncture and moxibustion treatment. Am J Forensic Med Pathol. 1992;13(4):338–41.
147. Wright RS, Kupperman JL, Liebhaber MI. Bilateral tension pneumothoraces after acupuncture. West J Med. 1991;154(1):102–3.
148. Miyamoto S, Ide T, Takemura N. Risks and causes of cervical cord and medulla oblongata injuries due to acupuncture. World Neurosurg. 2010;73(6):735–41.
149. White A. The safety of acupuncture techniques. J Altern Complement Med. 2007;13(1):9–10.
150. Macpherson H, Scullion A, Thomas KJ, Walters S. Patient reports of adverse events associated with acupuncture treatment: a prospective national survey. Qual Saf Health Care. 2004;13(5):349–55.
151. State Licensure Requirements [cited 2011 March 3]. http://www.nccaom.org/regulatory-affairs/state-licensure-map.
152. Acupuncture and Oriental Medicine Alliance. Ancient wisdom, new awareness, awakening American medicine. http://www.fda.gov/OHRMS/DOCKETS/ac/02/briefing/3839b1_14_tully.pdf.
153. Eley R, Gorman D, Gately J. Didgeridoos, songs and boomerangs for asthma management. Health Promot J Austr. 2010;21(1):39–44.
154. Thomas M, McKinley RK, Freeman E, Foy C, Prodger P, Price D. Breathing retraining for dysfunctional breathing in asthma: a randomised controlled trial. Thorax. 2003;58(2): 110–5.
155. Thomas M, McKinley RK, Mellor S, Watkin G, Holloway E, Scullion J, Shaw DE, Wardlaw A, Price D, Pavord I. Breathing exercises for asthma: a randomised controlled trial. Thorax. 2009;64(1):55–61.
156. Holloway E, Ram FS. Breathing exercises for asthma. Cochrane Database Syst Rev. 2004;(1):CD001277.
157. Ernst E. Breathing techniques—adjunctive treatment modalities for asthma? A systematic review. Eur Respir J. 2000;15(5):969–72.
158. Ritz T, Meuret AE, Wilhelm FH, Roth WT. Changes in pCO_2, symptoms, and lung function of asthma patients during capnometry-assisted breathing training. Appl Psychophysiol Biofeedback. 2009;34(1):1–6.
159. Huntley A, White AR, Ernst E. Relaxation therapies for asthma: a systematic review. Thorax. 2002;57(2):127–31.
160. Hackman RM, Stern JS, Gershwin ME. Hypnosis and asthma: a critical review. J Asthma. 2000;37(1):1–15.
161. Sabina AB, Williams AL, Wall HK, Bansal S, Chupp G, Katz DL. Yoga intervention for adults with mild-to-moderate asthma: a pilot study. Ann Allergy Asthma Immunol. 2005;94(5):543–8.
162. Cooper S, Oborne J, Newton S, Harrison V, Thompson Coon J, Lewis S, Tattersfield A. Effect of two breathing exercises (buteyko and pranayama) in asthma: a randomised controlled trial. Thorax. 2003;58(8):674–9.
163. Manocha R, Marks GB, Kenchington P, Peters D, Salome CM. Sahaja yoga in the management of moderate to severe asthma: a randomised controlled trial. Thorax. 2002;57(2):110–5.

164. Vedanthan PK, Kesavalu LN, Murthy KC, Duvall K, Hall MJ, Baker S, et al. Clinical study of yoga techniques in university students with asthma: a controlled study. Allergy Asthma Proc. 1998;19(1):3–9.
165. Birkel DA, Edgren L. Hatha yoga: improved vital capacity of college students. Altern Ther Health Med. 2000;6(6):55–63.
166. Singh V, Wisniewski A, Britton J, Tattersfield A. Effect of yoga breathing exercises (pranayama) on airway reactivity in subjects with asthma. Lancet. 1990;335(8702):1381–3.
167. Vempati R, Bijlani RL, Deepak KK. The efficacy of a comprehensive lifestyle modification programme based on yoga in the management of bronchial asthma: a randomized controlled trial. BMC Pulm Med. 2009;9:37.
168. Cooper S, Oborne J, Harrison T, Tattersfield A. Effect of mouth taping at night on asthma control—a randomised single-blind crossover study. Respir Med. 2009;103(6):813–9.
169. Hondras MA, Linde K, Jones AP. Manual therapy for asthma. Cochrane Database Syst Rev. 2005;(2):CD001002.
170. Guiney PA, Chou R, Vianna A, Lovenheim J. Effects of osteopathic manipulative treatment on pediatric patients with asthma: a randomized controlled trial. J Am Osteopath Assoc. 2005;105(1):7–12.
171. Bielory L, Russin J, Zuckerman GB. Clinical efficacy, mechanisms of action, and adverse effects of complementary and alternative medicine therapies for asthma. Allergy Asthma Proc. 2004;25(5):283–91.
172. Ernst E, Harkness E. Spinal manipulation: a systematic review of sham-controlled, double-blind, randomized clinical trials. J Pain Symptom Manage. 2001;22(4):879–89.
173. Bockenhauer SE, Julliard KN, Lo KS, Huang E, Sheth AM. Quantifiable effects of osteopathic manipulative techniques on patients with chronic asthma. J Am Osteopath Assoc. 2002;102(7):371–5; discussion 375.
174. Balon J, Aker PD, Crowther ER, Danielson C, Cox PG, O'Shaughnessy D, Walker C, Goldsmith CH, Duku E, Sears MR. A comparison of active and simulated chiropractic manipulation as adjunctive treatment for childhood asthma. N Engl J Med. 1998;339(15): 1013–20.
175. Rothwell DM, Bondy SJ, Williams JI. Chiropractic manipulation and stroke: a population-based case–control study. Stroke. 2001;32(5):1054–60.
176. Lisi AJ. Management of operation Iraqi freedom and operation enduring freedom veterans in a veterans health administration chiropractic clinic: a case series. J Rehabil Res Dev. 2010;47(1):1–6.
177. Rubinstein SM, Leboeuf-Yde C, Knol DL, de Koekkoek TE, Pfeifle CE, van Tulder MW. Predictors of adverse events following chiropractic care for patients with neck pain. J Manipulative Physiol Ther. 2008;31(2):94–103.
178. Gillespie BR. Case study in pediatric asthma: the corrective aspect of craniosacral fascial therapy. Explore. 2008;4(1):48–51.
179. Biodynamic Craniosacral Therapy Association of North America. Craniosacral therapy-what is craniosacral therapy?: Introduction to biodynamic craniosacral therapy [cited 2011 March 4]. http://www.craniosacraltherapy.org/Whatis.htm.
180. Mehl-Madrona L, Kligler B, Silverman S, Lynton H, Merrell W. The impact of acupuncture and craniosacral therapy interventions on clinical outcomes in adults with asthma. Explore. 2007;3(1):28–36.
181. Brygge T, Heinig JH, Collins P, Ronborg S, Gehrchen PM, Hilden J, Heegaard S, Poulsen LK. Reflexology and bronchial asthma. Respir Med. 2001;95(3):173–9.
182. Field T, Henteleff T, Hernandez-Reif M, Martinez E, Mavunda K, Kuhn C, Schanberg S. Children with asthma have improved pulmonary functions after massage therapy. J Pediatr. 1998;132(5):854–8.
183. Dennis J. Alexander technique for chronic asthma. Cochrane Database Syst Rev. 2000;(2): CD000995.
184. The Alexander Technique [cited 2011 March 4]. http://www.amsatonline.org/alexander-technique.

185. Wehner AP. Electro-aerosols, air ions and physical medicine. Am J Phys Med. 1969; 48(3):119–49.
186. Lipin I, Gur I, Amitai Y, Amirav I, Godfrey S. Effect of positive ionisation of inspired air on the response of asthmatic children to exercise. Thorax. 1984;39(8):594–6.
187. Warner JA, Marchant JL, Warner JO. Double blind trial of ionisers in children with asthma sensitive to the house dust mite. Thorax. 1993;48(4):330–3.
188. Nogrady SG, Furnass SB. Ionisers in the management of bronchial asthma. Thorax. 1983;38(12):919–22.
189. Jones DP, O'Connor SA, Collins JV, Watson BW. Effect of long-term ionized air treatment on patients with bronchial asthma. Thorax. 1976;31(4):428–32.
190. Ben-Dov I, Amirav I, Shochina M, Amitai I, Bar-Yishay E, Godfrey S. Effect of negative ionisation of inspired air on the response of asthmatic children to exercise and inhaled histamine. Thorax. 1983;38(8):584–8.
191. Blackhall K, Appleton S, Cates CJ. Ionisers for chronic asthma. Cochrane Database Syst Rev. 2003;(3):CD002986.
192. McCarney RW, Linde K, Lasserson TJ. Homeopathy for chronic asthma. Cochrane Database Syst Rev. 2004;(1):CD000353.
193. Reilly D, Taylor MA, Beattie NG, Campbell JH, McSharry C, Aitchison TC, Carter R, Stevenson RD. Is evidence for homoeopathy reproducible? Lancet. 1994;344(8937): 1601–6.
194. White A, Slade P, Hunt C, Hart A, Ernst E. Individualised homeopathy as an adjunct in the treatment of childhood asthma: a randomised placebo controlled trial. Thorax. 2003; 58(4):317–21.
195. Lewith GT, Watkins AD, Hyland ME, Shaw S, Broomfield JA, Dolan G, Holgate ST. Use of ultramolecular potencies of allergen to treat asthmatic people allergic to house dust mite: double blind randomised controlled clinical trial. BMJ. 2002;324(7336):520.
196. Reilly DT, Taylor MA, McSharry C, Aitchison T. Is homeopathy a placebo response? Lancet. 1986;2(8518):1272.
197. Pool R. Unbelievable results spark a controversy. Science. 1988;241(4864):407.
198. Davenas E, Beauvais F, Amara J, Oberbaum M, Robinzon B, Miadonna A, Tedeschi A, Pomeranz B, Fortner P, Belon P. Human basophil degranulation triggered by very dilute antiserum against IgE. Nature. 1988;333(6176):816–8.
199. Wilk M, Pachalska M, Lipowska M, Herman-Sucharska I, Makarowski R, Mirski A, et al. Speech intelligibility in cerebral palsy children attending an art therapy program. Med Sci Monit. 2010;16(5):CR222–31.
200. Madden JR, Mowry P, Gao D, Cullen PM, Foreman NK. Creative arts therapy improves quality of life for pediatric brain tumor patients receiving outpatient chemotherapy. J Pediatr Oncol Nurs. 2010;27(3):133–45.
201. Hamre HJ, Witt CM, Kienle GS, Meinecke C, Glockmann A, Willich SN, Kiene H. Anthroposophic therapy for children with chronic disease: a two-year prospective cohort study in routine outpatient settings. BMC Pediatr. 2009;9:39.
202. Kortesluoma RL, Punamaki RL, Nikkonen M. Hospitalized children drawing their pain: the contents and cognitive and emotional characteristics of pain drawings. J Child Health Care. 2008;12(4):284–300.
203. Pendleton SM, Cavalli KS, Pargament KI, Nasr SZ. Religious/spiritual coping in childhood cystic fibrosis: a qualitative study. Pediatrics. 2002;109(1):E8.
204. Beebe A, Gelfand EW, Bender B. A randomized trial to test the effectiveness of art therapy for children with asthma. J Allergy Clin Immunol. 2010;126(2):263–6; 266.e1.
205. Lehrer PM, Karavidas MK, Lu SE, Feldman J, Kranitz L, Abraham S, Sanderson W, Reynolds R. Psychological treatment of comorbid asthma and panic disorder: a pilot study. J Anxiety Disord. 2008;22(4):671–83.

Chapter 4
Integrative Therapies for People with Chronic Obstructive Pulmonary Disease

DorAnne M. Donesky

Abstract Chronic obstructive pulmonary disease (COPD) is an inflammatory illness distinguished by irreversible airflow limitation. It includes a spectrum of obstructive lung diseases, especially chronic bronchitis and emphysema, and despite optimal medical and pharmacological therapy, most people with COPD continue to suffer from symptoms of chronic, progressive dyspnea, cough, and fatigue. Patients must manage these symptoms themselves or with the support of caregivers on a day-to-day basis. Therefore, many patients turn to complementary and alternative therapies (CAM) for symptom relief. The purpose of this chapter is to review a wide variety of CAM therapies that have been described or tested in patients with COPD, including body-based practices such as massage, mind–body and movement practices such as acupuncture/acupressure or yoga, natural products such as aromatics and supplements, and whole medical systems such as Ayurveda and Traditional Chinese Medicine. The current state of the science concerning most CAM therapies for patients with COPD consists of awareness of therapies that patients anecdotally report to be beneficial, and exploratory pilot studies to document safety and efficacy. Many patients choose to use CAM therapies without consulting their medical doctor. Consequently, it is important for conventional medical providers to educate themselves about CAM options and inquire about each patient's CAM practices to ensure safety of the treatment regimen.

Keywords Chronic obstructive pulmonary disease • Complementary and alternative medicine • Self-management • Dyspnea

D.M. Donesky, PhD, RN (✉)
Department of Physiological Nursing, University of California,
2 Koret Way, N631K, San Francisco, CA 94143-0610, USA
e-mail: doranne@sbcglobal.net

L. Chlan and M.I. Hertz (eds.), *Integrative Therapies in Lung Health and Sleep*, Respiratory Medicine 4, DOI 10.1007/978-1-61779-579-4_4,

Chronic obstructive pulmonary disease (COPD) is an inflammatory illness distinguished by irreversible airflow limitation [1]. It includes a spectrum of obstructive lung diseases, especially chronic bronchitis and emphysema, that are characterized by chronic cough, progressive dyspnea, sputum production, and systemic consequences with advanced disease [2]. While mortality from other chronic diseases, including heart disease, cancer, and stroke has been decreasing, COPD ranks fourth as a cause of death in the world and is projected to become the third cause of death by 2030 [3, 4].

The goals of treatment for patients with COPD are maintenance of lung function, symptom management, prevention and early intervention of exacerbations, improvement of quality of life, and continuation of a meaningful life [2]. A comprehensive plan of care includes smoking cessation, optimal medication use including long-acting bronchodilators, prompt treatment of infections and exacerbations with antibiotics and corticosteroids, supplemental oxygen for hypoxic patients, education about symptom management and lifestyle modification, correction of aggravating factors such as sleep apnea, and exercise training [2]. Pulmonary rehabilitation programs are designed to adapt this comprehensive plan of care to an individualized program of health management for patients with COPD [5]. Despite optimal medical and pharmacological therapy, most people with COPD continue to suffer from symptoms of chronic, progressive dyspnea, cough, and fatigue [6]. Patients must manage these symptoms themselves or with the support of caregivers on a day-to-day basis [7]. Therefore, many patients turn to complementary and alternative therapies for symptom relief [8].

Complementary and alternative (CAM) therapies are defined as "a group of diverse medical and health care systems, practices, and products that are not generally considered part of conventional medicine" [9]. Complementary therapies are used with conventional medicine, and alternative therapies may be used instead of conventional medicine. Conventional medicine is typically taught in Western medical schools and practiced by medical doctors (MD physicians) and associated health professionals such as registered nurses, physical therapists, and psychologists. By contrast, CAM therapies often originate in ancient traditional health systems, take advantage of the health benefits of minimally processed plants and other natural substances, and/or focus on a holistic process of self-healing [10]. The distinction between conventional medicine and CAM therapies becomes blurred as research evidence supporting CAM therapies accumulates, and as allopathic health professionals add CAM therapies to their clinical recommendations for patients [9]. The term "integrative medicine" refers to the use of a combination of conventional and CAM therapies, based on evidence for safety and effectiveness [9].

Respiratory illness is one of the most common reasons why patients access CAM therapies [8, 11]. Patients with COPD are often attracted to CAM therapies because they suffer from a chronic illness with no known cure and their symptoms often are not controlled by conventional medicine [12]. Patients are more likely to use CAM therapies if they are well educated, have a holistic philosophy of health, experience cultural support for CAM therapies, and their symptoms are not controlled by conventional care [12, 13]. Although the literature supporting the safety and effectiveness of most CAM therapies for COPD is limited and the methodologies of research studies are often uncontrolled, this lack of evidence does not mean that CAM therapies are ineffective; it does mean that rigorous clinical investigation is needed [14]. Although the sample sizes are often small and the methodology is weak, there is a surprising amount of research literature that explores CAM therapies for patients with COPD [14].

The purpose of this chapter is to review the CAM therapies that have been described or tested in patients with COPD, published in the English language, and indexed in the PubMed or Embase databases. The CAM therapies are presented here according to the four CAM categories described by the National Center for Complementary and Alternative Medicine (NCCAM): (1) Body-Based practices that focus on the joints, soft tissues, circulatory, and lymphatic systems; (2) Mind–Body and Movement practices, such as meditation, yoga, and acupuncture, that promote physical, mental, emotional, and spiritual integration and well-being; (3) Natural Products, which include herbal medicines and dietary supplements; and (4) Whole Medical Systems, such as traditional healers, homeopathy, naturopathy, Ayurvedic, or traditional Chinese Medicine (TCM), that evolved from ancient cultures apart from conventional medicine. There are currently no published studies of manipulation of energy fields such as magnet therapy or healing touch in patients with COPD. Therefore, this category of CAM is not discussed in this chapter.

Body-Based Practices

Massage

Neuromuscular release massage therapy (NRMT) uses careful assessment of the tissues, and precise pressure on trigger points to increase blood flow, improve circulation, and release the pain related to muscle spasm. In diaphragmatic release, the massage therapist applies pressure to the diaphragm under the sternum and under the left and the right rib cage while the patient exhales into the therapist's hands. The effect of 24 weekly NRMT treatments on pulmonary function and quality of life was tested in five individuals with COPD [15]. The patients were able to tolerate the treatment and reported increased levels of energy and decreased dyspnea on weekly diaries by the midpoint of the study. They were able to participate in activities that they had given up because of their disease prior to the study. They experienced significant improvements in heart rate and oxygen saturation after massage therapy with greater improvement in the patients diagnosed with chronic bronchitis than in those with emphysema. Two of the participants continued with massage therapy at their own expense after completion of the study. The authors hypothesized that NRMT strengthens respiratory muscles, decreases muscle tension, and improves the efficiency of ventilation [15].

Neuromuscular Electrical Stimulation

Five studies have tested the feasibility and efficacy of neuromuscular electrical stimulation (NMES) of the lower extremities to treat muscle weakness for those who suffer from moderate to severe COPD. To overcome this, NMES of leg muscles, mainly the quadriceps muscle, seems to be of interest [16]. In the reported studies, pulse duration ranged from 200 to 400 μs and stimulation frequency ranged from 8 to 50 Hz. Intensities were progressively increased according to individual tolerance. The number of sessions ranged from 3 to 5 days/week for 4–6 weeks. No adverse effects, other than a mild exacerbation of COPD in two patients in one study [17], were reported which indicates that electrical stimulation is well tolerated by people with COPD. Improvement in muscle performance, muscle size, and exercise performance were reported in all studies of patients with severe COPD [17–20] but not in patients with moderate COPD [21]. In a small pilot study, NMES of the diaphragm did not enhance the benefits of diaphragmatic breathing [22]. Although further studies are needed to elucidate the optimal parameters and the types of patients that will benefit the most from this technique, NMES seems to be most appropriate in patients with advanced disease when the patient's ability to exercise is severely limited [16].

Osteopathic Manipulation

The use of osteopathic manipulation to treat people with COPD evokes much passion from osteopathic practitioners, but the research studies have not yet been forthcoming to fully support its use. Case reports and letters to editors indicate that osteopathic manipulation may be beneficial for people with COPD [23–26]. Several methodological descriptions of proposed studies of osteopathic manipulation as a treatment for people with COPD were proposed in the literature, but no published reports of study results were located [27–30].

A randomized controlled design was used to evaluate treatment of patients with COPD with seven standardized osteopathic manipulative techniques during one session compared to a sham control group [31]. Patients in the intervention group experienced worsening of air trapping, measured by the ratio of residual volume (RV) to total lung capacity (TLC), immediately after the session but reported subjective improvement in their breathing during a telephone interview a day later. Because the intervention was not standardized and multiple manipulative techniques were used in a single session, interactions between the techniques might have had a negative effect on the overall response.

In an observational study, 17 patients with COPD were consistently found to have paravertebral tissue abnormalities at the level of the right costotransverse articulation of the third thoracic spine segment. During acute exacerbations, the tissue was puffy to appearance and touch, erythematous, tender to deep palpation, and blanched after digital compression. Motion between the third and fourth thoracic segments was restricted, especially with left lateral flexion or rotation to the left. After a year of osteopathic manipulative therapy directed toward the mobilization of specific segments of the spinal column, TLC and residual volume improved, especially in patients whose baseline values were abnormal. There was no change in spirometry results [32].

Reflexology

Reflexology is a type of foot massage that is believed to stimulate blood supply and relieve tension in corresponding areas of the body. Patients with COPD who participated in a randomized controlled pilot study of reflexology reported improved sleep, better coping abilities, improved breathing, and feeling more relaxed after 4 weekly reflexology sessions. However, the only quantitative benefit was decreased heart rate immediately after the reflexology session. There were no differences between the intervention and control groups in quality of life or lung function [33]. This study demonstrates a common problem with CAM research: Qualitative interviews and anecdotal evidence point to positive benefits from CAM therapies, but those benefits are difficult to document with traditional instruments and methods used in controlled, valid, and reliable research endeavors. It is difficult to distinguish among the alternatives of whether (1) a benefit actually exists but the wrong outcomes were measured (Type 3 error), (2) a benefit exists for a specific subgroup but is not large enough to detect with traditional research methods, or (3) the benefit is actually a placebo effect.

Mind–Body and Movement Practices

Acupuncture/Acupressure

Six groups of investigators have explored the benefits of acupuncture and acupressure in patients with COPD; three groups focused on acupuncture alone [34–36], one group evaluated acupressure alone [37, 38], one group evaluated both acupuncture and acupressure [39–41], and one group assessed transcutaneous electrical nerve stimulation (TENS) at acupuncture points [42, 43]. An individualized treatment plan prepared by an experienced TCM physician was used in one study [34] while most studies used standardized treatment plans based on a combination of Western and Chinese medicine physiology [35, 36, 38, 40]. Although the research reports mention only minor adverse events such as minimal bruising and transient pain [35, 36], there have been case reports of pneumothorax caused by acupuncture needles [44, 45]. An exacerbation of symptoms early in treatment may indicate an ultimately positive response to treatment [46, 47].

Most acupuncture or acupressure intervention studies used cross-over [35, 39] or randomized designs [34, 35, 37, 38, 40–43] and duration of treatment ranged from one session [42] to 10 weeks [36]. Sham intervention, placebo, and usual care [36, 40] were commonly used as control groups. Sham interventions focused on intestinal movement and circulation [37, 38] or directed treatment to precisely localized regions where no acupuncture points are known to exist [41]. The placebo-control intervention consisted of a TENS unit attached to the skin that emitted a visual signal but no electrical current passed to the patient [35, 42, 43]. The most common outcomes measured were the six-minute walk distance, dyspnea, health-related quality of life measured by the St. George's Respiratory Questionnaire, and pulmonary function parameters. Study protocols and length of treatment were variable across studies, precluding direct comparisons and leading to equivocal results.

When compared directly, acupuncture has a stronger treatment effect than acupressure [40], but acupressure has an advantage in that it can be taught to patients and caregivers and is convenient and accessible for symptom relief during acute situations [40]. Acupressure is well tolerated with minimal adverse events and provides a low-cost tool that a patient with COPD can use to increase the sense of personal control over the symptoms and disability related to the disease. Adverse events related to acupuncture can be serious; however, an individualized acupuncture treatment program using nonreusable needles, designed and implemented by a trained and experienced TCM practitioner, may be more beneficial than acupressure with minimal risk of adverse events.

Biofeedback

Biofeedback for patients with COPD involves the use of visual or auditory cues of respiratory rate, respiratory pattern, oxygen saturation, or heart rate variability (defined as the increase and decrease in heart rate related to breathing phase). Uncontrolled repeated measures studies of biofeedback in patients with COPD suggest that biofeedback may be beneficial in slowing respiratory rate and increasing tidal volume, and in improving dyspnea, exercise performance, and quality of life [48–50].

A randomized controlled study of adding ventilatory feedback to an exercise training program found improvements in exercise duration and dynamic hyperinflation in patients who used ventilatory feedback during exercise, compared to those who either exercised without biofeedback or used biofeedback without exercise [51]. A group of physical therapists has described a "myofeedback" technique to assist in teaching diaphragmatic breathing and in reducing accessory muscle use with quiet breathing [52]. They attached electrodes to the lower rectus abdominis muscle which produced continuous audio and visual feedback, and facilitated the rapid adoption of abdominal breathing patterns. Audio and visual feedback from the sternocleidomastoid muscles during quiet breathing allowed patients to eliminate the use of accessory muscles within one 15-min training session.

Unconscious contraction of other neck and shoulder muscles related to anxiety produced a qualitatively distinct myofeedback sound and was also eliminated during the same training session.

Although the data regarding biofeedback are extremely limited, the technique appears promising and deserves further investigation. Unfortunately, the design of biofeedback systems requires substantial initial investment for development of monitoring systems that are designed for the needs of the patient with chronic lung disease—monitoring heart rate variability, hyperinflation, or exhaled carbon dioxide, for example, which may not be clinically relevant to other populations. This initial investment and technical expertise serves as a barrier to investigators who might otherwise be interested in evaluating biofeedback.

Breathing Strategies

There has been much controversy related to the positive effects of different types of breathing strategies for reducing dyspnea related to COPD [53]. Pursed lips breathing (PLB), diaphragmatic breathing, and a breathing pattern of prolonged exhalation are breathing techniques that are often taught to patients with COPD. Variations of these techniques have been taught in creative ways, such as playing the harmonica, singing, and blowing up balloons. These creative strategies offer the benefit of immediate visible or auditory feedback [54]. Controlled breathing techniques relieve dyspnea by their effects on dynamic hyperinflation, gas exchange, strength and endurance of respiratory muscles, the pattern of thoracoabdominal motion, and personal sense of control [55]. An evaluation of PLB, diaphragmatic breathing, and a combination of PLB with diaphragmatic breathing in people with COPD who had completed a pulmonary rehabilitation program found that these breathing techniques decreased respiratory rate and work of breathing, but were not adopted during spontaneous breathing [56].

Respiratory Muscle Training

Respiratory muscle training that includes inspiratory resistive breathing [57], respiratory muscle endurance training [58], or specific expiratory muscle training [59] has been shown to improve respiratory muscle strength and endurance, dyspnea, exercise performance, and quality of life. The evidence for the effect of inspiratory muscle training (IMT) on outcome variables including dyspnea was summarized in the American Association of Cardiovascular and Pulmonary Rehabilitation/American College of Chest Physicians Pulmonary Rehabilitation guidelines [60]. Overall, six investigations showed consistent improvements in inspiratory muscle function, increases in exercise performance, and reductions in dyspnea. Collectively, the positive results of the six new studies supported the findings of a meta-analysis [61] that IMT by itself significantly increased inspiratory muscle strength and endurance, significantly improved dyspnea related to daily activity and during exercise, and showed a nonsignificant trend for an increase in exercise capacity. The new studies used small samples and were performed at single institutions; therefore, the committee recommended that IMT be considered only in selected patients with COPD who have decreased inspiratory muscle strength and breathlessness despite receiving optimal medical therapy.

Pursed Lips Breathing

Some patients with shortness of breath have used PLB spontaneously and found this strategy to bring relief of their escalating dyspnea. More sophisticated laboratory studies and recent clinical studies have shown that PLB promotes slow and deeper breathing [62], improves oxygen saturation [63, 64], and decreases dyspnea [65, 66].

Diaphragmatic Breathing

Studies of diaphragmatic or abdominal breathing techniques vary considerably in technique, duration, and outcome variables [54, 67]. Variations include a focus on pushing out the epigastric region during inhalation, movement of the limbs while breathing, a 3–5 kg sandbag on the abdomen to aid exhalation while lying on the bed, and pacing the breath with walking or climbing stairs [68]. The physiological response to diaphragmatic breathing includes an increase in vital capacity and a decrease in respiratory rate, functional residual capacity, and O_2 consumption [69, 70]. These changes in lung function are postulated to result in a concomitant decrease in dyspnea. However, various investigators have studied the effect of diaphragmatic breathing on thoracoabdominal motion and found that this technique actually increases asynchronous and paradoxical breathing in patients with COPD [71, 72], especially during exercise in patients with severe disease [73]. Focusing on the movement of the lower rib cage, rather than on the abdomen, may minimize paradoxical breathing [74]. Electrical stimulation of the abdominal and thoracic muscles during exhalation as an adjunct to diaphragmatic breathing has been tested in patients with emphysema [22]. Although the subjects reported subjective improvement, there was no evidence of improvement in pulmonary function or gas exchange.

The true effect of diaphragmatic breathing on physiological alterations and symptoms is unknown [55, 75–77]. There is some evidence to suggest that the strength of the effect of diaphragmatic breathing is inversely related to disease severity [78]. Some patients with severe COPD are already very close to diaphragmatic fatigue with quiet breathing [54]. It has been suggested that people with COPD who have elevated respiratory rates, low tidal volumes that increase with diaphragmatic breathing, and abnormal arterial blood gases with adequate diaphragmatic movement may benefit [67]; patients with severe COPD may not benefit from diaphragmatic breathing [77]. A standardized methodology for the implementation of diaphragmatic breathing, based on a synthesis of the literature, is proposed by Cahalin et al. [67].

Paced Breathing

Patients who are short of breath have a tendency to take shallow breaths at a rapid rate [79–81]. This type of breathing pattern is associated with chronic carbon dioxide retention and inspiratory muscles weakness [82]. It increases dyspnea, and it also may escalate the anxiety or panic associated with increasing shortness of breath [83, 84]. Therefore, helping the patient practice and use a slow, deep breathing pattern [66, 85] has the expected outcomes of improving alveolar ventilation and oxygenation [86], preventing or correcting dynamic hyperinflation, and ultimately reducing the work of breathing [87]. A slow, deep breathing pattern becomes even more significant with the evidence that dynamic hyperinflation, with resulting restriction of tidal volume (V_T), is the primary contributor to dyspnea during exercise [88–90]. Although beneficial, care must be taken with slow, deep breathing, as it can induce respiratory muscle fatigue [76].

Investigators have found that patients can change their rate and depth of breathing through ventilatory feedback during exercise [51, 91]. Others have suggested that the traditional yoga pranayama technique of 4-4-8 can be modified for patients with COPD to a 4-2-7 pattern, that is, a count of 4 during inhalation, a count of 2 while holding the breath, with exhalation to a count of 7 while exhaling [92]. This pranayama technique can be practiced while mobilizing the diaphragm, lower chest, and then the upper chest in sequence during both phases of the breathing cycle [86]. The length of inhalation and exhalation can be modified to accommodate the patient's abilities, and music or distraction might be added if the patient is unable to count or needs greater relaxation. This pattern of breathing can be practiced in walking and stair climbing to pace inspiration and expiration [93]. Continual practice of this new breathing pattern, which includes reducing the respiratory rate, prolonging the expiratory time, and using a gentle forced expiration, may ultimately become unconscious and automatic for the patient. In acute dyspnea, breathing with the patient and counting expiration often supports the patient in slowing down their breathing pattern [94]. Specific step-by-step exercises to alter breathing rhythm are published elsewhere [95].

Creative Breathing Strategies

Creative breathing strategies that focus on slow, controlled exhalation may give patients more incentive to practice the breathing technique over time. For example, regularly blowing up a latex balloon for 8 weeks improved breathlessness in people with COPD [96]. Inhaling normally while standing in a warm swimming pool and exhaling with the nose and mouth under water improved pulmonary function after

2 months of 120 min/week practice [97]. Unpublished dissertations have explored wind instruments, harmonicas, recorders, or a senior center band for teaching breath control [54]. Props such as soap bubbles, a pinwheel, and a pipe and ball require substantial breath support and airflow, offer visual feedback of improvement, and provide a tangible reminder to practice regularly [54]. Thixotropy conditioning, consisting of inspiratory muscle contraction with airway occlusion at deflated chest wall volumes, depends on the principle that muscle response is partly affected by previous contraction history. In men with COPD and air trapping, the chest wall volume decreased after thixotropy conditioning [98].

Both breath support (the power behind the voice) and breath control (an energized air column while slowly emitting the air) are important for a good singing tone. In addition, breath support and control are necessary for a patient with COPD to successfully cope with dyspnea and maintain confidence in performing daily activities [54]. Quality of life, but not exercise performance, improved in studies of 12–24 sessions of a group singing intervention in patients with COPD [54, 99, 100]; subjective comments indicated improvements in breath control, posture, mood, and social support [54, 100]. Although dyspnea has been shown to increase briefly after a singing session [99], patients report improved breathlessness and more awareness of the breath after participating in a 6-week singing course [100]. Investigators observed that coughing and expectoration of sputum increased after singing sessions [54, 99].

Active exhalation, rib cage mobilization techniques, use of an abdominal belt to aid diaphragmatic function, and “conscious breathing” [101, 102] are all breathing techniques that have been explored, with varying degrees of benefit [55]. It is possible that a single held breath, like a yawn or a sigh, may more efficiently ventilate the lungs than a simple deep breath or multiple deep breaths [54].

Fresh Air and Fans

Patients with COPD have identified “fresh air” or the use of fans to provide a stream of cold air to the face and relieve dyspnea [103]. This clinical observation is supported by a laboratory study that investigated the effect of directing a flow of cold air against the cheek in normal subjects, causing a decrease in dyspnea [104]. More recently there has been a report that the use of a fan tested in an adequately powered crossover trial resulted in a significant improvement in breathlessness [105]. Two recent clinical trials report equivocal results; no statistical difference in dyspnea improvement was found between patients with dyspnea related to COPD or lung cancer randomized to use a handheld fan and those who received a wristband placebo [106]. However, in a crossover design, there was a significant improvement in dyspnea when using a handheld fan directed to the face, compared to a fan directed to the leg [107]. A fan that allows the patient to breathe circulating cold air may be one of the most effective non-pharmacological strategies available for acute or chronic dyspnea. This treatment is inexpensive, free of side effects, and can be applied almost anywhere [108].

Guided Imagery

Guided imagery is a gentle technique that engages the senses and focuses the imagination. It can be used to elicit the positive feelings of a favorite place or time, experience a positive health or sports outcome, or perceive physical or emotional healing. The goal of guided imagery is to reduce stress and connect the mind, body, and spirit in a sense of peace and tranquility. People with chronic bronchitis, who participated in a 4-week pilot study of weekly guided imagery sessions facilitated by a therapist and two 15-min taped sessions per day at home, experienced improvement in perceived quality of life [109]. During the guided imagery sessions, participants were seated with eyes closed and asked to visualize a scene for an hour as a standard script was read in a well-modulated voice.

Inpatients in a pulmonary rehabilitation unit in Hong Kong were randomly assigned to either 7 weekly sessions of listening to a 30-min guided imagery audiotape or 30 min of sitting quietly in the same quiet room with lights dimmed. The guided imagery audiotape provided instructions for constructing a pleasant mental picture while breathing gently from the abdomen and listening to soft music in the background. During the final session, oxygen saturation significantly improved compared to the resting control group, and line graphs of heart rate and skin conductance decreased during the session [110]. The authors concluded that guided imagery should be selectively offered to patients who are interested in adopting a new coping technique and that the psychological effects of guided imagery relaxation should be evaluated in future studies. Guided imagery is successfully used by clinicians, especially in pulmonary rehabilitation programs, to increase the patients' tolerance for intensity and duration of exercise.

Hydrotherapy

Hydrotherapy for people with COPD has been tested as either a breathing exercise where the patient stands in warm mineral water and inhales normally, then exhales into the water [97, 111, 112], or as a location for calisthenics [113, 114]. The hydrotherapy breathing exercises have consistently shown an improvement in FEV_1/FVC ratio, and decreased pCO_2. They were more effective when performed 120 rather than 20 min/week [97], and were more effective than a similar breathing exercise performed on land [112]. The authors conclude that this exercise would be easy for patients with deep Japanese-style soaking bathtubs to perform at home.

Two groups in Sweden have tested exercise training in group pool sessions. One group tested a 15-min exercise session on land and then reproduced a similar exercise session in the pool, led by the same physical therapist [113]. A few patients experienced some transient dyspnea and fear when they were first lowered into the therapy pool. Otherwise, there were no adverse events associated with pool training, and all patients achieved their target heart rate during both pool and land exercise.

A second research team randomized subjects to either land or water high-intensity exercise groups, three 45-min sessions per week for 12 weeks, and compared the results to a nonrandomized control group [114]. The high-intensity interval exercise programs included both strength and endurance exercises, and music was used to guide the intensity of the exercise program. Both exercise groups increased exercise performance parameters, and the water group also improved health-related quality of life measures. These exercise groups did not require any equipment other than the supervision of the leader. Group calisthenic exercise classes, either in the gym or in the pool, could be used to provide variety for patients with COPD who need to exercise regularly but get bored with using the same exercise all the time.

Therapy in water may have several physiological benefits for people with COPD [111]. Cardiac output may increase by the combined effects of increased cardiac preload related to improved venous return and decreased afterload caused by the weightlessness of being in water. Exposure to mineral hot springs, which is a common treatment in Europe and Japan, may increase mucolysis through the exposure to hydrogen sulfate, may coat the skin surface with materials dissolved in the spring water which prevents heat from radiating, and may keep the body warm for a longer period of time compared to plain water. The hydraulic pressure on the abdomen may decrease dead space during exhalation. Exhaling into water may prevent small airways from collapsing [112]. Some evidence suggests that exhalation under water may boost immune function or suppress infection [112].

Hypnosis

A brief case report suggests that hypnotically induced relaxation with suggestions of well-being and muscle relaxation was helpful in reducing dyspnea for one woman with COPD during periods of anxiety [115]. Hypnotic relaxation may also improve the breathing of anxious patients with COPD during ventilator weaning trials [116]. Hypnosis has been shown to decrease ventilatory drive and decrease response to CO_2 without decreasing metabolic rate in healthy adults breathing carbon-dioxide rich air [117]. A similar study has not been performed in patients with COPD who have elevated pCO_2.

Laughter

Because hyperinflation is an important cause of dyspnea in patients with COPD laughter, which increases the exhalation time, might be expected to improve hyperinflation and dyspnea. In a proof-of-concept trial, a group humor intervention triggered regular laughter in patients with COPD [118]. Breathing assessment with LifeShirt™ real-time assessment and plethysmography revealed that residual volume decreased after the laughter intervention although intense laughter worsened hyperventilation. In an unpublished dissertation, Lebowitz also found that laughter increased air trapping, especially in people with less-severe disease. In addition, a humor-focused personality style was associated with positive psychological and health attributes [119].

Mindfulness Meditation

A subgroup of meditative practices known as mindfulness meditation is receiving attention as a type of CAM therapy for people with chronic diseases and symptoms. Mindfulness meditation is defined as paying total attention to the present moment with a non-judgmental awareness of the inner and/or outer experiences [120]. A recent systematic review of the neurobiological and clinical features of mindfulness meditation found that clinically, mindfulness-based stress reduction was efficacious for subjects with chronic medical conditions and for healthy subjects [121]. However, the low quality designs of current studies made it difficult to establish whether clinical outcomes were due to specific or nonspecific effects. A study of mindfulness meditation in patients with COPD provided evidence that results may be due to nonspecific effects. When compared to a control group, an 8-week mindfulness-based breathing and relaxation therapy course for 86 men with COPD did not improve any health-related outcomes such as dyspnea, mindfulness, or health-related quality of life [122].

Music

Music can be used to distract a patient from their shortness of breath during exercise [123–126], or to promote relaxation and decrease dyspnea and anxiety during acute dyspnea episodes [127, 128]. Thornby et al. [125] found that at every level of treadmill exercise, perceived "respiratory effort" was lower in patients with COPD while listening to music than while listening to gray noise or silence. Patients also performed significantly more exercise while listening to music. In a study of 24 COPD patients in a home walking program, subjects who listened to music while walking had improved functional performance and decreased perceptions of dyspnea, whereas control subjects experienced decline in functional performance and dyspnea [123]. Patients with COPD who listened to music while walking improved positive affect, decreased global dyspnea scores, and specifically decreased the affective but not the intensity dimension of dyspnea [126].

The benefits of music are not limited to walking. When compared to an attention control group, groups who listened to either fast- or slow-tempo music during 4 weeks of upper extremity exercise training experienced significant improvement in upper extremity functional performance compared to an exercise-only control group [124]. Listening to music while resting has been documented as an adjunct therapy in patients hospitalized because of a COPD exacerbation [128] and as a dyspnea management strategy [127]. Singh et al. [128] compared the effectiveness of music to progressive muscle relaxation (PMR) in hospitalized COPD patients experiencing an acute exacerbation. After two 30-min intervention sessions within the same day, both groups had significant reductions in perceived dyspnea, heart and respiratory rates, and anxiety. Using a repeated measures one group design, 24 participants who listened to slow instrumental music when experiencing situational dyspnea experienced reduced dyspnea and anxiety immediately after a music session, although there was no significant durable change in dyspnea and anxiety over 5 weeks [127].

Several of the studies of distraction with music during exercise noted significant improvement in exercise intensity in addition to decreased dyspnea during auditory distraction [123, 125]. However, other investigators who used crossover designs to evaluate the effect of walking with or without music on dyspnea, anxiety, and six-minute walk distance reported no objective benefits to the use of music during exercise [129, 130]. The patients' reports of enjoying the music while walking may have positive implications for adherence to exercise [131]. The benefits of listening to music while exercising suggests that this technique should be implemented to support pulmonary rehabilitation [126]. When selecting music as a therapeutic strategy, pitch, tempo, personal preference, type of music, and sensitivity to music in general are issues that must be considered. Music must be carefully selected to counteract dyspnea and anxiety, and to support the therapeutic goal of either relaxation or distraction during exercise [127].

Posture

Patients should always be encouraged to assume the position that is most comfortable for them, even during acute dyspnea when health professionals or family members may think they should assume a different "more comfortable" position. A position that is often helpful in reducing dyspnea is the head down and leaning-forward position with arms supported while either standing or sitting. This postural relief is thought to be due to an improvement in the mechanical efficiency of the diaphragm and optimal functioning of the accessory muscles [132]. The seated leaning-forward position is hypothesized to restore diaphragmatic function and decrease hyperinflation. It has been reported to reduce abdominal and accessory muscle tension in people with COPD [133]. The position was found to be the optimum posture when compared to five other positions for patients with COPD at the beginning and 5 days into an exacerbation, based on maximal inspiratory pressures and subjective relief of dyspnea [134]. However, comparison between a slumped and upright sitting position for people with COPD found no difference in pulmonary function, breathing frequency, heart rate, or oxygen saturation between the two positions at rest [135].

Arm position has been shown to influence pulmonary function and lung volumes; inspiratory capacity decreases when the arms are raised unsupported above the head, compared to 90° or less [136]. This finding supports the common recommendation to do upper body strengthening exercises to increase tolerance for arm tasks above 90° of shoulder flexion, and to support the arms in a neutral position to counteract dyspnea and optimize lung mechanics. Bracing the arms while standing improves maximal respiratory pressures and respiratory muscle endurance in patients with COPD [137]. In several research studies, the use of a rolling walker (rollator), which braces the arms and provides stability of balance, increased six-minute walking distance and oxygen saturation in individuals with COPD [138–140].

Progressive Muscle Relaxation

PMR has been shown to reduce dyspnea and anxiety immediately after sessions [128, 141] and at the conclusion of 4 weekly training sessions [142]. Although results did not reach statistical significance, listening to a prerecorded PMR tape for 25 min/week produced consistent improvements in anxiety and depression when added to a comprehensive pulmonary rehabilitation program [143]. A protocol that combines PMR with guided imagery and PLB decreased heart rate and respiratory rate, but not blood pressure, in one case report of a woman with COPD [144].

A relaxation maneuver consisting of pressure on wedge-shaped wooden plates placed over the accessory respiratory muscles for 20 min, twice a day, for 4–6 weeks, improved inspiratory capacity and airway obstruction in male patients with COPD [145]. Muscle pain was a common side effect of treatment. Although the authors recommended that this maneuver be included in respiratory treatment programs, no additional studies comparing this intervention to a control group have been published.

Tai Chi

Tai Chi is a type of exercise focused on meditation and well-being and appears to be associated with improvements in psychological well-being including reduced stress, anxiety, depression, and mood disturbance [146]. A recent pilot study of Tai Chi in ten patients with COPD found significant improvement in quality of life compared to a usual care control group, excellent adherence to the study protocol, and indicated that a randomized clinical trial of Tai Chi would be feasible for patients with COPD [147].

Trager Psychophysical Integration

Trager Psychophysical Integration (TPI) uses a series of gentle, painless, passive rocking and shaking movements to reduce tension, decrease anxiety, and restore mobility in tense, restricted areas of the body [148, 149]. Milton Trager advocated use of TPI for patients with emphysema, to break up "holding patterns" and "restrictions" in the abdomen, chest, and mind [148]. An exploratory study of four 20-min TPI sessions over 2 weeks in patients with chronic lung disease demonstrated improvement in forced vital capacity, decreased respiratory rate, and increased chest expansion after treatment compared to a crossover control condition [149]. Forced expiratory volume in one second (FEV_1) did not change significantly during the study. Subjective reports of improvement included improved sleep, increased energy, and less dyspnea. The authors suggest that improvements were related to increased chest wall mobility, decreased anxiety and tension, and increased general relaxation [149].

Yoga

With its focus on achieving slow and deeper breathing, improved breath control, and improved stress management and physical fitness, yoga would be expected to promote relaxation and reduction in dyspnea or distress related to dyspnea in people with COPD. Reductions in dyspnea without physiological changes from greater "aerobic fitness" have been attributed to patients' increased feeling of control over their breathing, a response shift in the perception of the symptom, or a decrease in anxiety, which often enhances dyspnea [150–152].

To date, there are five studies of variable quality that have tested the effects of yoga on pulmonary outcomes in patients with COPD. These studies have shown significant reductions in dyspnea [153], "easier control" of dyspnea attacks and decreased dyspnea-related distress [154, 155], improvements in respiratory pattern [156], and improved exercise performance [154, 155]. None of the studies of yoga for patients with COPD have identified any safety concerns.

Two early investigators using a case series and a matched group design with male participants who had COPD or chronic bronchitis studied the effect of yoga breathing exercises over time on a measure of dyspnea. In one study more participants in a yoga program compared to a physiotherapy group stated that they had "easier control" of their dyspnea attacks [155]. In another there were significant reductions in dyspnea measured with a visual analog scale at week 4, but not at week 2 [153]. Although both studies included a small number of males and used nonvalidated measures of dyspnea, their findings provided preliminary evidence that yoga may be an alternative exercise to relieve dyspnea, especially in advanced disease when impaired mobility prohibits walking, swimming, or biking. A third study of men with COPD compared a 12-week yoga group to a physical therapy group and a usual care group [157]. Patients in the yoga group experienced significant reductions in respiratory rate and heart rate, possibly due to increased vagal tone, compared to the usual care group. The physical therapy group experienced an intermediate response. Spirometry values did not change during the study. More recently we compared the safety, feasibility, and efficacy of a yoga program developed primarily for people with COPD to a usual care group [154]. Participants with moderate to severe COPD safely participated in a 12-week yoga program, tolerated more activity with significantly less distress related to dyspnea, and improved their functional performance.

Natural Products

Aromatics

Aromatics (i.e., Vicks' VapoRub®) consisting of eucalyptol, camphor, menthol, and turpentine applied to the chest are used as a home remedy for congestion and cough. The common wisdom is that aromatics have healing properties and clear the lungs of mucus. Hasani et al. [158] used a within-subject crossover design to study the effects of menthol application to the chest in previous or current smokers with chronic bronchitis. Tracheobronchial clearance was significantly increased after menthol administration, as compared to baseline or petrolatum (Vaseline®) administration, for 1 h after administration. Sputum wet weight and frequency of coughing were significantly increased in the menthol group. Accelerated clearance of sputum is postulated to decrease the likelihood and severity of lung infections, although these were not measured in this study.

Supplements

Antioxidant Vitamins

Antioxidant therapy is believed to be beneficial for people with COPD. Oxidative stress from exposure to smoking, environmental pollution, infections, and exercise damages DNA and other cell and tissue components, and is an important factor in the pathogenesis of many diseases, including COPD [159]. Maintenance of the balance between the toxic effects of oxidants and the antioxidant defense systems is especially important in the oxygen-rich environment of the lungs with its large surface area and blood supply [160, 161]. The oxidative stress from cigarette smoking stimulates neutrophils and macrophages, increasing the production of proteases and other oxidants, and resulting in the development of chronic inflammation and emphysema in the lung [161]. A population study of people with chronic airflow limitation in New York evaluated seven serum antioxidants and corresponding dietary antioxidants, four oxidative stress markers, and pulmonary function parameters [162]. They found that the antioxidants that included retinol, beta-carotene, and vitamin C were positively associated with forced expiratory volume in one second (FEV_1%), and serum biomarkers of oxidative stress were negatively associated with $FEV_1\%$, supporting the hypothesis that antioxidant/oxidant imbalance is associated with chronic airflow limitation.

Antioxidants are the source of many potential medications as well as dietary supplements. As such, they qualify as both Western medicine and CAM therapy. Antioxidants can be classified as either enzymatic or nonenzymatic. Enzymatic antioxidant medications that have been tested in patients with COPD include mucolytics such as *N*-acetyl-L-cysteine (NAC) and PDE4 inhibitors such as Roflumilast. Vitamin E/alpha-tocopherol, vitamin C, vitamin A/beta-carotene, selenium, and glutathione are some of the most common nonenzymatic antioxidants in the human body [163]. Malondialdehyde (MDA) is a lipid peroxidation product that is commonly measured as an indicator of oxidative stress.

Epidemiological and cross-sectional studies have shown a positive effect of antioxidants like vitamins A, C, and E on ventilatory function in patients with COPD [164, 165]. However, one prospective study did not support that relationship [166]. Another prospective study found a relationship between COPD mortality and intake of fruit and vitamin E [167]. Vitamin E and vitamin C supplementation for 12 weeks improved the resistance of DNA to oxidative challenge, but did not change spirometry values in people with COPD [168]. Baseline evaluation of 29,133 male current or previous smokers found a strong association between high serum levels of beta-carotene and alpha-tocopherol, or high dietary intake of beta-carotene or vitamin E, and low prevalence of COPD symptoms of cough, phlegm, and dyspnea [161]. High intake and serum levels of retinol were associated with low prevalence of dyspnea but not other COPD symptoms. A subsequent randomized, placebo-controlled study of these men, with a median follow-up of 6.1 years, found that supplementation by beta-carotene and/or alpha-tocopherol was not associated with any reduction in COPD symptoms [161].

A large cross-sectional analysis of both men and women who had not previously been diagnosed with obstructive lung disease found that plasma vitamin C levels were inversely related to obstructive lung disease based on spirometry [169]. There was an interaction between plasma vitamin C and smoking: Smokers with the lowest levels of plasma vitamin C had much higher likelihood of having obstruction on their spirometry [169].

In a sample of patients with severe lung disease awaiting lung transplantation, serum retinol (vitamin A) was positively associated with increased weight and serum tocopherols (vitamin E) were significantly higher in underweight patients compared to normal-weight people with COPD [170]. Vitamin E supplementation with 400 IU twice daily for 8 weeks in addition to standard treatment for men with COPD did not result in any additional clinical benefit when compared to a placebo-control group [171]. Results were similar in a group of 15 patients with COPD who took 400 IU of vitamin E daily for 12 weeks and were compared to 20 healthy nonsmokers. In the same study, subjects with COPD initially had higher levels of MDA, a product of lipid peroxidation, than healthy controls and supplementation with vitamin E decreased MDA levels significantly [172]. Because smokers have lower plasma levels of alpha-tocopherol (vitamin E) compared to controls, supplementation with vitamin E is postulated to be beneficial for preventing free radical injury and development of COPD in the future as well as slow the rate of damage to lung tissue [172].

Vitamins E and C may work together synergistically to prevent oxidative damage to cell membranes [173]. The NHANES III study explored the relationships between both the dietary intake and serum levels of vitamin C, vitamin E, beta-carotene (precursor to vitamin A), and selenium, which they identified as the major dietary antioxidant nutrients [174]. They found that all four antioxidants, measured by either serum or dietary intake, were independently associated with lung function. The combined effect of all four nutrients on lung function was greater than the effect of any of the individual nutrients, but less than the additive effect when each nutrient was analyzed separately. They note that dietary intake of the three vitamins is highly correlated since they come from many of the same food sources and this could explain the absence of a synergistic effect. In addition, they found that each antioxidant had a different interaction with smoking status. Because each of the antioxidants has a different mechanism of action, some oxidants may be targeted more to either smoking or nonsmoking-type of oxidant stress, and the level of oxidant burden may affect the effectiveness of the antioxidant function [174].

Oxidative stress is increased and antioxidant enzymes are reduced during periods of exercise and during COPD exacerbations [175]. Exercise increases levels of MDA, a marker of oxidative stress, in people with COPD, but not in healthy controls [159]. After 1 month of antioxidant therapy with vitamin E and C supplementation, treadmill exercise time increased significantly and MDA was no longer increased after exercise [159]. Twelve weeks of either vitamin C or vitamin E supplementation did not lessen DNA damage to blood cells in patients with COPD but DNA breakage after oxidative challenge was significantly reduced in patients who took vitamin supplements compared to baseline while the placebo group showed no effect [168]. The investigators found that supplementation with either vitamin elevated the plasma levels of both vitamins after 12 weeks and hypothesized that the two vitamins may interact in vivo by vitamin C recycling the vitamin E radical and sparing the destruction of both vitamins [168].

In a study of vitamins A, C, and E in COPD patients during stable periods and during COPD exacerbations, serum concentrations of vitamin C did not differ from healthy controls [163]. However, MDA levels were higher in patients than in healthy controls, and MDA levels were higher in exacerbations than in stable periods, suggesting that oxidative stress is always present in people with COPD but intensified during periods of exacerbation. Both vitamins A and E serum levels were lower during exacerbations than during stable periods, and vitamin E levels in stable patients were lower than controls, indicating that these vitamins might influence the disease process.

Although increased oxidative stress is pivotal for the pathogenesis and progression of COPD, successful treatment with antioxidants has been elusive [171, 176]. "An effective wide-spectrum antioxidant therapy that has good bioavailability and potency is urgently needed to control the localized oxidative and inflammatory processes that occur in the pathogenesis of COPD" [177]. Most oxidative tissue damage may have already taken place by the time antioxidant therapy is administered, and late-stage therapeutic interventions may be unable to reverse existing pathology [176]. Perhaps antioxidant supplementation would be more effective if it were focused on preventive therapy in at-risk groups such as smokers and during COPD exacerbation, rather than after the patient has already developed irreversible disease [178]. Early identification of subgroups that will respond to antioxidant therapy is an important priority for future research.

Coenzyme Q10

Coenzyme Q10 (CoQ10) is a substance naturally occurring in mitochondria that facilitates energy production and metabolism. The presence of CoQ10 improves oxygen delivery to the muscles, increasing energy production, and improves the function of skeletal, cardiac, and respiratory muscles. Patients with COPD exhibit a low serum level of CoQ10 compared to healthy subjects [179] and CoQ10 levels are significantly correlated with body weight and obesity [180]. The percentage of oxidized CoQ10 in patients with COPD is much higher than in healthy subjects, but low in patients with COPD who receive supplemental oxygen, suggesting that the use of oxygen limits the oxidative damage of COPD [181]. Patients who received 50 mg of CoQ10 (ubidecarenone) daily during pulmonary rehabilitation for 4 weeks experienced improved maximal oxygen consumption, compared to a control group [182].

Patients with COPD who also have exercise-induced hypoxemia have further reductions in CoQ10 levels during exercise, compared to people with COPD who do not become hypoxemic during exercise [180]. After oral administration of 90 mg daily of CoQ10 for 8 weeks, partial pressure of oxygen and incremental treadmill time increased significantly although oxygen consumption during exercise did not change [180]. This pattern may have been due to improved oxygenation of the peripheral tissue combined with improved cardiac output.

Elevated CoQ10 levels are associated with hypothyroid disorders, particularly low-T3 syndrome. Patients with COPD who also have low T3 levels have significantly higher CoQ10 serum levels when compared to people with COPD who have normal T3 levels, indicating that they may experience true hypothyroidism and not simply an adaptation to chronic illness [183].

Non-antioxidant Vitamins

A study of micronutrient intake in Swedish COPD patients found that the intake of folic acid and vitamin D did not meet recommended levels [184]. Perhaps the intake of fruit and vegetables was decreased because of food preferences, dental problems, or digestive difficulties. Vitamin D is usually thought to be beneficial for bone health, but its effect on inflammation, microbes, the immune system, and skeletal muscle function may be helpful in treating chronic lung disease as well [185]. COPD exacerbations are the most common during the winter months, when serum levels of vitamin D are the lowest [186]. Lung function may be related to vitamin D levels [187]. However, even with generous supplementation, patients with chronic lung disease are often deficient of vitamin D. Fortunately, vitamin D supplementation is inexpensive and safe so until definitive studies on the value of vitamin D supplementation for patients with COPD are done, it is not harmful to take vitamin D supplements.

The reduction in serum folic acid that is associated with COPD may contribute to the increased cardiovascular risk in patients with COPD by causing hyperhomocysteinaemia [188]. A case-control cross-sectional study of 42 patients with COPD and 29 control subjects found that COPD patients had reduced plasma concentrations of B vitamins, especially vitamin B6 and folic acid. Patients with COPD also had elevated homocysteine levels compared to the matched control group, a finding that is not surprising since B vitamins are essential cofactors in homocysteine metabolism. This finding, combined with higher levels of heart failure, triglyceridemia, and hypertension in patients with COPD, suggests that patients with COPD are more likely to experience metabolic syndrome, which is a strong risk factor for cardiovascular disease [188].

Ergogenic Aids

Ergogenic aids are supplements that improve exercise capacity, reduce fatigue, and stimulate muscle protein synthesis [189]. Ergogenic supplementation such as anabolic steroids, creatine, L-carnitine, branched-chain amino acids (leucine, isoleucine, and valine which serve as an important energy substrate), and human growth hormone has each been considered for use in people with COPD, with limited initial evidence of benefit [189]. Most of the research on ergogenic aids has focused on anabolic steroids, which consistently improve lean body mass in people with COPD [189]. Liver disease and prostate cancer must be ruled out before considering anabolic steroid therapy, as these conditions can be accelerated by the use of anabolic steroids [189].

Because COPD is associated with muscle wasting and loss of muscle function, creatine supplementation has been tested as a means to enhance muscle function and mass. Creatine is an easily obtained nutritional supplement that is used by the body for energy generation, especially in the initial stages of exercise when metabolism is high. A systematic review of three published randomized controlled trials of creatine supplementation as an adjunct to exercise therapy in people with COPD [190–192] concluded that it had no significant benefits in exercise capacity, quality of life, or muscle strength [193]. However, the effects of creatine may be overwhelmed by the benefits of pulmonary rehabilitation in the trials that have been done [193]. The heterogeneity of the causes of myopathy, including caloric imbalance, deconditioning, effects of steroid treatment, and systemic inflammation [194], combined with the heterogeneity of the subgroups of people with COPD may mask beneficial effects of creatine that would only be recognizable with much larger studies and subgroup analyses [191].

L-carnitine is naturally produced in the body to support energy production. L-carnitine supplementation reduced lactate concentration and improved exercise tolerance in a small pilot study, but did not modify airflow obstruction or muscle mass in people with COPD during a 6-week pulmonary rehabilitation program [195].

Melatonin

People with COPD who have difficulty sleeping often are reluctant to use benzodiazapines and other medications because of the side effect of respiratory depression and worsened nocturnal hypoxemia. Melatonin provides a good option, as it induces normal sleep that includes rapid eye movement, has minimal side effects, and may enhance the immune response [196]. Melatonin is a hormone produced from serotonin in the pineal gland, a small organ near the cerebellum deep inside the brain. Serum melatonin levels are higher during the night and low during the day, stimulated by light exposure to the retina of the eye. A randomized placebo-controlled study of 30 outpatients with COPD found that 3 mg of Melatonin taken 1 h before bedtime improved sleep [197]. A pilot study if patients with respiratory failure in a pulmonary intensive care unit showed that treatment with melatonin improved duration and quality of sleep [196].

Probiotics

Probiotics, microbes that are beneficial to the host, are often given in conjunction with antibiotic treatment to prevent antibiotic-associated diarrhea. Because people with COPD frequently take repeated courses of antibiotics for recurrent exacerbations, it follows that probiotics would be beneficial for people with COPD. However, research evidence does not support the benefit of probiotics for people with COPD. In a randomized trial of a multispecies probiotic containing nine different strains compared to an identical placebo control, patients with COPD who had a history of frequent antibiotic use experienced no beneficial effect of a 2-week course of probiotics on the bacterial composition, frequency, or consistency of stool [198]. There were also no differences in bacterial profiles between patients who developed diarrhea and those who did not. The authors suggest that the bacterial flora may be altered by frequent antibiotic use, and a longer probiotic treatment time may be necessary to experience benefits.

Diet

COPD is associated with systemic muscle wasting, increased resting energy metabolism related to chronic inflammation, and progressive weight loss. The reason for malnutrition in patients with COPD is not understood [199], but may be related to early activation of anaerobic metabolism [199] or impaired gas exchange [200].

Dietary assessment of outpatients with stable COPD has shown that the most underweight people with COPD have higher calorie and protein intake levels compared to normal or overweight people with COPD [201]. In a Swedish study, underweight patients with COPD had caloric intake well above recommended levels, but protein intake did not meet the recommendations for people with COPD [184]. Intake of poly-unsaturated fatty acids was below recommended levels, but intake of saturated fatty acids exceeded recommendations. In that study, weight loss in patients with COPD followed exacerbations in a step-wise fashion. Problems related to nutrition, including lack of appetite, fear of gaining weight, dyspnea while eating, depression, dental problems, nausea, and early satiety, are common concerns for people with COPD [202]. These problems are more common in current smokers and in women. A study of a dietary intervention consisting of five scheduled consultations with a dietician over the course of a year and unlimited additional availability of diet consultations for people with COPD showed small but significant improvements in caloric intake, exercise capacity, and nutrient intake, especially in patients who were underweight [203].

Because increasing energy intake with caloric supplementation is difficult to achieve among people with severe COPD, it is important to intervene early in people with COPD who are at risk for weight loss [204]. It is possible that a focus on dietary change rather than supplementation would be more beneficial for people with COPD, but this has not yet been studied [204, 205]. Patients with COPD who were given high-protein supplement drinks during 8 weeks of pulmonary rehabilitation maintained their serum albumin and improved their Fischer ratio (an indicator of amino acid imbalance associated with muscle catabolism) compared to patients with COPD in the rehab program who did not take protein supplements [206]. Both groups significantly improved their six-minute walk distance and quality of life, as measured by the Chronic Respiratory Disease Questionnaire. The authors suggest that high-quality protein supplementation may spare respiratory muscle dysfunction and nutritional management is an essential component of care for people with COPD.

Dietary supplements are used by 42% of people with COPD in Japan, which is similar to the general population (43%) [207]. Men are most likely to use energy drinks, and women are most likely to use multivitamins or vinegar. Younger age, comorbidities, and severe disease are associated with less dietary supplement use in Japanese patients with COPD [207]. Patients with COPD in Australia use dietary supplements at a similar rate (41%), with vitamin and mineral preparations more common than herbal preparations [8].

A study of 793 men in Holland (92% current or previous smokers) who were followed for 25 years found no significant difference in beta-carotene, vitamin C, or selenium intake in men who were diagnosed with chronic lung disease compared to men without lung disease during the follow-up period [166]. However, intake of apples and pears was significantly lower among men who were diagnosed with lung disease, possibly because of the high level of flavonoids, a plant pigment that may have antioxidant and other bioactive properties, in those fruits, antioxidant. The incidence of lung disease was higher among abstainers than among consumers of alcohol [166]. The intake of black tea and fresh fruits and vegetables was higher in healthy controls than in people diagnosed with COPD in a cross-sectional study, possibly due to antioxidant properties in those foods [208]. Intake of fresh fruit is associated with higher FEV_1 levels in both smokers and nonsmokers [209]. However, a randomized, double-blinded trial of pomegranate juice compared to placebo drink did not show any improvement in hematologic indices, blood chemistry, pulmonary function, or bioavailability of pomegranate metabolites in the intervention group [210]. People in Chinese societies believe that "cooling foods" such as bean sprouts, asparagus, cucumber, and citrus, exacerbate the symptoms of COPD [211]. People with COPD who live in Taiwan ate fewer fruit and vegetables, especially those classified as "cooling foods," compared to healthy people in a case-control study [211].

Several foods are hypothesized to be beneficial for people with COPD based on in vitro and animal studies, but human studies have not yet been done. Polyphenols and flavonols are plant foods with antioxidant and anti-inflammatory properties [160, 212]. Examples include curcumin (turmeric), green tea, fruit, and resveratrol (from red wine). Green tea has antioxidant properties primarily from EGCG (epigallocatechin-3-gallate) and green tea consumption may be beneficial for people with COPD [213]. Curcumin is an anti-inflammatory and antioxidant substance found in turmeric, a spice commonly used in Indian curries [214].

Omega-3 polyunsaturated fatty acids (PUFAs), found in cold water oily fish such as salmon, herring, mackerel, anchovies, and sardines, have a natural anti-inflammatory effect. Cross-sectional studies point to a protective effect of dietary fish oils in smokers—higher dietary fish oil consumption is associated with less likelihood of diagnosis of COPD [215–217]. A prospective study of COPD mortality found no relationship with fish consumption [167]. Dyspnea and oxygen saturation during 6 MW, and sputum Leukotriene B4, TNF-alpha, and IL-8 levels improved in patients with COPD taking omega-3 PUFA-rich supplements, compared to patients taking a non-rich supplement over a 2-year interval [218]. This evidence suggests that nutritional support with omega-3 PUFAs may be a valuable treatment for people with COPD.

Whole Medical Systems

Medicinal plants for treating respiratory diseases have been used for centuries in Indian Ayurveda and in TCM. Seventy medicinal plants that may be beneficial for chronic lung diseases have been identified, and of these, 28 plants have been studied in either patients or animal models with COPD [219]. Many of the research articles supporting the use of these plants are published in languages other than English, limiting the adoption of these therapies in English-speaking countries. However, recent reviews [219, 220] are drawing attention to the possible benefits of these medicinal plants. The goal of TCM is to achieve health by balancing opposing energies and to allow the life force (qi, pronounced "chee") to flow freely [221]. The organs of the body are considered to be complex networks with qi flowing through the organ systems via meridians. Therapy is designed to stimulate the body's own healing abilities.

A systematic review published in 2006 identified 14 RCTs of herbal medicines [220]. In general, the quality of the RCTs was poor, with five reporting that they were double blinded, one reporting an appropriate method of blinding, three reporting an appropriate method of randomization, five describing details of droupouts and withdrawals, and two controlled by placebo. Eight of the 14 RCTs were published in Chinese, two in German, and four in English. Each of the 14 RCTs studied a different herbal medicine. Ten of the RCTs studied an herbal mixture, and four studied a monotherapy. Only five trials included information on adverse events, although herb–drug interactions are a serious concern [222]. Data on standardization of the extract is not readily available for these traditional Chinese herbal medicines. Outcome measures are not standardized in most of these studies [220].

"Warming kidney regime" is a TCM protocol that includes two primary drugs ("Pellet of Warming Kidney-yang" and "Pellet of Nourishing Kidney-yin"), combined with a compound of Chinese medical herbs for bronchitis, and "Pellet of Radix Phytolaccae Compound" for acute attacks. The drugs are used preventatively from early autumn through the spring. The ratio of drugs used is personalized to each patient depending on their symptoms, and drugs are not given during the summer months. Most of the 522 patients with chronic bronchitis treated over 11 years in a Shanghai medical college were found to have deficiency of Kidney-yang, consistent with the TCM theory that chronic illness damages the kidney [223]. Evaluation of both endocrine and immunology changes during warming "kidney regime treatment" found that cellular immunity did not change but pituitary and thyroid function improved.

Bufei Keli granules, which are intended to invigorate the lung, reinforce the kidney, and increase immunity, are a combination of four Chinese medicinal materials that are taken three times a day for 30 days to prevent relapse of chronic bronchitis [224]. According to TCM, chronic bronchitis is a qi deficiency syndrome with the primary symptoms of frequent colds, loose stools, cough, pale or enlarged tongue, and pulse abnormalities. The minor symptoms include shortness of breath, lassitude, abdominal distension, puffy complexion, expectoration, dyspnea, and dizziness. One year after treatment, patients with chronic bronchitis had fewer colds and exacerbations were shorter and less severe compared to a control group treated with a placebo granules [224].

Chronic bronchitis is also treated by a combination of Ma Xing Shi Gan Tang which is a combination of ephedra and three other herbs, and Er Chen Tang which is made from two TCM drugs [225]. Patients with chronic bronchitis were treated with either a formula of TCM drugs designed to remove phlegm-dampness from the lungs and facilitate the flow of lung-qi to relieve cough, with a formula designed to clear away phlegm-heat congestion and resolve phlegm, or with a formula designed to replenish qi, nourish yin, and arrest cough through the flow of lung-qi. Antibiotics were used for people with elevated WBC counts. After 2 weeks of treatment, marked improvement was achieved in 73% of patients [225].

An example of the added value TCM can bring to standard Western medicine involves the evaluation of osteoporosis in patients with COPD [226]. According to TCM evaluation, patients with COPD can have either a deficiency of the lung and spleen (TDLS) or a deficiency of the lung, spleen, and kidney (TDLSK). According to TCM, the kidney and bone are closely related so it follows that osteoporosis would be more likely in patients with the TDLSK type of COPD. Symptoms of TDLS include spontaneous sweating, shortness of breath, low voice, exacerbation related to weather, cough, sputum, and poor appetite. Symptoms of TDLSK include difficulty in inhalation, dizziness, tinnitus, soreness and weakness in the knees, pale complexion, chills, cold limbs, and night sweating. In a study of 26 men with COPD who were diagnosed by two TCM physicians, 15 patients with TDLSK were more likely to have osteoporosis than those with TDLS, although bone density in TDLS was also decreased compared to healthy subjects [226]. This distinction opens up the possibility that patients with TDLS might benefit from preventive TCM kidney treatment before their disease develops into TDLSK, with the goal of preventing bone loss and fractures.

Tanreqing injection is the TCM therapy for patients with an acute exacerbation of COPD [227]. Tanreqing intravenous injection or inhalation therapy is a standardized product that consists of five herbs. It has antibacterial, antiviral, and anti-inflammatory properties, and improves airway secretions. A systematic review found 14 randomized clinical trials that compared Tanreqing injection as an adjunct to conventional Western medicine vs. Western medical treatment alone for treatment of acute exacerbation of COPD [227]. These studies, all of which were performed in China, consistently reported improvement in FEV_1, pO_2, pCO_2, and length of hospital stay in patients who received the Tanreqing injection. Only two of the 14 studies were deemed to have a low risk of bias and all of the studies had relatively small sample sizes, but these results indicate that larger, more rigorous randomized clinical trials of Tanreqing are warranted.

Ginseng is beneficial for COPD [228], probably by improving respiratory muscle strength and endurance, although it interacts with many common drugs. Ginseng seems to shift energy production toward aerobic metabolism and improve airflow in both the major bronchi and periphery of the lungs. No side effects from ginseng use were observed in a study of 92 adults with COPD [228].

Hochuekkito (Chinese name Bu-Zong-Yi-Qi-Tang; no English translation) is a traditional Japanese mixture of ten herbs that may have some anti-inflammatory properties. A randomized pilot study of 35 patients with stable COPD showed significant improvement in C-reactive protein, TNF-alpha, and serum prealbumin after treatment with 2.5 g of Hocheukkito given three times daily with meals for 6 months [229].

Pelargonium sidoides (EPs 7630) has been tested in a sample of patients with acute bronchitis [230] and in a sample of people with bronchitis that included about 10% of the sample who had a bronchitis exacerbation of COPD [231]. Assessment of typical bronchitis symptoms such as coughing, wheezing, expectoration, pain with coughing, and dyspnea was much improved after 2 days, and 70% of patients were clearly improved or symptom-free 1 week later [231]. Gastrointestinal complaints were the primary adverse event, reported by 11 people (5%). No serious adverse events occurred.

In a randomized trial of DCBT 1234-Lung KR herbal formulation, men with COPD in India were found to have improved respiratory symptoms, FEV_1, and oxygen saturation compared to placebo and to a group treated with oral respiratory medications [232]. The active ingredients of DCBT 1234-Lung KR include Bryonia which is a homeopathic remedy used to treat bronchitis; drosera which has mucolytic, muscle relaxant, and antibiotic properties; and ipecac which can be used as an expectorant. The possibility of heavy metal poisoning with long-term use of plant-based ayurvedic medications is a concern, so serum levels of heavy metals should be monitored [233].

Myrtol Standardized is a European product sold under the name of "Gelomyrtol forte." It consists of a combination of limonene, which comes from citrus peels, cineole, found in eucalyptus oil with a camphor-like smell, and alpha-pinene which is found in rosemary and pine oils and used for clearing bronchial secretions and anti-inflammatory effects. In studies of alveolar macrophages from patients with COPD [234], and compared to placebo, antibiotic, and mucolytic control groups in patients with acute [235] and chronic bronchitis [236, 237], myrtol standardized consistently improved inflammation, cough, and sputum symptoms and protected against acute exacerbations.

Cineole alone, one of the components of Myrtol standardized and the primary component of eucalyptus oil, has antimicrobial, anti-inflammatory, and immune stimulating effects [238]. It has been shown to decrease frequency, duration, and severity of exacerbations as well as improve airflow obstruction, reduce dyspnea, and improve health status, in patients with COPD [239]. Cineole is well tolerated with minimal side effects and relatively low cost.

Ginkgo biloba is an herb with antioxidant and anti-inflammatory properties that is used medicinally in Europe for a variety of conditions. An in vitro study showed that ginkgo biloba extract protects the human pulmonary artery endothelial cells from damage caused by cigarette smoke [240]. Studies in animal models of asthma and acute lung injury suggest that ginkgo biloba may have additional beneficial pulmonary effects [241–243]; those benefits have not yet been studied in patients with COPD.

Petasites is a plant with spasmolytic properties that is used as a TCM herb and is also used in Europe to treat gastrointestinal problems and asthma. The plant has been found to have phosphodiesterase-inhibiting qualities, similar to anti-inflammatory medications that are in development for treatment of COPD [244]. A study of Petasites 600 mg daily in patients with chronic obstructive bronchitis found consistent improvement in FEV_1 and methacholine challenge [245].

Conclusion

The current state of the science concerning most CAM therapies for patients with COPD consists of awareness of therapies that patients anecdotally report to be beneficial, and exploratory pilot studies to document safety and efficacy. Some potentially helpful interventions, such as spiritual support or energy therapies, have not been the subject of peer-reviewed publication. Many patients choose to use CAM therapies without consulting their medical doctor. Consequently, it is important for conventional medical providers to educate themselves about CAM options and inquire about each patient's CAM practices to ensure safety of the treatment regimen.

There are many challenges to overcome in evaluating nonpharmacological and CAM therapies [246]. Although the classic randomized clinical trial may not be an appropriate design to evaluate all CAM therapies [247], researchers and clinicians must learn enough about these therapies to assure safety and minimize negative interactions with other therapies.

References

1. Fabbri L, Pauwels RA, Hurd SS. Global strategy for the diagnosis, management, and prevention of chronic obstructive pulmonary disease: GOLD executive summary updated 2003. COPD. 2004;1(1):105–41; discussion 103–4.
2. Celli BR. Update on the management of COPD. Chest. 2008;133(6):1451–62.
3. Halpin DM, Miravitlles M. Chronic obstructive pulmonary disease: the disease and its burden to society. Proc Am Thorac Soc. 2006;3(7):619–23.
4. Jemal A, Ward E, Hao Y, Thun M. Trends in the leading causes of death in the United States, 1970–2002. JAMA. 2005;294(10):1255–9.
5. Nici L, Donner C, Wouters E, et al. American Thoracic Society/European Respiratory Society statement on pulmonary rehabilitation. Am J Respir Crit Care Med. 2006;173(12):1390–413.
6. Bausewein C, Booth S, Gysels M, Kuhnbach R, Haberland B, Higginson IJ. Understanding breathlessness: cross-sectional comparison of symptom burden and palliative care needs in chronic obstructive pulmonary disease and cancer. J Palliat Med. 2010;13(9):1109–18.
7. Booth S, Silvester S, Todd C. Breathlessness in cancer and chronic obstructive pulmonary disease: using a qualitative approach to describe the experience of patients and carers. Palliat Support Care. 2003;1(4):337–44.
8. George J, Ioannides-Demos LL, Santamaria NM, Kong DC, Stewart K. Use of complementary and alternative medicines by patients with chronic obstructive pulmonary disease. Med J Aust. 2004;181(5):248–51.
9. NCCAM. What is complementary and alternative medicine? NCCAM Publication #D347; 2010.
10. Mason S, Tovey P, Long AF. Evaluating complementary medicine: methodological challenges of randomised controlled trials. BMJ. 2002;325(7368):832–4.
11. Abadoglu O, Cakmak E, Kuzucu Demir S. The view of patients with asthma or chronic obstructive pulmonary disease (COPD) on complementary and alternative medicine. Allergol Immunopathol (Madr). 2008;36(1):21–5.
12. Testerman JK, Morton KR, Mason RA, Ronan AM. Patient motivations for using complementary and alternative medicine. Complement Health Pract Rev. 2004;9(2):81–92.
13. Astin JA. Why patients use alternative medicine: results of a national study. JAMA. 1998;279(19):1548–53.
14. Lewith GT. Respiratory illness: a complementary perspective. Thorax. 1998;53(10):898–904.
15. Beeken JE, Parks D, Cory J, Montopoli G. The effectiveness of neuromuscular release massage therapy in five individuals with chronic obstructive lung disease. Clin Nurs Res. 1998;7(3):309–25.

16. Roig M, Reid WD. Electrical stimulation and peripheral muscle function in COPD: a systematic review. Respir Med. 2009;103(4):485–95.
17. Neder JA, Sword D, Ward SA, Mackay E, Cochrane LM, Clark CJ. Home based neuromuscular electrical stimulation as a new rehabilitative strategy for severely disabled patients with chronic obstructive pulmonary disease (COPD). Thorax. 2002;57(4):333–7.
18. Bourjeily-Habr G, Rochester CL, Palermo F, Snyder P, Mohsenin V. Randomised controlled trial of transcutaneous electrical muscle stimulation of the lower extremities in patients with chronic obstructive pulmonary disease. Thorax. 2002;57(12):1045–9.
19. Vivodtzev I, Pepin JL, Vottero G, et al. Improvement in quadriceps strength and dyspnea in daily tasks after 1 month of electrical stimulation in severely deconditioned and malnourished COPD. Chest. 2006;129(6):1540–8.
20. Zanotti E, Felicetti G, Maini M, Fracchia C. Peripheral muscle strength training in bed-bound patients with COPD receiving mechanical ventilation: effect of electrical stimulation. Chest. 2003;124(1):292–6.
21. Dal Corso S, Napolis L, Malaguti C, et al. Skeletal muscle structure and function in response to electrical stimulation in moderately impaired COPD patients. Respir Med. 2007;101(6):1236–43.
22. Becklake MR, Mc GM, Goldman HI, Braudo JL. A study of the effects of physiotherapy in chronic hypertrophic emphysema using lung function tests. Dis Chest. 1954;26(2):180–91.
23. Allen TW, Kelso AF. Osteopathic research and respiratory disease. J Am Osteopath Assoc. 1980;79(6):360.
24. Howell RK, Kappler RE. The influence of osteopathic manipulative therapy on a patient with advanced cardiopulmonary disease. J Am Osteopath Assoc. 1973;73(4):322–7.
25. Mall R. An evaluation of routine pulmonary function tests as indicators of responsiveness of a patient with chronic obstructive lung disease to osteopathic health care. J Am Osteopath Assoc. 1973;73(4):327–33.
26. Masarsky CS, Weber M. Chiropractic management of chronic obstructive pulmonary disease. J Manipulative Physiol Ther. 1988;11(6):505–10.
27. Engel RM, Vemulpad S. Progression to chronic obstructive pulmonary disease (COPD): could it be prevented by manual therapy and exercise during the “at risk” stage (stage 0)? Med Hypotheses. 2009;72(3):288–90.
28. Engel RM, Vemulpad SR. Immediate effects of osteopathic manipulative treatment in elderly patients with chronic obstructive pulmonary disease. J Am Osteopath Assoc. 2008;108(10):541–2. author reply 542.
29. Foellner RP, Taylor RM, Marjan G, Kelso AF. Proposed study to evaluate the effect of osteopathic manipulative therapy in the treatment of the emphysema patient. J Am Osteopath Assoc. 1968;67(9):1075–6.
30. Kappler RE. A proposed cooperative study of osteopathic management of chronic obstructive lung disease. J Am Osteopath Assoc. 1970;69(10):1037–9.
31. Noll DR, Degenhardt BF, Johnson JC, Burt SA. Immediate effects of osteopathic manipulative treatment in elderly patients with chronic obstructive pulmonary disease. J Am Osteopath Assoc. 2008;108(5):251–9.
32. Howell RK, Allen TW, Kappler RE. The influence of osteopathic manipulative therapy in the management of patients with chronic obstructive lung disease. J Am Osteopath Assoc. 1975;74(8):757–60.
33. Wilkinson IS, Prigmore S, Rayner CF. A randomised-controlled trail examining the effects of reflexology of patients with chronic obstructive pulmonary disease (COPD). Complement Ther Clin Pract. 2006;12(2):141–7.
34. Jobst K, Chen JH, McPherson K, et al. Controlled trial of acupuncture for disabling breathlessness. Lancet. 1986;2(8521–22):1416–9.
35. Lewith GT, Prescott P, Davis CL. Can a standardized acupuncture technique palliate disabling breathlessness: a single-blind, placebo-controlled crossover study. Chest. 2004;125(5):1783–90.

36. Suzuki M, Namura K, Ohno Y, et al. The effect of acupuncture in the treatment of chronic obstructive pulmonary disease. J Altern Complement Med. 2008;14(9):1097–105.
37. Wu HS, Lin LC, Wu SC, Lin JG. The psychologic consequences of chronic dyspnea in chronic pulmonary obstruction disease: the effects of acupressure on depression. J Altern Complement Med. 2007;13(2):253–61.
38. Wu HS, Wu SC, Lin JG, Lin LC. Effectiveness of acupressure in improving dyspnoea in chronic obstructive pulmonary disease. J Adv Nurs. 2004;45(3):252–9.
39. Maa SH, Gauthier D, Turner M. Acupressure as an adjunct to a pulmonary rehabilitation program. J Cardiopulm Rehabil. 1997;17(4):268–76.
40. Maa SH, Sun MF, Hsu KH, et al. Effect of acupuncture or acupressure on quality of life of patients with chronic obstructive asthma: a pilot study. J Altern Complement Med. 2003;9(5):659–70.
41. Maa SH, Tsou TS, Wang KY, Wang CH, Lin HC, Huang YH. Self-administered acupressure reduces the symptoms that limit daily activities in bronchiectasis patients: pilot study findings. J Clin Nurs. 2007;16(4):794–804.
42. Lau KS, Jones AY. A single session of Acu-TENS increases FEV1 and reduces dyspnoea in patients with chronic obstructive pulmonary disease: a randomised, placebo-controlled trial. Aust J Physiother. 2008;54(3):179–84.
43. Ngai SP, Jones AY, Hui-Chan CW, Ko FW, Hui DS. Effect of 4 weeks of Acu-TENS on functional capacity and beta-endorphin level in subjects with chronic obstructive pulmonary disease: a randomized controlled trial. Respir Physiol Neurobiol. 2010;173(1):29–36.
44. von Riedenauer WB, Baker MK, Brewer RJ. Video-assisted thorascopic removal of migratory acupuncture needle causing pneumothorax. Chest. 2007;131(3):899–901.
45. Whale C, Hallam C. Tension pneumothorax related to acupuncture. Acupunct Med. 2004;22(2):101. author reply 101–2.
46. Jobst KA. A critical analysis of acupuncture in pulmonary disease: efficacy and safety of the acupuncture needle. J Altern Complement Med. 1995;1(1):57–85.
47. Jobst KA. Acupuncture in asthma and pulmonary disease: an analysis of efficacy and safety. J Altern Complement Med. 1996;2(1):179–206; discussion 110–207.
48. Giardino ND, Chan L, Borson S. Combined heart rate variability and pulse oximetry biofeedback for chronic obstructive pulmonary disease: preliminary findings. Appl Psychophysiol Biofeedback. 2004;29(2):121–33.
49. Sitzman J, Kamiya J, Johnston J. Biofeedback training for reduced respiratory rate in chronic obstructive pulmonary disease: a preliminary study. Nurs Res. 1983;32(4):218–23.
50. Tiwary RS, Lakhera SC, Kain TC, Sinha KC. Effect of incentive breathing on lung functions in chronic obstructive pulmonary disease (COPD). J Assoc Physicians India. 1989;37(11):689–91.
51. Collins EG, Langbein WE, Fehr L, et al. Can ventilation-feedback training augment exercise tolerance in patients with chronic obstructive pulmonary disease? Am J Respir Crit Care Med. 2008;177(8):844–52.
52. Johnston R, Lee K. Myofeedback: a new method of teaching breathing exercises in emphysematous patients. Phys Ther. 1976;56(7):826–31.
53. Gigliotti F, Romagnoli I, Scano G. Breathing retraining and exercise conditioning in patients with chronic obstructive pulmonary disease (COPD): a physiological approach. Respir Med. 2003;97(3):197–204.
54. Engen RL. The singer's breath: implications for treatment of persons with emphysema. J Music Ther. 2005;42(1):20–48.
55. Gosselink R. Controlled breathing and dyspnea in patients with chronic obstructive pulmonary disease (COPD). J Rehabil Res Dev. 2003;40(5 Suppl 2):25–33.
56. Jones AY, Dean E, Chow CC. Comparison of the oxygen cost of breathing exercises and spontaneous breathing in patients with stable chronic obstructive pulmonary disease. Phys Ther. 2003;83(5):424–31.
57. de Andrade AD, Silva TN, Vasconcelos H, et al. Inspiratory muscular activation during threshold therapy in elderly healthy and patients with COPD. J Electromyogr Kinesiol. 2005;15(6):631–9.

58. Koppers RJ, Vos PJ, Boot CR, Folgering HT. Exercise performance improves in patients with COPD due to respiratory muscle endurance training. Chest. 2006;129(4):886–92.
59. Weiner P, McConnell A. Respiratory muscle training in chronic obstructive pulmonary disease: inspiratory, expiratory, or both? Curr Opin Pulm Med. 2005;11(2):140–4.
60. Ries AL, Bauldoff GS, Carlin BW, et al. Pulmonary rehabilitation: joint ACCP/AACVPR evidence-based clinical practice guidelines. Chest. 2007;131(5 Suppl):4S–2.
61. Lotters F, van Tol B, Kwakkel G, Gosselink R. Effects of controlled inspiratory muscle training in patients with COPD: a meta-analysis. Eur Respir J. 2002;20(3):570–6.
62. Breslin EH. The pattern of respiratory muscle recruitment during pursed-lip breathing. Chest. 1992;101(1):75–8.
63. Faager G, Stahle A, Larsen FF. Influence of spontaneous pursed lips breathing on walking endurance and oxygen saturation in patients with moderate to severe chronic obstructive pulmonary disease. Clin Rehabil. 2008;22(8):675–83.
64. Tiep BL, Burns M, Kao D, Madison R, Herrera J. Pursed lips breathing training using ear oximetry. Chest. 1986;90(2):218–21.
65. Bianchi R, Gigliotti F, Romagnoli I, et al. Patterns of chest wall kinematics during volitional pursed-lip breathing in COPD at rest. Respir Med. 2007;101(7):1412–8.
66. Nield MA, Soo Hoo GW, Roper JM, Santiago S. Efficacy of pursed-lips breathing: a breathing pattern retraining strategy for dyspnea reduction. J Cardiopulm Rehabil Prev. 2007;27(4):237–44.
67. Cahalin LP, Braga M, Matsuo Y, Hernandez ED. Efficacy of diaphragmatic breathing in persons with chronic obstructive pulmonary disease: a review of the literature. J Cardiopulm Rehabil. 2002;22(1):7–21.
68. Yan Q, Sun Y. Quantitative research for improving respiratory muscle contraction by breathing exercise. Chin Med J (Engl). 1996;109(10):771–5.
69. Campbell E, Friend J. Action of breathing exercises in pulmonary emphysema. Lancet. 1955;1:325–9.
70. Miller WF. A physiologic evaluation of the effects of diaphragmatic breathing training in patients with chronic pulmonary emphysema. Am J Med. 1954;17:471–7.
71. Sackner MA, Gonzalez HF, Jenouri G, Rodriguez M. Effects of abdominal and thoracic breathing on breathing pattern components in normal subjects and in patients with chronic obstructive pulmonary disease. Am Rev Respir Dis. 1984;130(4):584–7.
72. Willeput R, Vachaudez JP, Lenders D, Nys A, Knoops T, Sergysels R. Thoracoabdominal motion during chest physiotherapy in patients affected by chronic obstructive lung disease. Respiration. 1983;44(3):204–14.
73. Delgado HR, Braun SR, Skatrud JB, Reddan WG, Pegelow DF. Chest wall and abdominal motion during exercise in patients with chronic obstructive pulmonary disease. Am Rev Respir Dis. 1982;126(2):200–5.
74. Sharma V. Diaphragmatic breathing training: further investigation needed. Phys Ther. 2005;85(4):366–7. author reply 367–8.
75. Dechman G, Wilson CR. Evidence underlying breathing retraining in people with stable chronic obstructive pulmonary disease. Phys Ther. 2004;84(12):1189–97.
76. Gosselink R. Breathing techniques in patients with chronic obstructive pulmonary disease (COPD). Chron Respir Dis. 2004;1(3):163–72.
77. Lewis LK, Williams MT, Olds T. Short-term effects on outcomes related to the mechanism of intervention and physiological outcomes but insufficient evidence of clinical benefits for breathing control: a systematic review. Aust J Physiother. 2007;53(4):219–27.
78. Vitacca M, Clini E, Bianchi L, Ambrosino N. Acute effects of deep diaphragmatic breathing in COPD patients with chronic respiratory insufficiency. Eur Respir J. 1998;11(2):408–15.
79. Ferrari K, Goti P, Duranti R, et al. Breathlessness and control of breathing in patients with COPD. Monaldi Arch Chest Dis. 1997;52(1):18–23.
80. Gallo-Silver L, Pollack B. Behavioral interventions for lung cancer-related breathlessness. Cancer Pract. 2000;8(6):268–73.
81. Kawut SM, Mandel M, Arcasoy SM. Two faces of progressive dyspnea. Chest. 2000;117(5): 1500–4.

82. Gorini M, Misuri G, Corrado A, et al. Breathing pattern and carbon dioxide retention in severe chronic obstructive pulmonary disease. Thorax. 1996;51(7):677–83.
83. Dudgeon DJ, Lertzman M, Askew GR. Physiological changes and clinical correlations of dyspnea in cancer outpatients. J Pain Symptom Manage. 2001;21(5):373–9.
84. Gift AG, Cahill CA. Psychophysiologic aspects of dyspnea in chronic obstructive pulmonary disease: a pilot study. Heart Lung. 1990;19(3):252–7.
85. Spahija J, de Marchie M, Grassino A. Effects of imposed pursed-lips breathing on respiratory mechanics and dyspnea at rest and during exercise in COPD. Chest. 2005;128(2):640–50.
86. Pomidori L, Campigotto F, Amatya TM, Bernardi L, Cogo A. Efficacy and tolerability of yoga breathing in patients with chronic obstructive pulmonary disease: a pilot study. J Cardiopulm Rehabil Prev. 2009;29(2):133–7.
87. Macklem PT. Therapeutic implications of the pathophysiology of COPD. Eur Respir J. 2010;35(3):676–80.
88. Belman MJ, Botnick WC, Shin JW. Inhaled bronchodilators reduce dynamic hyperinflation during exercise in patients with chronic obstructive pulmonary disease. Am J Respir Crit Care Med. 1996;153:967–75.
89. O'Donnell DE, McGuire M, Samis L, Webb KA. The impact of exercise reconditioning on breathlessness in severe chronic airflow limitation. Am J Respir Crit Care Med. 1995;152: 2005–13.
90. O'Donnell DE, Revill SM, Webb KA. Dynamic hyperinflation and exercise intolerance in chronic obstructive pulmonary disease. Am J Respir Crit Care Med. 2001;164(5):770–7.
91. Collins E, Fehr L, Bammert C, et al. Effect of ventilation-feedback training on endurance and perceived breathlessness during constant work-rate leg-cycle exercise in patients with COPD. J Rehabil Res Dev. 2003;40(5 Suppl 2):35–44.
92. Sharma V. Personal communication; 2004.
93. Frownfelter D, Massery M. Facilitating ventilation patterns and breathing strategies. In: Frownfelter D, Dean E, editors. Cardiovascular and pulmonary physical therapy: evidence and practice. 4th ed. St. Louis: Mosby; 2006. p. 377–404.
94. Carrieri-Kohlman V. Dyspnea in the weaning patient: assessment and intervention. AACN Clin Issues Crit Care Nurs. 1991;2(3):462–73.
95. Petty TL, Burns M, Tiep BL. Essentials of pulmonary rehabilitation: a do it yourself guide to enjoying life with chronic lung disease. 2nd ed. http://www.perf2ndwind.org/Essentials.html; 2005.
96. Chauhan AJ, McLindon JP, Dillon P, Sawyer JP, Gray L, Leahy BC. Regular balloon inflation for patients with chronic bronchitis: a randomised controlled trial. BMJ. 1992;304(6843): 1668–9.
97. Kurabayashi H, Machida I, Handa H, Akiba T, Kubota K. Comparison of three protocols for breathing exercises during immersion in 38 degrees C water for chronic obstructive pulmonary disease. Am J Phys Med Rehabil. 1998;77(2):145–8.
98. Izumizaki M, Kakizaki F, Tanaka K, Homma I. Immediate effects of thixotropy conditioning of inspiratory muscles on chest-wall volume in chronic obstructive pulmonary disease. Respir Care. 2006;51(7):750–7.
99. Bonilha AG, Onofre F, Vieira ML, Prado MY, Martinez JA. Effects of singing classes on pulmonary function and quality of life of COPD patients. Int J Chron Obstruct Pulmon Dis. 2009;4:1–8.
100. Lord VM, Cave P, Hume VJ, et al. Singing teaching as a therapy for chronic respiratory disease—a randomised controlled trial and qualitative evaluation. BMC Pulm Med. 2010;10:41.
101. Hendricks G. Conscious breathing: breathwork for health, stress release and personal mastery. New York: Bantan Books; 1995.
102. Lewis D. Free your breath, free your life: how conscious breathing can relieve stress, increase vitality, and help you live more fully. Boston: Shambhala Publications; 2004.
103. Carrieri V, Janson-Bjerklie S. Strategies patients use to manage the sensation of dyspnea. West J Nurs Res. 1986;8:284–305.

104. Schwartzstein RM, Lahive K, Pope A, Weinberger SE, Weiss JW. Cold facial stimulation reduces breathlessness induced in normal subjects. Am Rev Respir Dis. 1987;136(1): 58–61.
105. Galbraith S, Perkins P, Lynch A, Booth S. Does a handheld fan improve intractable breathlessness? Proceedings of the EAPC research forum. Trondheim, Norway; 2008.
106. Bausewein C, Booth S, Gysels M, Kuhnbach R, Higginson IJ. Effectiveness of a hand-held fan for breathlessness: a randomized phase II trial. BMC Palliat Care. 2010;9:22.
107. Galbraith S, Fagan P, Perkins P, Lynch A, Booth S. Does the use of a handheld fan improve chronic dyspnea? A randomized, controlled, crossover trial. J Pain Symptom Manage. 2010;39(5):831–8.
108. Hansen-Flaschen J. Advanced lung disease: palliation and terminal care. Clin Chest Med. 1997;18(3):645–55.
109. Moody LE, Fraser M, Yarandi H. Effects of guided imagery in patients with chronic bronchitis and emphysema. Clin Nurs Res. 1993;2(4):478–86.
110. Louie SW. The effects of guided imagery relaxation in people with COPD. Occup Ther Int. 2004;11(3):145–59.
111. Kurabayashi H, Kubota K, Machida I, Tamura K, Take H, Shirakura T. Effective physical therapy for chronic obstructive pulmonary disease. Pilot study of exercise in hot spring water. Am J Phys Med Rehabil. 1997;76(3):204–7.
112. Kurabayashi H, Machida I, Tamura K, Iwai F, Tamura J, Kubota K. Breathing out into water during subtotal immersion: a therapy for chronic pulmonary emphysema. Am J Phys Med Rehabil. 2000;79(2):150–3.
113. Perk J, Perk L, Boden C. Cardiorespiratory adaptation of COPD patients to physical training on land and in water. Eur Respir J. 1996;9(2):248–52.
114. Wadell K, Sundelin G, Henriksson-Larsen K, Lundgren R. High intensity physical group training in water—an effective training modality for patients with COPD. Respir Med. 2004;98(5):428–38.
115. Acosta-Austan F. Tolerance of chronic dyspnea using a hypnoeducational approach: a case report. Am J Clin Hypn. 1991;33(4):272–7.
116. Acosta F. Weaning the anxious ventilator patient using hypnotic relaxation: case reports. Am J Clin Hypn. 1987;29(4):272–80.
117. Sato P, Sargur M, Schoene RB. Hypnosis effect on carbon dioxide chemosensitivity. Chest. 1986;89(6):828–31.
118. Brutsche MH, Grossman P, Muller RE, et al. Impact of laughter on air trapping in severe chronic obstructive lung disease. Int J Chron Obstruct Pulmon Dis. 2008;3(1):185–92.
119. Lebowitz KR. The effects of humor on cardiopulmonary functioning, psychological well-being, and health status among older adults with chronic obstructive pulmonary disease. Department of Psychology, Ohio State University; 2002.
120. Ludwig DS, Kabat-Zinn J. Mindfulness in medicine. JAMA. 2008;300(11):1350–2.
121. Chiesa A, Serretti A. Mindfulness based cognitive therapy for psychiatric disorders: a systematic review and meta-analysis. Psychiatry Res. 2011;187(3):441–53.
122. Mularski RA, Munjas BA, Lorenz KA, et al. Randomized controlled trial of mindfulness-based therapy for dyspnea in chronic obstructive lung disease. J Altern Complement Med. 2009;15(10):1083–90.
123. Bauldoff GS, Hoffman LA, Zullo TG, Sciurba FC. Exercise maintenance following pulmonary rehabilitation: effect of distractive stimuli. Chest. 2002;122(3):948–54.
124. Bauldoff GS, Rittinger M, Nelson T, Doehrel J, Diaz PT. Feasibility of distractive auditory stimuli on upper extremity training in persons with chronic obstructive pulmonary disease. J Cardiopulm Rehabil. 2005;25(1):50–5.
125. Thornby MA, Haas F, Axen K. Effect of distractive auditory stimuli on exercise tolerance in patients with COPD. Chest. 1995;107(5):1213–7.
126. von Leupoldt A, Taube K, Schubert-Heukeshoven S, Magnussen H, Dahme B. Distractive auditory stimuli reduce the unpleasantness of dyspnea during exercise in patients with COPD. Chest. 2007;132(5):1506–12.

127. McBride S, Graydon J, Sidani S, Hall L. The therapeutic use of music for dyspnea and anxiety in patients with COPD who live at home. J Holist Nurs. 1999;17(3):229–50.
128. Singh VP, Rao V, Prem V, Sahoo RC, Keshev Pai K. Comparison of the effectiveness of music and progressive muscle relaxation for anxiety in COPD—a randomized controlled pilot study. Chron Respir Dis. 2009;6(4):209–16.
129. Brooks D, Sidani S, Graydon J, McBride S, Hall L, Weinacht K. Evaluating the effects of music on dyspnea during exercise in individuals with chronic obstructive pulmonary disease: a pilot study. Rehabil Nurs. 2003;28(6):192–6.
130. Pfister T, Berrol C, Caplan C. Effects of music on exercise and perceived symptoms in patients with chronic obstructive pulmonary disease. J Cardiopulm Rehabil. 1998;18(3):228–32.
131. Bauldoff GS. Music: more than just a melody. Chron Respir Dis. 2009;6(4):195–7.
132. Sharp JT, Drutz WS, Moisan T, et al. Postural relief of dyspnea in severe chronic obstructive pulmonary disease. Am Rev Respir Dis. 1980;122:201–13.
133. Barach AL. Chronic obstructive lung disease: postural relief of dyspnea. Arch Phys Med Rehabil. 1974;55(11):494–504.
134. O'Neill S, McCarthy DS. Postural relief of dyspnoea in severe chronic airflow limitation: relationship to respiratory muscle strength. Thorax. 1983;38(8):595–600.
135. Landers MR, McWhorter JW, Filibeck D, Robinson C. Does sitting posture in chronic obstructive pulmonary disease really matter? An analysis of 2 sitting postures and their effect [corrected] on pulmonary function. J Cardiopulm Rehabil. 2006;26(6):405–9.
136. McKeough ZJ, Alison JA, Bye PT. Arm positioning alters lung volumes in subjects with COPD and healthy subjects. Aust J Physiother. 2003;49(2):133–7.
137. Cavalheri V, Camillo CA, Brunetto AF, Probst VS, Ramos EM, Pitta F. Effects of arm bracing posture on respiratory muscle strength and pulmonary function in patients with chronic obstructive pulmonary disease. Rev Port Pneumol. 2010;16(6):887–91.
138. Honeyman P, Barr P, Stubbing DG. Effect of a walking aid on disability, oxygenation, and breathlessness in patients with chronic airflow limitation. J Cardiopulm Rehabil. 1996;16(1):63–7.
139. Probst VS, Troosters T, Coosemans I, et al. Mechanisms of improvement in exercise capacity using a rollator in patients with COPD. Chest. 2004;126(4):1102–7.
140. Solway S, Brooks D, Lau L, Goldstein R. The short-term effect of a rollator on functional exercise capacity among individuals with severe COPD. Chest. 2002;122(1):56–65.
141. Renfroe KL. Effect of progressive relaxation on dyspnea and state anxiety in patients with chronic obstructive pulmonary disease. Heart Lung. 1988;17(4):408–13.
142. Gift AG, Moore T, Soeken K. Relaxation to reduce dyspnea and anxiety in COPD patients. Nurs Res. 1992;41(4):242–6.
143. Lolak S, Connors GL, Sheridan MJ, Wise TN. Effects of progressive muscle relaxation training on anxiety and depression in patients enrolled in an outpatient pulmonary rehabilitation program. Psychother Psychosom. 2008;77(2):119–25.
144. Broussard R. Using relaxation for COPD. Am J Nurs. 1979;79(11):1962–3.
145. Fujimoto K, Kubo K, Miyahara T, et al. Effects of muscle relaxation therapy using specially designed plates in patients with pulmonary emphysema. Intern Med. 1996;35(10):756–63.
146. Wang C, Bannuru R, Ramel J, Kupelnick B, Scott T, Schmid CH. Tai Chi on psychological well-being: systematic review and meta-analysis. BMC Complement Altern Med. 2010; 10:23.
147. Yeh GY, Roberts DH, Wayne PM, Davis RB, Quilty MT, Phillips RS. Tai chi exercise for patients with chronic obstructive pulmonary disease: a pilot study. Respir Care. 2010;55(11):1475–82.
148. Cavanaugh C. Beyond relaxation: the work of Milton Trager. Yoga J. 1982;46(5):20–5.
149. Witt PL, MacKinnon J. Trager psychophysical integration. A method to improve chest mobility of patients with chronic lung disease. Phys Ther. 1986;66(2):214–7.
150. Carrieri-Kohlman V, Gormley JM, Douglas MK, Paul SM, Stulbarg MS. Exercise training decreases dyspnea and the distress and anxiety associated with it. Monitoring alone may be as effective as coaching. Chest. 1996;110(6):1526–35.

151. Kidd P, Parshall MB, Wojcik S, Struttmann T. Assessing recalibration as a response-shift phenomenon. Nurs Res. 2004;53(2):130–5.
152. Wilson IB. Clinical understanding and clinical implications of response shift. In: Schwartz CE, Sprangers MAG, editors. Adaptation to changing health: response shift in quality-of-life research. Washington: American Psychological Association; 2000. p. 159–74.
153. Behera D. Yoga therapy in chronic bronchitis. J Assoc Physicians India. 1998;46(2):207–8.
154. Donesky-Cuenco D, Nguyen HQ, Paul S, Carrieri-Kohlman V. Yoga therapy decreases dyspnea-related distress and improves functional performance in people with chronic obstructive pulmonary disease: a pilot study. J Altern Complement Med. 2009;15(3):225–34.
155. Tandon MK. Adjunct treatment with yoga in chronic severe airways obstruction. Thorax. 1978;33(4):514–7.
156. Pomidori L, Campigotto F, Amatya TM, Bernardi L, Cogo A. Efficacy and tolerability of yoga breathing in patients with chronic obstructive pulmonary disease: a pilot study. J Cardiopulm Rehabil Prev. 2009;29(2):133–7.
157. Kulpati DD, Kamath RK, Chauhan MR. The influence of physical conditioning by yogasanas and breathing exercises in patients of chronic obstructive lung disease. J Assoc Physicians India. 1982;30(12):865–8.
158. Hasani A, Pavia D, Toms N, Dilworth P, Agnew JE. Effect of aromatics on lung mucociliary clearance in patients with chronic airways obstruction. J Altern Complement Med. 2003;9(2):243–9.
159. Agacdiken A, Basyigit I, Ozden M, et al. The effects of antioxidants on exercise-induced lipid peroxidation in patients with COPD. Respirology. 2004;9(1):38–42.
160. Rahman I, Kilty I. Antioxidant therapeutic targets in COPD. Curr Drug Targets. 2006;7(6): 707–20.
161. Rautalahti M, Virtamo J, Haukka J, et al. The effect of alpha-tocopherol and beta-carotene supplementation on COPD symptoms. Am J Respir Crit Care Med. 1997;156(5):1447–52.
162. Ochs-Balcom HM, Grant BJ, Muti P, et al. Antioxidants, oxidative stress, and pulmonary function in individuals diagnosed with asthma or COPD. Eur J Clin Nutr. 2006;60(8):991–9.
163. Tug T, Karatas F, Terzi SM. Antioxidant vitamins (A, C and E) and malondialdehyde levels in acute exacerbation and stable periods of patients with chronic obstructive pulmonary disease. Clin Invest Med. 2004;27(3):123–8.
164. Devereux G, Seaton A. Why don't we give chest patients dietary advice? Thorax. 2001;56 Suppl 2:ii15–22.
165. Tabak C, Smit HA, Rasanen L, et al. Dietary factors and pulmonary function: a cross sectional study in middle aged men from three European countries. Thorax. 1999;54(11):1021–6.
166. Miedema I, Feskens EJ, Heederik D, Kromhout D. Dietary determinants of long-term incidence of chronic nonspecific lung diseases. The Zutphen Study. Am J Epidemiol. 1993;138(1):37–45.
167. Walda IC, Tabak C, Smit HA, et al. Diet and 20-year chronic obstructive pulmonary disease mortality in middle-aged men from three European countries. Eur J Clin Nutr. 2002;56(7):638–43.
168. Wu TC, Huang YC, Hsu SY, Wang YC, Yeh SL. Vitamin E and vitamin C supplementation in patients with chronic obstructive pulmonary disease. Int J Vitam Nutr Res. 2007;77(4):272–9.
169. Sargeant LA, Jaeckel A, Wareham NJ. Interaction of vitamin C with the relation between smoking and obstructive airways disease in EPIC Norfolk. European prospective investigation into cancer and nutrition. Eur Respir J. 2000;16(3):397–403.
170. Forli L, Pedersen JI, Bjortuft O, Blomhoff R, Kofstad J, Boe J. Vitamins A and E in serum in relation to weight and lung function in patients with advanced pulmonary disease. Int J Vitam Nutr Res. 2002;72(6):360–8.
171. Nadeem A, Raj HG, Chhabra SK. Effect of vitamin E supplementation with standard treatment on oxidant-antioxidant status in chronic obstructive pulmonary disease. Indian J Med Res. 2008;128(6):705–11.
172. Daga MK, Chhabra R, Sharma B, Mishra TK. Effects of exogenous vitamin E supplementation on the levels of oxidants and antioxidants in chronic obstructive pulmonary disease. J Biosci. 2003;28(1):7–11.

173. Menzel DB. Antioxidant vitamins and prevention of lung disease. Ann N Y Acad Sci. 1992;669:141–55.
174. Hu G, Cassano PA. Antioxidant nutrients and pulmonary function: the Third National Health and Nutrition Examination Survey (NHANES III). Am J Epidemiol. 2000;151(10):975–81.
175. Gumral N, Naziroglu M, Ongel K, et al. Antioxidant enzymes and melatonin levels in patients with bronchial asthma and chronic obstructive pulmonary disease during stable and exacerbation periods. Cell Biochem Funct. 2009;27(5):276–83.
176. Jindal SK. Does vitamin E supplementation help in COPD? Indian J Med Res. 2008;128(6):686–7.
177. Rahman I. Oxidative stress and gene transcription in asthma and chronic obstructive pulmonary disease: antioxidant therapeutic targets. Curr Drug Targets Inflamm Allergy. 2002;1(3):291–315.
178. Rahman I. Antioxidant therapeutic advances in COPD. Ther Adv Respir Dis. 2008;2(6): 351–74.
179. Tanrikulu AC, Abakay A, Evliyaoglu O, Palanci Y. Coenzyme Q10, copper, zinc, and lipid peroxidation levels in serum of patients with chronic obstructive pulmonary disease. Biol Trace Elem Res. 2011;143:659–67.
180. Fujimoto S, Kurihara N, Hirata K, Takeda T. Effects of coenzyme Q10 administration on pulmonary function and exercise performance in patients with chronic lung diseases. Clin Investig. 1993;71(8 Suppl):S162–6.
181. Wada H, Hagiwara S, Saitoh E, et al. Increased oxidative stress in patients with chronic obstructive pulmonary disease (COPD) as measured by redox status of plasma coenzyme Q10. Pathophysiology. 2006;13(1):29–33.
182. Satta A, Grandi M, Landoni CV, et al. Effects of ubidecarenone in an exercise training program for patients with chronic obstructive pulmonary diseases. Clin Ther. 1991;13(6):754–7.
183. Mancini A, Corbo GM, Gaballo A, et al. Relationships between plasma CoQ10 levels and thyroid hormones in chronic obstructive pulmonary disease. Biofactors. 2005;25(1–4):201–4.
184. Andersson I, Gronberg A, Slinde F, Bosaeus I, Larsson S. Vitamin and mineral status in elderly patients with chronic obstructive pulmonary disease. Clin Respir J. 2007;1(1):23–9.
185. Janssens W, Lehouck A, Carremans C, Bouillon R, Mathieu C, Decramer M. Vitamin D beyond bones in chronic obstructive pulmonary disease: time to act. Am J Respir Crit Care Med. 2009;179(8):630–6.
186. Hughes DA, Norton R. Vitamin D and respiratory health. Clin Exp Immunol. 2009;158(1):20–5.
187. Gilbert CR, Arum SM, Smith CM. Vitamin D deficiency and chronic lung disease. Can Respir J. 2009;16(3):75–80.
188. Fimognari FL, Loffredo L, Di Simone S, et al. Hyperhomocysteinaemia and poor vitamin B status in chronic obstructive pulmonary disease. Nutr Metab Cardiovasc Dis. 2009;19(9):654–9.
189. Villaca DS, Lerario MC, Dal Corso S, Neder JA. New treatments for chronic obstructive pulmonary disease using ergogenic aids. J Bras Pneumol. 2006;32(1):66–74.
190. Deacon SJ, Vincent EE, Greenhaff PL, et al. Randomized controlled trial of dietary creatine as an adjunct therapy to physical training in chronic obstructive pulmonary disease. Am J Respir Crit Care Med. 2008;178(3):233–9.
191. Faager G, Soderlund K, Skold CM, Rundgren S, Tollback A, Jakobsson P. Creatine supplementation and physical training in patients with COPD: a double blind, placebo-controlled study. Int J Chron Obstruct Pulmon Dis. 2006;1(4):445–53.
192. Fuld JP, Kilduff LP, Neder JA, et al. Creatine supplementation during pulmonary rehabilitation in chronic obstructive pulmonary disease. Thorax. 2005;60(7):531–7.
193. Al-Ghimlas F, Todd DC. Creatine supplementation for patients with COPD receiving pulmonary rehabilitation: a systematic review and meta-analysis. Respirology. 2010;15(5):785–95.
194. Griffiths TL, Proud D. Creatine supplementation as an exercise performance enhancer for patients with COPD? An idea to run with. Thorax. 2005;60(7):525–6.
195. Borghi-Silva A, Baldissera V, Sampaio LM, et al. L-carnitine as an ergogenic aid for patients with chronic obstructive pulmonary disease submitted to whole-body and respiratory muscle training programs. Braz J Med Biol Res. 2006;39(4):465–74.

196. Shilo L, Dagan Y, Smorjik Y, et al. Effect of melatonin on sleep quality of COPD intensive care patients: a pilot study. Chronobiol Int. 2000;17(1):71–6.
197. Nunes DM, Mota RM, Machado MO, Pereira ED, Bruin VM, Bruin PF. Effect of melatonin administration on subjective sleep quality in chronic obstructive pulmonary disease. Braz J Med Biol Res. 2008;41(10):926–31.
198. Koning CJ, Jonkers D, Smidt H, et al. The effect of a multispecies probiotic on the composition of the faecal microbiota and bowel habits in chronic obstructive pulmonary disease patients treated with antibiotics. Br J Nutr. 2009;103(10):1452–60.
199. Kutsuzawa T, Shioya S, Kurita D, Haida M, Ohta Y, Yamabayashi H. Muscle energy metabolism and nutritional status in patients with chronic obstructive pulmonary disease. A 31P magnetic resonance study. Am J Respir Crit Care Med. 1995;152(2):647–52.
200. Sridhar MK, Carter R, Lean ME, Banham SW. Resting energy expenditure and nutritional state of patients with increased oxygen cost of breathing due to emphysema, scoliosis and thoracoplasty. Thorax. 1994;49(8):781–5.
201. Keim NL, Luby MH, Braun SR, Martin AM, Dixon RM. Dietary evaluation of outpatients with chronic obstructive pulmonary disease. J Am Diet Assoc. 1986;86(7):902–6.
202. Gronberg AM, Slinde F, Engstrom CP, Hulthen L, Larsson S. Dietary problems in patients with severe chronic obstructive pulmonary disease. J Hum Nutr Diet. 2005;18(6):445–52.
203. Slinde F, Gronberg AM, Engstrom CR, Rossander-Hulthen L, Larsson S. Individual dietary intervention in patients with COPD during multidisciplinary rehabilitation. Respir Med. 2002;96(5):330–6.
204. Brug J, Schols A, Mesters I. Dietary change, nutrition education and chronic obstructive pulmonary disease. Patient Educ Couns. 2004;52(3):249–57.
205. Schols AM. Nutritional and metabolic modulation in chronic obstructive pulmonary disease management. Eur Respir J Suppl. 2003;46:81s–6.
206. Kubo H, Honda N, Tsuji F, Iwanaga T, Muraki M, Tohda Y. Effects of dietary supplements on the Fischer ratio before and after pulmonary rehabilitation. Asia Pac J Clin Nutr. 2006;15(4):551–5.
207. Hirayama F, Lee AH, Binns CW, Taniguchi H. Dietary supplementation by Japanese patients with chronic obstructive pulmonary disease. Complement Ther Med. 2009;17(1):37–43.
208. Celik F, Topcu F. Nutritional risk factors for the development of chronic obstructive pulmonary disease (COPD) in male smokers. Clin Nutr. 2006;25(6):955–61.
209. Strachan DP, Cox BD, Erzinclioglu SW, Walters DE, Whichelow MJ. Ventilatory function and winter fresh fruit consumption in a random sample of British adults. Thorax. 1991;46(9):624–9.
210. Cerda B, Soto C, Albaladejo MD, et al. Pomegranate juice supplementation in chronic obstructive pulmonary disease: a 5-week randomized, double-blind, placebo-controlled trial. Eur J Clin Nutr. 2006;60(2):245–53.
211. Lin YC, Wu TC, Chen PY, Hsieh LY, Yeh SL. Comparison of plasma and intake levels of antioxidant nutrients in patients with chronic obstructive pulmonary disease and healthy people in Taiwan: a case-control study. Asia Pac J Clin Nutr. 2010;19(3):393–401.
212. Rahman I. Antioxidant therapies in COPD. Int J Chron Obstruct Pulmon Dis. 2006;1(1): 15–29.
213. Sartor L, Pezzato E, Garbisa S. (–)Epigallocatechin-3-gallate inhibits leukocyte elastase: potential of the phyto-factor in hindering inflammation, emphysema, and invasion. J Leukoc Biol. 2002;71(1):73–9.
214. Venkatesan N, Punithavathi D, Babu M. Protection from acute and chronic lung diseases by curcumin. Adv Exp Med Biol. 2007;595:379–405.
215. Schwartz J, Weiss ST. The relationship of dietary fish intake to level of pulmonary function in the first National Health and Nutrition Survey (NHANES I). Eur Respir J. 1994;7(10): 1821–4.
216. Shahar E, Folsom AR, Melnick SL, et al. Dietary n-3 polyunsaturated fatty acids and smoking-related chronic obstructive pulmonary disease. Atherosclerosis Risk in Communities Study Investigators. N Engl J Med. 1994;331(4):228–33.

217. Sharp DS, Rodriguez BL, Shahar E, Hwang LJ, Burchfiel CM. Fish consumption may limit the damage of smoking on the lung. Am J Respir Crit Care Med. 1994;150(4):983–7.
218. Matsuyama W, Mitsuyama H, Watanabe M, et al. Effects of omega-3 polyunsaturated fatty acids on inflammatory markers in COPD. Chest. 2005;128(6):3817–27.
219. Ram A, Balachandar S, Vijayananth P, Singh VP. Medicinal plants useful for treating chronic obstructive pulmonary disease (COPD): current status and future perspectives. Fitoterapia. 2011;82(2):141–51.
220. Guo R, Pittler MH, Ernst E. Herbal medicines for the treatment of COPD: a systematic review. Eur Respir J. 2006;28(2):330–8.
221. A.D.A.M. Inc. What is traditional Chinese medicine? http://www.umm.edu/altmed/articles/traditional-chinese-000363.htm
222. Izzo AA, Ernst E. Interactions between herbal medicines and prescribed drugs: a systematic review. Drugs. 2001;61(15):2163–75.
223. Shen ZY, Jiang XH, Zha LL, et al. Studies on the use of warming kidney regime in senile chronic bronchitis. J Tradit Chin Med. 1983;3(4):295–302.
224. Liu Y, Wang N, Liu G, Yan H. Clinical observation in 31 cases of chronic bronchitis at remission stage treated with bufei keli. J Tradit Chin Med. 2003;23(4):246–50.
225. Zhu Y, Liu X. Treatment of chronic bronchitis with modified ma xing shi gan tang and er chen tang. J Tradit Chin Med. 2004;24(1):12–3.
226. Wang G, Li TQ, Mao B, et al. Relationship between bone mineral density and syndrome types described in traditional Chinese medicine in chronic obstructive pulmonary disease: a preliminary clinical observation. Am J Chin Med. 2005;33(6):867–77.
227. Zhong Y, Mao B, Wang G, et al. Tanreqing injection combined with conventional Western medicine for acute exacerbations of chronic obstructive pulmonary disease: a systematic review. J Altern Complement Med. 2010;16(12):1309–19.
228. Gross D, Shenkman Z, Bleiberg B, Dayan M, Gittelson M, Efrat R. Ginseng improves pulmonary functions and exercise capacity in patients with COPD. Monaldi Arch Chest Dis. 2002;57(5–6):242–6.
229. Shinozuka N, Tatsumi K, Nakamura A, Terada J, Kuriyama T. The traditional herbal medicine Hochuekkito improves systemic inflammation in patients with chronic obstructive pulmonary disease. J Am Geriatr Soc. 2007;55(2):313–4.
230. Chuchalin AG, Berman B, Lehmacher W. Treatment of acute bronchitis in adults with a pelargonium sidoides preparation (EPs 7630): a randomized, double-blind, placebo-controlled trial. Explore (NY). 2005;1(6):437–45.
231. Matthys H, Heger M. EPs 7630-solution—an effective therapeutic option in acute and exacerbating bronchitis. Phytomedicine. 2007;14 Suppl 6:65–8.
232. Murali PM, Rajasekaran S, Paramesh P, et al. Plant-based formulation in the management of chronic obstructive pulmonary disease: a randomized double-blind study. Respir Med. 2006; 100(1):39–45.
233. Balamugesh T. Plant-based formulation in COPD. Respir Med. 2006;100(7):1294. author reply 1295.
234. Rantzsch U, Vacca G, Duck R, Gillissen A. Anti-inflammatory effects of myrtol standardized and other essential oils on alveolar macrophages from patients with chronic obstructive pulmonary disease. Eur J Med Res. 2009;14(4):205–9.
235. Matthys H, de Mey C, Carls C, Rys A, Geib A, Wittig T. Efficacy and tolerability of myrtol standardized in acute bronchitis. A multi-centre, randomised, double-blind, placebo-controlled parallel group clinical trial vs. cefuroxime and ambroxol. Arzneimittelforschung. 2000;50(8):700–11.
236. Meister R, Wittig T, Beuscher N, de Mey C. Efficacy and tolerability of myrtol standardized in long-term treatment of chronic bronchitis. A double-blind, placebo-controlled study. Study Group Investigators. Arzneimittelforschung. 1999;49(4):351–8.
237. Ulmer WT, Schott D. Chronic obstructive bronchitis. Effect of Gelomyrtol forte in a placebo-controlled double-blind study. Fortschr Med. 1991;109(27):547–50.

238. Sadlon AE, Lamson DW. Immune-modifying and antimicrobial effects of eucalyptus oil and simple inhalation devices. Altern Med Rev. 2010;15(1):33–47.
239. Worth H, Schacher C, Dethlefsen U. Concomitant therapy with Cineole (Eucalyptole) reduces exacerbations in COPD: a placebo-controlled double-blind trial. Respir Res. 2009;10:69.
240. Hsu CL, Wu YL, Tang GJ, Lee TS, Kou YR. Ginkgo biloba extract confers protection from cigarette smoke extract-induced apoptosis in human lung endothelial cells: role of heme oxygenase-1. Pulm Pharmacol Ther. 2009;22(4):286–96.
241. Babayigit A, Olmez D, Karaman O, et al. Effects of Ginkgo biloba on airway histology in a mouse model of chronic asthma. Allergy Asthma Proc. 2009;30(2):186–91.
242. Haines DD, Varga B, Bak I, et al. Summative interaction between astaxanthin, Ginkgo biloba extract (EGb761) and vitamin C in suppression of respiratory inflammation: a comparison with ibuprofen. Phytother Res. 2011;25(1):128–36.
243. Tang Y, Xu Y, Xiong S, et al. The effect of Ginkgo Biloba extract on the expression of PKCalpha in the inflammatory cells and the level of IL-5 in induced sputum of asthmatic patients. J Huazhong Univ Sci Technolog Med Sci. 2007;27(4):375–80.
244. Shih CH, Huang TJ, Chen CM, Lin YL, Ko WC. S-petasin, the main sesquiterpene of Petasites formosanus. Inhibits phosphodiesterase activity and suppresses ovalbumin-induced airway hyperresponsiveness. Evid Based Complement Alternat Med. 2009;29:29.
245. Ziolo G, Samochowiec L. Study on clinical properties and mechanisms of action of Petasites in bronchial asthma and chronic obstructive bronchitis. Pharm Acta Helv. 1998;72(6): 378–80.
246. Bausewein C, Booth S, Gysels M, Higginson I. Non-pharmacological interventions for breathlessness in advanced stages of malignant and non-malignant diseases. Cochrane Database Syst Rev. 2008;16(2):CD005623.
247. Smith GC, Pell JP. Parachute use to prevent death and major trauma related to gravitational challenge: systematic review of randomised controlled trials. BMJ. 2003;327(7429): 1459–61.

Chapter 5
Integrative Therapies for People with Interstitial Lung Disease, Idiopathic Pulmonary Fibrosis, and Pulmonary Arterial Hypertension

Kathleen Oare Lindell, Kevin F. Gibson, and Hunter C. Champion

Abstract There have been minimal evidence-based studies on the role of complementary and alternative medicine (CAM) in patients with interstitial lung disease. Clinical experience demonstrates that patients often use complementary and alternative medical approaches independently without medical advice or guidance. The use of CAM, while biologically plausible, may unknowingly expose the patient to harmful side effects with or without interactions with their prescribed medications. Further research is necessary to determine the role of CAM in patients with interstitial lung diseases.

Keywords Interstitial lung disease • Idiopathic pulmonary fibrosis • Pulmonary arterial hypertension • Sarcoidosis • Autoimmune-related lung disease

Interstitial Lung Disease

Interstitial lung diseases (ILD) are characterized by progressive inability to maintain normal blood oxygen levels due to impaired transfer of gas across the alveolar-capillary membrane [1]. ILD includes a variety of conditions, all of which share the common characteristics of lung scarring and progressive loss of the normal gas transfer ability [2]. Patients experience a progressive loss of functional ability and ultimately die from respiratory failure. More than 150 clinical diagnostic entities are associated with ILD [3].

K.O. Lindell, PhD, RN (✉) • K.F. Gibson, MD • H.C. Champion, MD, PhD, FAHA
Department of Pulmonary, Allergy and Critical Care Medicine,
Dorothy P. and Richard P. Simmons Center for Interstitial Lung Disease,
University of Pittsburg, Pittsburgh, PA, USA
e-mail: indellko@upmc.edu

L. Chlan and M.I. Hertz (eds.), *Integrative Therapies in Lung Health and Sleep*,
Respiratory Medicine 4, DOI 10.1007/978-1-61779-579-4_5,

The major abnormality in ILD is disruption of the distal lung parenchyma causing lung injury that is reflected pathologically by inflammation and/or fibrosis. While the incidence is difficult to determine, it has been estimated that ILD represents approximately 15% of patients seen by pulmonologists nationwide [4].

While there are greater than 100 distinct types of ILD, those most frequently encountered clinically include idiopathic pulmonary fibrosis (IPF), sarcoidosis, and connective tissue-related ILD. In all of these conditions, the lung parenchyma is the primary area of involvement and most patients present with nonspecific respiratory symptoms, including cough and dyspnea. An accurate prognosis and optimal treatment strategies depend on accurately discriminating between many diagnostic possibilities [5].

Three pivotal parameters that aid in diagnosis of ILD include clinical context, tempo of the disease process, and radiologic findings. Diagnostic studies should include high resolution computed tomography (HRCT) of chest, pulmonary function studies (spirometry, lung volumes, and diffusing capacity), lab tests (include serologic testing), echocardiogram, test for gastroesophageal reflux (GERD), bronchoscopy (BAL), and open lung biopsy, usually accomplished by video-assisted thoracoscopic surgery (VATS) [5].

IPF is the most common idiopathic interstitial pneumonia with no known cause or proven therapy at this time. Typically the disease is a gradually progressive disease, with a median survival of approximately 3 years [6, 7].

While the disease sarcoidosis was reported more than 100 years ago, the cause remains unknown. Sarcoidosis has been found in all ethnicities in varying frequencies. The natural course of the disease is highly variable, often not requiring therapy. All patients diagnosed with sarcoidosis should be screened for disease in other organs, especially the lung, heart, and eyes. Fibrosis associated with sarcoidosis may result in permanent pulmonary injury and ultimately determines the prognosis of the disease [8].

Connective tissue diseases (CTDs), excluding systemic lupus erythematosus, may imitate IPF. It is estimated that up to 15–20% of patients who present with a chronic ILD either have an underlying CTD or go on to develop a clinical picture consistent with CTD. Patients with CTD-related ILD survive longer than those patients diagnosed with IPF. Patients who have a lung biopsy consistent with a pattern of nonspecific interstitial pneumonia (NSIP) should have a high suspicion for a CTD. Once the diagnosis of a CTD is made, treatment regimes such as cyclophosphamide for scleroderma have been shown to decrease dyspnea and improve quality of life for patients at 1 year [9].

Exercise and ILD

Patients with ILD experience dyspnea on exertion and poor health-related quality of life (HRQoL). Exercise training has been found to improve exercise capacity and HRQoL in patients with chronic obstructive pulmonary disease (COPD), but its role in patients with ILD is unclear. The physiological basis for exercise training in patients with COPD differs from patients with ILD on which exercise performance is closely associated with circulatory impairment and exercise-induced hypoxemia [10]. Patients with IPF often demonstrate greater abnormalities of exercise-induced hypoxemia than patients with other forms of ILD. It is an important research goal to find out whether exercise is good for ILD patients in general.

Quality of Life and ILD

Patients with current symptoms of sarcoidosis and patients with IPF report the most impairment in the domains of physical health and level of independence for their quality of life. Patients with current symptoms of sarcoidosis report reduced physical functioning relative to their health status. Patients with IPF report impairment in all aspects of health status. In patients with current symptoms of sarcoidosis, the major symptom is fatigue, and IPF dyspnea, cough, and exercise intolerance have the most negative impact on patients' lives [11].

Studies aimed at assessing QoL or health status in other ILD are scarce or non-existent. Gaps in the literature include lack of evidence-based nursing studies and limited psychosocial assessment and interventions. Other variables to be considered include the impact of oxygen therapy and pulmonary rehabilitation, the impact of psychosocial aspects, the role of care partners, and the role of complementary and alternative therapy for ILD.

A review of the literature revealed no current publications looking at the role of CAM research in patients with ILD. The role of CAM has been researched in patients with other chronic disease [12, 13] as well as in patients with chronic lung diseases, i.e, cystic fibrosis [14], COPD [15, 16], and chronic asthma [17].

Pulmonary Hypertension in ILD

It is clear that a high percentage of ILD patients have pulmonary hypertension (PH) that contributes greatly to symptoms, disability, and mortality. The prevalence of PH is variable among the different types of ILD. A study of 79 patients with advanced IPF undergoing pre-lung transplant evaluation showed a PH prevalence of 31.6% by right heart catheterization [18]. Another study estimated a rate of 84% in 88 consecutive IPF patients screened by transthoracic echocardiography [19]. Additionally, the prevalence of PH appears to increase as patients deteriorate while awaiting lung transplantation [20, 21]. PH is also prevalent in patients with scleroderma lung disease and estimates range between 4.9 and 26.7% [22]. PH has also been shown to be associated with sarcoidosis, especially when ILD is present (up to 73.8%) [23]. PH has long been known to increase the morbidity and mortality in patients with CLD. In IPF and sarcoidosis, higher PAP was correlated with lower diffusing capacity, lower 6-min walk distance, and increased risk of death. Moreover, patients with scleroderma and PH have a lower response to PH therapy and worse outcome when compared to patients with idiopathic pulmonary arterial hypertension [24, 25].

While CAM treatments have not been directly tested in patients with ILD and/or PH, it is clear from our own experience that many patients extrapolate the findings and perceptions of CAM from other cardiovascular conditions and use these agents for their own conditions. We should recognize that 25–50% of Americans in the general population use some form of CAM (including herbal preparations) [26]. It is important to consider the use of CAM in patients with PH, especially given the potential for herb/drug and herb/herb interactions. Since some United States Food and Drug Administration (FDA)-approved therapies for PH carry a risk of elevated liver enzymes, it is important to consider the potential for exacerbation of liver function test elevations with concomitant treatment or that the herb may be the cause by itself. Given the commonality of symptoms and volume management difficulties, many patients with PH use CAM that are most commonly associated with the treatment of heart failure and other cardiovascular diseases. Here, we will discuss some of these therapies that we have observed patients use in PH as they relate to cardiovascular disease and, importantly, the potential for drug/herb interactions with medications that are commonly used in the treatment of PH.

Coenzyme Q10 (CoQ10; Ubiquinone)

Coenzyme Q10 (CoQ10) is a vitamin-like, fat-soluble quinone found in high concentrations in the mitochondria of the heart, liver, and kidney, where it is important for cellular mitochondrial respiration. CoQ10 acts in part as a redox link between flavoproteins and cytochromes, which are needed for oxidative phosphorylation and adenosine triphosphate (ATP) synthesis and as such, it is essential for energy production [26, 27]. It also has antioxidant, free radical scavenging, and membrane stabilizing properties [27].

Although not specifically tested in PH, the ubiquitous use of CoQ10 in congestive heart failure, angina, and hypertension has led to relatively extensive use in the PH community. It is postulated that a deficiency of CoQ10 contributes to the disease process and levels of the protein correlates with the clinical severity of heart failure [26, 28–31]. Although commonly used in the treatment of congestive heart failure in Italy and Japan, the data to support its use are not conclusive. A meta-analysis of eight randomized trials in congestive heart failure using CoQ10 from 1984 to 1994 demonstrated an improvement in cardiac output, stroke volume, and left ventricular ejection fraction [32]. However, this meta-analysis was unable to address clinical end points such as hospitalization or mortality [32]. More recently, CoQ10 has been studied in patients treated with a contemporary congestive heart failure treatment regimen. Watson et al. performed a randomized, double-blind, crossover trial of 30 patients with an left ventricular ejection fraction $<35\%$ (mean, $26 \pm 6\%$), all of whom were on maximum tolerated dose of ACEI and most of whom were given diuretics and digoxin and randomized to receive 33 mg of CoQ10 three times a day or placebo for 12 weeks [33]. The investigators found no improvement in ejection fraction, wedge pressure, cardiac index, or quality of life scores after 3 months of treatment. These data were echoed in another 6-month study [34].

While it is reasonable to conclude CoQ10 is safe, it is impossible to draw conclusions about efficacy especially in PH. It is also important to consider potential drug interactions with CoQ10 including, but not limited to, additive blood pressure-lowering effects with antihypertensive agents and vitamin K-like procoagulant effects that lowers INR on patients treated with warfarin (as is often the case with PH) [35–37].

L-Carnitine

Like CoQ10, carnitine is commonly used in heart failure and increasingly being used in patients with PH. Carnitine is a quaternary amine, synthesized from methionine and lysine and found mainly in skeletal and heart muscle, where it plays a key role in energy production [38]. Thus, it is believed that carnitine supplementation can improve mitochondrial function in patients with congestive heart failure. There is a paucity of information as to the role of carnitine in congestive heart failure in adults [39, 40]. Rizos studied the effects of carnitine in 80 adults, aged 48–50 years, with non-ischemic cardiomyopathy, NYHA classes III to IV, and left ventricular ejection fraction <35%. Patients were randomized to receive either L-Carnitine (2 g/day) or placebo and observed for 3 years. Results included nonsignificantly lower mortality rates with treatment (1 vs. 6 deaths in the placebo group) and improved hemodynamics and maintenance of sinus rhythm [39, 40]. To date, this is the largest trial of carnitine in cardiomyopathy, with the longest follow-up. Like CoQ10, there is no reason to believe that carnitine therapy is unsafe in PH, but the data in PH specifically are lacking despite its biological plausibility.

Hawthorn (Crataegus)

Traditional Chinese medicine has used the leaf and flower of the *Crataegus* plant (Hawthorn) for treating congestive heart failure and other cardiovascular diseases [26, 38]. More recently, the pharmacologically active constituents (flavonoids and procyanidins) have been isolated, leading to a standardized concentration of procyanidins (18%) [26, 38]. Owing to its inotropic activity, *Crataegus* Special Extract WS1442 is widely used in Germany for treatment of mild heart failure and is thought to have a wider therapeutic window and less renal clearance, thus giving it an advantage over digoxin [41]. Although the pharmacological action of WS1442 is unknown, several mechanisms have been postulated, including cAMP-independent positive inotropy, digoxin-like effect, vasodilation, and antioxidative and anti-inflammatory properties [42]. Most *Crataegus* studies in humans have been conducted in patients with congestive heart failure and for a short duration. In a meta-analysis published in 1996, in NYHA class I–III heart failure, *Crataegus* extract yielded improvement in symptoms beyond placebo, with no increase in adverse events [43]. Side effects include nausea, gastrointestinal upset, fatigue, sweating, palpitations, and agitation [26]. Moreover, there are potential additive effects with other agents such as digoxin, coronary vasodilators (nitrates, adenosine, theophylline), and herbal cardiac glycosides like oleander and Siberian ginseng.

Potential Drug Interactions with Agents Commonly Used in PH

Regardless of the type of complementary therapy, it is critical to consider any agent may have a drug interaction with drugs traditionally used in the treatment of ILD and/or PH. With this in mind, caregivers should always ask patients about the use of CAM and consider these agents as potential causes of adverse events in this patient population. Below, we identify and discuss common drug interactions.

Warfarin and Antiplatelet Therapy

Warfarin is often used in PH to prevent clot in the lung in situ or when patients have concomitant medical issues that are common in this patient population (atrial fibrillation, pulmonary embolism, deep venous thrombosis). It is well known that many herbs interact with warfarin or alter platelet function such that the risk of bleeding is potentially increased in patients treated with warfarin or conventional antiplatelet therapy while using these herbal agents [26]. In many cases, the potential for increased bleeding is hypothetical; however, there have been numerous case reports of increased bleeding tendency in patients taking herbal supplements with or without the concomitant use of warfarin [26]. Because of what is known about the effects of these herbs on platelet function and markers of coagulation, their use should be avoided in patients requiring warfarin or other conventional antiplatelet therapy. A few of these herbs that we have observed in our own clinic and their effect on coagulation are included in Table 5.1.

Amiodarone

Amiodarone is primarily used for treatment of atrial fibrillation, and less frequently for life-threatening ventricular arrhythmias. Amiodarone has many potential adverse effects, including photosensitivity, hepatotoxicity, pulmonary fibrosis, and

Table 5.1 Common biologically based complementary and alternative medicine therapies used in patients with heart failure and potentially PH: indications and potential interactions with standard pharmacotherapy

Biological agent	CAM properties/uses	Potential drug interactions
Vitamin E	Antioxidant: prevention of cardiovascular disease. Data unclear on efficacy in CHF	Increased bleeding with antithrombotic and antiplatelet agents
Coenzyme Q10	Antioxidant and free radical scavenger; used to treat heart failure and other cardiovascular disorders	Procoagulant: lowers INR in patients on stable warfarin dose
Hawthorn (*Crataegus* species) L-carnitine	Treatment of heart failure and arrhythmias. Involved in cellular energy production, supplement in nutritional deficiency, possible role in heart failure	Digoxin-like effects Limited data on drug interactions
Garlic	Antispasmodic, antiseptic, promotes leukocytosis, hypocholesterolemic, vasoactive properties	Inhibits epinephrine-induced in vitro platelet aggregation small study showing inhibition of ex vivo platelet aggregation

thyroid disorders. Its metabolism is complex, and multiple drug/drug interactions, including but not limited to some statins, warfarin, and digoxin, are well known. With this in mind, great care should be taken to avoid herbal remedies that may further interact with amiodarone.

Digoxin

Numerous herbs have been identified as containing digoxin-like substances, and therefore they may potentiate digoxin effects. Digoxin is commonly used in PH in an effort to improve right ventricular contractility, and potential interactions with CAM should be carefully considered.

Conclusion

While there is significant plausible biological evidence and relatively small clinical trials that would support the use of CAM in patients with PH, the potential for drug/drug, drug/CAM, and CAM/CAM interactions should be carefully considered, especially if an unexpected adverse event is encountered. Moreover, it is important that patients be cautioned about these potential interactions prior to the use of herbal remedies. In addition, a careful questioning of patients with regard to which CAM they may be using is as important as their prescription medications.

These considerations underscore the great need for larger studies to be conducted specifically in patients with ILD and/or PH in order to substantiate efficacy and safety.

References

1. American Thoracic Society; European Respiratory Society. American Thoracic Society/European Respiratory Society International Multidisciplinary Consensus Classification of the Idiopathic Interstitial Pneumonias. Am J Respir Crit Care Med. 2002;165(2):277–304.
2. American Thoracic Society. Idiopathic pulmonary fibrosis: diagnosis and treatment. International consensus statement. American Thoracic Society (ATS), and the European Respiratory Society (ERS). Am J Respir Crit Care Med. 2000;161(2 Pt 1):646–64.
3. King Jr TE. Clinical advances in the diagnosis and therapy of the interstitial lung diseases. Am J Respir Crit Care Med. 2005;172(3):268–79.
4. Schwarz M, King TE. Interstitial lung disease. In: Cosgrove G, Schwaz MI, editors. Approach to the evaluation and diagnosis of interstitial lung disease. 5th ed. Shelton, CT: People's Medical Publishing House-USA; 2011.
5. Ryu JH, Daniels CE, Hartman TE, Yi ES. Diagnosis of interstitial lung diseases. Mayo Clin Proc. 2007;82(8):976–86.
6. Raghu G, Collard HR Egan JJ, Martinez FJ, Behr J, et al. on behalf of the ATS/ERS/JRS/ALAT Committee on Idiopathic Pulmonary Fibrosis. An official ATS/ERS/JRS/ALAT statement: idiopathic pulmonary fibrosis: evidence-based guidelines for diagnosis and management. Am J Respirat Crit Care Med 2011;183:788–824.
7. Lindell KO, Jacobs SS. Idiopathic pulmonary fibrosis. Am J Nurs 2003;103(4):32–42; quiz 43.
8. Judson M. Sarcoidosis: clinical presentation, diagnosis, and approach to treatment. Am J Med Sci. 2008;335(1):26–33.
9. Tzelepis G, Toya SP, Moutsopoulos HM. Occult connective tissue diseases mimicking idiopathic interstitial pneumonias. Eur Respir J. 2008;31:11–20.
10. Holland AE, Hill CJ, Conron M, Munro P, McDonald CF. Short-term improvement in exercise capacity and symptoms following exercise training in interstitial lung disease. Thorax. 2008;63(6):549–94.
11. De Vries J, Drent M. Quality of life and health status in interstitial lung diseases. Curr Opin Pulm Med. 2006;12(5):354–8.
12. Saydah SH, Eberhardt MS. Use of complementary and alternative medicine among adults with chronic diseases: United States 2002. J Altern Complement Med. 2006;12(8):805–12.
13. Metcalfe A, Williams J, McChesney J, Patten SB, Jetté N. Use of complementary and alternative medicine by those with a chronic disease and the general population—results of a national population based survey. BMC Complement Altern Med. 2010;18:10–58.
14. Anbar RD, Murthy VV. Reestablishment of hope as an intervention for a patient with cystic fibrosis awaiting lung transplantation. J Altern Complement Med. 2010;16(9):1007–10.
15. Mularski RA, Munjas BA, Lorenz KA, Sun S, Robertson SJ, Schmelzer W, Kim AC, Shekelle PG. Randomized controlled trial of mindfulness-based therapy for dyspnea in chronic obstructive lung disease. J Altern Complement Med. 2009;15(10):1083–90.
16. Davis CL, Lewith GT, Broomfield J, Prescott P. A pilot project to assess the methodological issues involved in evaluating acupuncture as a treatment for disabling breathlessness. J Altern Complement Med. 2001;7(6):633–9.
17. Maa S, Sun MF, Hsu KH, Hung TJ, Chen HC, Yu CT, Wang CH, Lin HC. Effect of acupuncture or acupressure on quality of life of patients with chronic obstructive asthma; a pilot study. J Altern Complement Med. 2003;9(5):659–70.

18. Lettieri CJ, Nathan SD, Barnett SD, Ahmad S, Shorr AF. Prevalence and outcomes of pulmonary arterial hypertension in advanced idiopathic pulmonary fibrosis. Chest. 2006;129(3):746–52.
19. Nadrous HF, Pelikka PA, Krowka MJ, Swanson KL, Chaowalit N, Decker PA, Ruy JH. Pulmonary hypertension in patients with idiopathic pulmonary fibrosis. Chest. 2005;128(4):2393–9.
20. Nathan SD. Pulmonary hypertension in interstitial lung disease. Int J Clin Pract Suppl. 2008;160:21–8.
21. Shorr AF, Wainright JL, Cors CS, Lettieri CJ, Nathan SD. Pulmonary hypertension in patients with pulmonary fibrosis awaiting lung transplant. Eur Respir J. 2007;30(4):715–21.
22. Proudman SM, Stevens WM, Sahhar J, Celemajer D. Pulmonary arterial hypertension in systemic sclerosis: the need for early detection and treatment. Intern Med J. 2007;37(7):485–94.
23. Shigemitsu H, Nagai S, Sharma OP. Pulmonary hypertension and granulomatous vasculitis in sarcoidosis. Curr Opin Pulm Med. 2007;13(5):434–8.
24. Girgis RE, Mathai SC, Krishnan JA, Wigley FM, Hassoun PM. Long-term outcome of bosentan treatment in idiopathic pulmonary arterial hypertension and pulmonary arterial hypertension associated with the scleroderma spectrum of diseases. J Heart Lung Transplant. 2005;24(10): 1626–31.
25. Polomis D, Runo JR, Meyer KC. Pulmonary hypertension in interstitial lung disease. Curr Opin Pulm Med. 2008;14(5):462–9.
26. Kelly L, Miller MD, Richard S, Liebowitz MD, Newby LK. Complementary and alternative medicine in cardiovascular disease: a review of biologically based approaches. Am Heart J. 2004;147(3):401–11.
27. Pepping J. Coenzyme Q10. Am J Health Syst Pharm. 1999;56:519–20.
28. Folkers K, Vadhanavikit S, Mortensen SA. Biochemical rationale and myocardial tissue data on the effective therapy of cardiomyopathy with coenzyme Q10. Proc Natl Acad Sci USA. 1985;82:901–4.
29. Mortensen SA. Perspectives on therapy of cardiovascular disease with coenzyme Q10 (ubiquinone). Clin Investig. 1993;71(Suppl):S116–23.
30. Langsjoen PH, Langsjoen PH, Folkers K. Long-term efficacy and safety of coenzyme Q10 therapy for idiopathic dilated cardiomyopathy. Am J Cardiol. 1990;65:521–3.
31. Morisco C, Trimarco B, Condorelli M. Effect of coenzyme Q10 therapy in patients with congestive cardiac failure: a long term multicenter randomized study. Clin Investig. 1993;71(Suppl): S134–6.
32. Soja AM, Mortensen SA. Treatment of CHF with CoQ10 illuminated by meta-analyses of clinical trials. Mol Aspects Med. 1997;18(Suppl):S159–68.
33. Watson PS, Scalia GM, Galbraith A, et al. Lack of effect of coenzyme Q on left ventricular function in patients with congestive heart failure. J Am Coll Cardiol. 1999;33:1549–52.
34. Khatta M, Alexander BS, Krichten CM, et al. The effect of coenzyme Q10 in patients with congestive heart failure. Ann Intern Med. 2000;132:636–40.
35. Combs AB, Porter TH, Folkers K. Anticoagulant activity of naphthoquinone analog of vitamin K and an inhibitor of coenzyme Q10-enzyme systems. Res Commun Chem Pathol Pharmacol. 1976;13:109–14.
36. Landbo C, Almdal TP. Interaction between warfarin and coenzyme Q10. Ugeskr Laeger. 1998;160:3226–7.
37. Spigset O. Reduced effect of warfarin caused by ubidecarenone. Lancet. 1994;344:1372–3.
38. Jellin JM, Gregory PJ, Batz F, et al. Pharmacist's letter/presciber's letter natural medicine comprehensive database. 5th ed. Stockton, CA: Therapeutic Research Faculty; 2003. p. 379–82.
39. Rizos I. Three-year survival of patients with heart failure caused by dilated cardiomyopathy and L-carnitine administration. Am Heart J. 2000;139:S130–3.
40. Jeejeebhoy F, Keith M, Freeman M, et al. Nutritional supplementation with Myo Vive repletes essential cardiac myocyte nutrients and reduces left ventricular size in patients with left ventricular dysfunction. Am Heart J. 2002;143:1092–100.
41. Krzeminski T, Chatterjee SS. Ischemia and early reperfusion induced arrhythmias: beneficial effects of an extract of *Crataegus oxyacantha L.* Pharm Pharmacol Lett. 1993;3:45–8.

42. Holubarsch CJ, Colucci WS, Meinertz T, et al. Survival and prognosis: investigation of crataegus extract WS 1442 in congestive heart failure (SPICE) rationale, study design and study protocol. Eur J Heart Fail. 2000;2:431–7.
43. Wiehmayr T, Ernst E. Die therapeutische Wirksamkeit von Crataegus. Fortschr Med. 1996;1–2:27–9.

Chapter 6
Integrative Therapies for People with Cystic Fibrosis*

Claire A. Butler and Scott C. Bell

Abstract Cystic fibrosis (CF) is the most common lethal autosomal inherited disorder affecting Caucasian populations. Due to improved treatments and multidisciplinary team care, the life expectancy of patients with CF has increased dramatically in the last 2 decades. Medical therapy for the majority of patients consists of regular sputum clearance, mucolytic therapy, antibiotics, pancreatic enzyme replacement, nutritional support, and anti-inflammatory agents such as azithromycin. Review by complementary and alternative medicine (CAM) therapists and the utilization of CAM medicines is common in people with CF and healthcare practitioners should encourage discussion with their patients about the use of such therapies. Data to date on the effectiveness of CAM therapy in CF are limited; therefore, adequately powered and carefully designed studies are required to enhance knowledge of the correct role of such therapies. Collaborations between academic centers established to evaluate CAM therapies with CF researchers would provide excellent opportunity to enhance the study of the role of CAM.

Keywords Cystic fibrosis • Complementary medicine • Alternative medicines • Holistic therapy

*Conflict of Interest Statement: Neither author has a financial or other interest in any of the products discussed in this chapter.

C.A. Butler, MB, BCh, BAO, MRCP • S.C. Bell, MBBS, MD, FRACP (✉)
Department of Thoracic Medicine, The Prince Charles Hospital, Rode Road,
Chermside Brisbane, QLD 4032, Australia
e-mail: scottbell@health.gld.gov.au

L. Chlan and M.I. Hertz (eds.), *Integrative Therapies in Lung Health and Sleep*,
Respiratory Medicine 4, DOI 10.1007/978-1-61779-579-4_6,

Introduction and Overview

Cystic fibrosis (CF) is the most common lethal autosomal recessive inherited disorder in Caucasian populations. Earlier diagnosis, institution of intensive therapies, and multidisciplinary care have contributed to improved life expectancy over the past 20 years. According to the Cystic Fibrosis Foundation Patient Registry (USA), the median age of survival has increased from 27 years in 1985 to 36 years in 2009 [1].

There are over 1,800 known mutations in the CF gene, which encodes for the cystic fibrosis transmembrane conductance regulator (CFTR), a chloride channel expressed on epithelial surfaces of the airway, gastrointestinal tract, the liver, and the male reproductive tract.

Dysfunction of the CFTR gene results in many effects including, but not limited to, chronic respiratory infection and the development of bronchiectasis, rhinosinusitis, and nasal polyposis; pancreatic insufficiency; distal intestinal obstruction (meconium ileus in neonates); and male infertility [2]. The majority of mortality and disease morbidity is due to chronic suppurative lung disease. While *Haemophilus influenzae* and *Staphylococcus aureus* are common in childhood, the most common bacterial infection after childhood is *Pseudomonas aeruginosa* causing chronic infection in ~80% of adults with CF [3]. Chronic bronchial infection results in an exuberant inflammatory response, leading to the development of bronchiectasis and gas trapping, and ultimately respiratory insufficiency [4].

There has been a large increase in the numbers of adults with CF over the past 3 decades, approaching 50% of the total CF population [5]. With increasing age, there are increasing rates of nonpulmonary complications including CF-related diabetes, metabolic bone disease, multiresistant bacteria, and complications of therapy including drug allergy and toxicity [6]. Lung transplantation is an established therapy for those patients with end stage lung disease and is one of the most common indications for that procedure [7].

Treatment Principles

Specialized, multidisciplinary approach to care for patients with CF is thought to have contributed to improved survival over the past 2 decades [8]. The preservation of lung function is associated with frequent review in specialist centers [9]. Currently available therapies address the "secondary" effects of CFTR dysfunction, but several trials currently underway incorporate therapies which aim to improve the function of the CFTR-regulated chloride ion channel [10]. Therapeutic options available for the common manifestations of CF are outlined in Table 6.1 [4, 9–25] and consist of airway clearance techniques; mucolytic agents such as hypertonic saline, mannitol, and recombinant deoxyribonuclease (rhDNase); antibiotic therapy (both maintenance and for treatment of exacerbations); anti-inflammatory drugs such as azithromycin and nonsteroidal anti-inflammatory agents; and nutritional support. However, the treatments which have emerged in the past 20 years may be dwarfed

Table 6.1 Therapeutic approaches for cystic fibrosis

CFTR dysfunction	CFTR potentiators [10]
	CFTR correctors [11]
	CFTR gene transfer
Abnormal dehydrated mucus	Airways clearance, i.e., physiotherapy supported techniques and independent techniques (including active cycle of breathing, autogenic drainage, flutter, and Acapella® [4, 12])
	Inhaled hypertonic saline [13, 14]
	Inhaled recombinant deoxyribonuclease (rhDNase) [15]
Inflammation	High-dose oral ibuprofen [16, 17]
	Maintenance azithromycin [18, 19]
	Inhaled corticosteroids (limited role) [20]
Infection	Intravenous or oral antibiotics for exacerbations [9, 21]
	Nebulized antibiotics for health maintenance (e.g., tobramycin, colomycin, aztreonam) [22–24]
Progressive bronchiectasis and end-stage respiratory failure	Lung transplantation
Nutrition	Pancreatic enzyme replacement therapy (PERT) [25]
	Fat-soluble vitamin replacement [25]
	Nutritional energy support (high energy, high protein supplementation)
	Enteral nutritional support

by new therapies in the coming decade, such as drugs which improve the function of the CFTR. This provides hope for further improvements in life span and quality of life for people with CF.

Search Strategy

Both authors searched Medline (between 15th and 31st May 2011), Google Scholar, and the Cochrane Library for reviews pertinent to holistic therapies in CF with the search terms "complementary medicine and therapies," "alternative medicine and therapies," "holistic therapies," "nutritional supplements," "herbal," "Chinese medicines," "massage," "acupuncture," "chiropractic," "biofeedback," "creative arts," "garlic," "curcumin," "antioxidants," "probiotics," and "homeopathy" with "cystic fibrosis."

Overview of Studies of Utilization of Complementary and Alternative Medicine in CF

The overall use of complementary and alternative medicine (CAM) and CAM therapists by the general population has increased over recent years as assessed by random telephone poll calls to 1,539 adults in the United States and due to patient nondisclosure may actually be underestimated [26]. The American Academy of Pediatrics defined CAM as "strategies that have not met the standards of clinical effectiveness, either through randomized controlled trials (RCTs) or through the consensus of the biomedical community" [27].

Despite encouraging improvements in outcomes for people with CF, chronic symptoms including, but not limited to, chest discomfort, cough, and breathlessness persist even with maximal medical therapy, and it is not surprising that they may try other modalities to improve symptom control. A number of studies have addressed the CAM usage and patient review by CAM therapists in adults and children with CF.

An early study of 402 children and adults with CF with a median age of 18 years demonstrated 66% of the study population used at least one nonmedical modality, and two-thirds of these had a religious basis [28]. The majority reported the use of nonmedical modalities as beneficial, especially participation in group prayer and the use of religious articles. Notably, the cost of such practices was small and generally less than US $200 in the patient's lifetime [28].

Tanase assessed the use of CAM in pediatric patients with CF and reported that 77% of the responders (50.5% of the patients who received the questionnaire) used some form of CAM inclusive of prayer, and one-third employed more than one form of CAM [29]. The most popular therapy (49% of patients) was "body–mind medicine" which included prayer, deep breathing exercises, meditation, and herbs among others [29]. Interventions such as massage, homeopathy, and yoga were utilized to a lesser extent. Only half of the patients had informed their doctor regarding their use of CAM. Another study of the use of CAM in children with chronic medical conditions included 22 patients with CF [30]. Of these children, 4 (18.2%) were using CAM, which was similar to use of this modality in patients with other chronic disease such as spina bifida and Duchenne muscular dystrophy. The most popular forms of CAM were massage, dietary, and herbal therapies [30].

A study by Burrows in 2002 investigated the use of CAM in 83 adult patients with CF by the use of a self-reported questionnaire which was developed with the guidance of a CAM practitioner, a sociologist and a patient focus group [31]. The mean age of the participants was 27 years and almost two-thirds had visited a CAM practitioner in their lifetime and 26% were currently consulting a CAM practitioner. Lifetime and current use of CAM therapy were also high (70 and 45%, respectively). A significantly higher proportion of women had consulted a CAM practitioner or had ever taken CAM therapies [31]. Table 6.2 shows the most frequently used complementary and alternative therapies used by the patients in this study [31]. The most common CAM therapists were masseuse, naturopaths, and chiropractors (Fig. 6.1) [31]. One in ten patients spent more than US $550 annually to receive these consultations and to purchase CAM therapies. While 68% of patients believed conventional medicine provided greater benefit than CAM, 15% felt that CAM provided equal benefit to medications prescribed by their CF center [31]. Thirty-nine percent of patients in this study had informed their doctor regarding the use of CAM though the majority (82%) felt their team would support CAM use.

Table 6.2 Most commonly utilized complementary and alternative medicines (Adapted from Burrows et al. [31]; with permission from the *Journal of Pharmacy Practice and Research*)

Garlic and horseradish
Vitamin C
Naturopath herbal mixtures
Echinacea
Herbal teas
Chinese herbal mixtures
Fish oils
Acidophilus
Aromatherapy oils
B group vitamins
Colloidal silver
Coenzyme Q
Ambratose
Goldenseal
Evening primrose oil

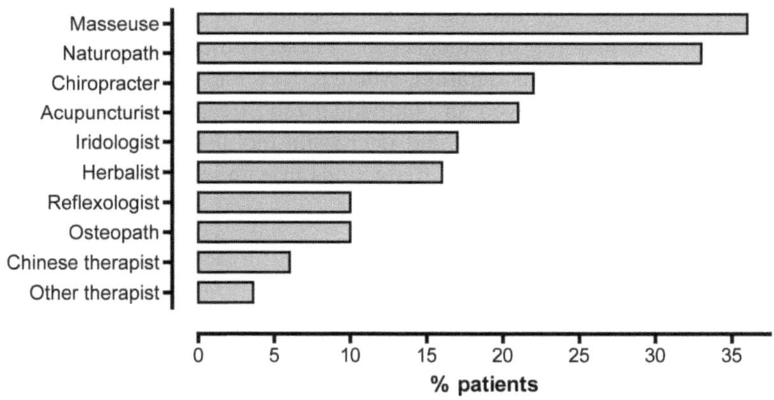

Fig. 6.1 Complementary and alternative medicine therapists consulted by cystic fibrosis patients in the study by Burrows et al. [31] (adapted with permission from the *Journal of Pharmacy Practice and Research*)

Specific Approaches

For each of the various subcategories of CAM discussed below, the theory behind the use will be discussed followed by a summary of previous research in that area.

Manipulative Body and Based Practices

Massage

Physiotherapists commonly employ massage techniques on patients with CF to promote soft tissue and fascial relaxation and to improve circulation [32]. It is well known that patients with CF suffer pain in many areas but chest, back, and abdominal pain predominate [33, 34]. There have been a number of RTCs assessing the use of massage as part of therapy for chronic lung disease such as asthma, many with encouraging results, including two studies in patients with CF.

Parent-administered massage for children with CF has been assessed as part of a trial with reading as a control intervention [35]. In the "massage" group, children received a 20-min session prior to bedtime for 1 month. Parents were trained to provide a standard massage regime performed each evening, and adherence was checked with regular phone calls and a demonstration of the massage at outpatient clinic. Both children and parents completed a questionnaire designed to assess anxiety levels. Children in the massage group demonstrated reduced anxiety levels and improved peak flow readings [35], which were accompanied by a reduction in parental anxiety.

A study from Australia recruited 105 adults with CF with the aim to assess the impact of a single massage and mobilization session on discomfort and ease of breathing [36]. The majority of patients (90%) described chronic musculoskeletal pain of greater than 3 months duration, whereas 10% had acute pain (less than 3 days duration). Patients received an "individualized" treatment from the physiotherapist consisting of "spinal joint and intercostal mobilization" and "soft tissue therapy and remedial massage" [36]. Reductions in pain levels and breathlessness were reported [36].

Chiropractic Therapy

This highly utilized form of alternative therapy is generally employed for chronic back pain and spinal manipulation for relief of pain [37]. Evidence for its role in CF management is lacking and only one study was identified.

In the report by Stern et al. examining use of CAM in patients with CF, 14% reported use of chiropractic services and 65% of those patients reported an improvement in symptoms, most commonly an improvement in pain [38]. Care must be taken to avoid bone fractures with chiropractic therapy, as many patients with CF have metabolic bone disease and reduced bone density [38].

Acupuncture

Acupuncture is a treatment modality derived from Chinese Medicine practice and involves the use of needles, which are purported to restore the flow of energy or "Qi" [32]. The risk of serious adverse event is low at 0.55 per 10,000 patients [39].

Performing a blinded investigation of acupuncture is impossible [32]. Studies of the role of acupuncture in CF are limited. A study of acupuncture for management of pain in 30 CF patients with an average age of 26.7 years who were referred for acupuncture treatments primarily for chest pain (38%) or back pain (21%) demonstrated significantly reduced pain scores (visual analogue score) immediately following an isolated acupuncture session [40]. Similarly, a small study of nine patients in the United Kingdom reported improvements in chest pain score (visual analogue pain scale) and improved overall well-being and relaxation, without serious adverse events [41].

Mind–Body Practices

Hope

Patients with CF are known to have an increased incidence of depression and anxiety compared to healthy individuals [42, 43]. A study of 670 German patients with CF who completed the Hospital Anxiety and Depression Scale (HADS) identified increased anxiety scores in 20% of patients and evidence of depression in 10% [44]. Older patients were more likely to experience anxiety and depression and women were more likely to experience anxiety than men [44]. Previous research has demonstrated improved outcomes for a range of chronic diseases in patients with an optimistic attitude and good "coping" skills [45]. This appears to be particularly relevant in patients with chronic lung conditions (inclusive of a proportion of patients with CF) who are waiting for lung transplantation where psychosocial intervention (education about stress, relaxation, and problem solving) led to improved quality of life [46].

Biofeedback

Delk et al. compared the efficacy of biofeedback-assisted breathing retraining (BRT) sessions with a placebo consisting of biofeedback-assisted relaxation training [47]. They enrolled 26 patients (aged 10–41 years) who underwent eight sessions over a 4-week period, after which lung function was measured and compared with baseline. The BRT group were taught pursed lip and diaphragmatic breathing using an incentive spirometer, and those in the "placebo" group were trained in relaxation techniques using relaxation tapes and hand warming with temperature biofeedback, i.e., instruction in breathing techniques were omitted [47]. Patients in the BRT group had an increase in FEV_1 of 32% compared with 9% in the relaxation only group. A reduction in air trapping, increased muscle strength, and enhanced motivation were suggested by the authors as potential factors [47]. A recent Cochrane review of 13 studies addressing various behavioral and educational interventions in patients with CF, which incorporated this study, concluded that the results showed a significant effect of physiotherapy and biofeedback [48].

Hypnosis

A study of 12 patients with CF assessed the effect of self-hypnosis on psychological factors such as anxiety and a marker of lung function, peak expiratory flow rate [49]. They found a significant improvement in peak expiratory flow rate following hypnosis in this small group of patients. A study of pulmonologist-taught self-hypnosis over one or two sessions in 49 patients with CF (mean age 18 years) noted 86% use of this modality to assist with relaxation and relief of pain [50]. Subjective efficacy of the intervention was assessed by the patient's response to a number of "open-ended questions." Sixteen of the patients continued with hypnosis for more than 6 months.

Creative Arts

Grasso assessed the effect on enjoyment of chest physiotherapy of a "treatment music" tape, which had been specifically composed by a music therapist, compared with a no music and "familiar" music crossover [51]. Twenty-one children under the age of 2 years old were randomized to the "treatment music" tape for 12 weeks ($n=10$) or the no tape (for 6 weeks)/familiar music (for 6 weeks) arm ($n=11$). The specially tailored music tape led to increased children's enjoyment (as assessed by the parent) and increased the parental enjoyment [51].

Trained singers are known to have enhanced lung capacity which is thought to be due to diaphragmatic breathing and improved respiratory muscle strength [52, 53]. A recent Cochrane review attempted to evaluate the effects of the addition of singing to a patient's usual treatment regime; however, no trials met the selection criteria for inclusion in the meta-analysis [54].

Vitamin, Mineral, and Herbal Products

Garlic

The term adjuvant therapy for antibiotics was coined by Hurley et al. in their recent Cochrane review [55]. This review identified three studies involving adjuvant therapies for antibiotics involving β-carotene, garlic, and zinc supplementation and did not identify any significant improvement in lung function, quality of life, or rates of pulmonary exacerbations [55].

Garlic extract possesses interesting properties that are relevant to CF pathobiology. Many patients with CF become chronically infected with *P. aeruginosa* [56, 57]. *Pseudomonas* populations possess a "signaling" mechanism, called quorum sensing, which promotes impaired neutrophil function and other host immune functions [57]. Garlic has been shown in vitro to inhibit quorum sensing, and increase *P. aeruginosa* killing by neutrophils in in vitro experiments [58, 59]. A recent study reported reduced expression of a number of *Pseudomonas* quorum sensing, genes, and virulence factors in response to garlic, in addition to a significant reduction in biofilm growth and bacterial attachment [60].

In a RCT of garlic supplementation vs. placebo in 26 patients with a median age of 18 years who had moderate obstructive lung disease and chronic *P. aeruginosa* infection, there was a nonsignificant trend toward improved lung function and weight gain in the active treatment group; however, the small sample size must be taken into account [61]. The main adverse effect was halitosis!

Ginseng

Ginseng is a commonly utilized Chinese herb with reported anti-inflammatory properties and an ability to improve clearance of bacteria in animal models [62–64]. In an in vitro study by Song et al., ginseng did not demonstrate reduction in *P. aeruginosa* growth; in fact, the lowest strength of ginseng (1.25%) appeared to increase bacterial growth [65]. However, the authors did note anti-quorum sensing activity at a concentration of 5% ginseng, though they were uncertain as to whether this might have been due to an effect of one of the other ingredients contained in ginseng extract [65].

Curcumin

Dysfunctional CFTR underpins the clinical symptoms characteristic of CF. Curcumin, a component of turmeric, is a sarcoplasmic/endoplasmic reticulum calcium (SERCA) pump inhibitor. In 2004, Egan et al. described curcumin fed to homozygous Δ(delta)F508 CFTR mice led to a correction of nasal potential difference (marker of chloride epithelial transport) and prolonged survival [66]. Another study reported enhanced activation of CFTR channels by curcumin in an in vitro model using cells transfected with a number of different CFTR mutations [67]. One group reported that curcumin-induced suppression of calreticulin, a negative regulator of CFTR, led to upregulation of wild-type, though not p508del CFTR [68]. However, this effect was not duplicated by Song et al. among others, and therefore, the role of curcumin in cystic fibrosis therapy is undecided [69]. More recent research has suggested an additive role for curcumin to genistein (an isoflavone) in increasing the channel activity of another CFTR mutation-G551D [70]. To date, no human studies have investigated the in vivo effects of this spice.

Antioxidants

Oxidative stress is thought to lead to pulmonary dysfunction in patients with CF, and persistent infection and activation of the inflammatory cascade diminishes antioxidant stores in the body [71, 72]. Antioxidant levels also decrease with age in CF [32, 72]. Due to pancreatic insufficiency and malabsorption and despite dietary supplementation, some patients with CF will have impaired absorption of fat-soluble vitamins, including vitamin E, which is a known antioxidant compound [73].

At present there is limited knowledge regarding the efficacy of ingested antioxidants in CF. Although supplementation of various micronutrients (such as Vitamin C, selenium, and β-carotene) led to improvement in biomarkers such as antioxidant enzyme function and plasma supplement levels, a Cochrane review was unable to determine any clinically meaningful improvements in lung function or quality of life [74]. One study of omega-3 supplementation in CF showed an improvement in pulmonary function, although a Cochrane review involving three such studies was unable to demonstrate a definite favorable effect of this supplement [75, 76].

Probiotics

Probiotics are live bacteria, such as lactobacilli, and are widely used for medical conditions including irritable bowel syndrome and gastroenteritis [32]. Due to recurrent antibiotic exposure in CF patients, the gut microflora can be disturbed [77].

A reduction in intestinal inflammation in a small number of patients with CF receiving the probiotic strain, *Lactobacillus rhamnosus* GG, was reported in a pilot study by Bruzzese et al. Interestingly, children with CF had high baseline stool levels of calprotectin, a marker of intestinal inflammation that is also found to be increased in inflammatory bowel disease [78]. Treatment with probiotics for 4 weeks significantly reduced calprotectin levels in the ten children with CF, but despite the suggestion of reduced intestinal inflammation, the levels were still above the normal range. The same research group studied five children with CF after probiotic treatment, and also noted a significant decrease in rectal nitric oxide, another marker of intestinal inflammation [78].

An RCT crossover study by Bruzzese et al. reported in 2007 enrolled 19 children with CF and pancreatic insufficiency [77]. Children received *L. rhamnosus* GG (or placebo) for 6 months then cross over after a 4-week washout period. A reduction in pulmonary exacerbations and hospital admissions and an increase in % predicted FEV_1 and body weight were noted in the active treatment arm compared to placebo [77]. Another study investigated the effect of a 6-month treatment with mixed probiotics (*Lactobacillus acidphilus, Lactobacillus bulgaricus, Bifidobacterium bifidum, Streptococcus thermophiles*) in ten patients with CF [79]. The mean age of the group was 26 years and baseline FEV_1 (% predicted) was 63.8%. The researchers reported a reduction in exacerbation rate compared to that noted in the 2 years prior to treatment and 6 months posttreatment (none of the patients experienced an exacerbation during the treatment period) although there was no change in lung function or body mass index [79].

Homeopathy

While homeopathic therapies are utilized by patients with CF [31], there are no published studies of this form of complementary medicine.

Summary and Conclusions and Directions for Future Research

Evaluation by CAM therapists and the utilization of CAM medicines is common in people with CF. Open communication between the CF physician and CF pharmacist with the CF patients (and their families) should allow improved understanding of the use of such therapies within the CF clinic and provide an opportunity for discussions about motivation for use and evaluation of any adverse effects and or potential interactions with other therapies.

Studies reporting positive outcome measures are limited to date, despite several classes of therapy having good rationale for their potential beneficial effects. The lack of clinical studies into CAM and CF means that the efficacy of these interventions is unable to be accurately assessed. Furthermore, there is likely to be publication bias, as studies with positive results are more likely to be selected for publication than those that are negative [32]. Adequately powered and carefully designed studies are required to enhance knowledge of the role of CAM therapies in CF, especially as many are expensive and potential toxicities and drug interactions are poorly understood. Collaborations between academic centers established to evaluate CAM therapies with CF researchers would provide excellent opportunity to enhance the study of the role of CAM.

References

1. Cystic Fibrosis Foundation Patient Registry. 2009 Annual data report. Bethesda, MD: Cystic Fibrosis Foundation; 2009.
2. De Boeck K, Wilschanski M, Castellani C, et al. Cystic fibrosis: terminology and diagnostic algorithms. Thorax. 2006;61:627–35.
3. Anon. Cystic Fibrosis Foundation Patient Registry. 2009 Annual data report. Bethesda, MD: Cystic Fibrosis Foundation; 2009.
4. O'Sullivan BP, Freedman SD. Cystic fibrosis. Lancet. 2009;373:1891–904.
5. Cystic Fibrosis Foundation. 2010 Annual Report. Bethesda, Maryland: Cystic Fibrosis Foundation; 2010.
6. Yankaskas JR, Marshall BC, Sufian B, Simon RH, Rodman D. Cystic fibrosis adult care: consensus conference report. Chest. 2004;125 Suppl 1:1S–39.
7. Christie JD, Edwards LB, Kucheryavaya AY, et al. The registry of the international society for heart and lung transplantation: twenty-seventh official adult lung and heart-lung transplant report-2010. J Heart Lung Transpl. 2010;29(10):1104–18.
8. Mahadeva R, Webb K, Westerbeek RC, et al. Clinical outcome in relation to care in centres specialising in cystic fibrosis: cross sectional study. BMJ. 1998;316(7147):1771–5.
9. Johnston C, Butler SM, Konstan MW, Morgan W, Wohl ME. Factors influencing outcomes in cystic fibrosis: a centre-based analysis. Chest. 2003;123:20–7.

10. Accurso FJ, Rowe SM, Clancy JP, et al. Effect of VX-770 in persons with cystic fibrosis and the G551D-CFTR mutation. N Engl J Med. 2010;363(21):1991–2003.
11. http://www.vrtx.com/current-projects/drug-candidates/VX-809.html. 2011. Accessed 06/07/2011, 2011.
12. Pryor JA, Tannenbaum E, Scott SF, et al. Beyond postural drainage and percussion: airway clearance in people with cystic fibrosis. J Cyst Fibros. 2010;9:187–92.
13. Donaldson SH, Bennett WD, Zeman KL, Knowles MR, Tarran R, Boucher RC. Mucus clearance and lung function in cystic fibrosis with hypertonic saline. N Engl J Med. 2006;354:241–50.
14. Elkins MR, Robinson M, Rose BR, et al. A controlled trial of long-term inhaled hypertonic saline in patients with cystic fibrosis. N Engl J Med. 2006;354(3):229–40.
15. Fuchs HJ, Borowitz DS, Christiansen DH, Group TPS, et al. Effect of aerosolized recombinant human DNase on exacerbations of respiratory symptoms and on pulmonary function in patients with cystic fibrosis. N Engl J Med. 1994;331:637–42.
16. Konstan MW, Byard PJ, Hoppel CL, Davis PB. Effect of high-dose ibuprofen in patients with cystic fibrosis. N Engl J Med. 1995;332:848–54.
17. Lands LC, Milner R, Cantin AM, Manson D, Corey M. High-dose ibuprofen in cystic fibrosis: Canadian safety and effectiveness trial. J Pediatr. 2007;151:249–54.
18. Saiman L, Marshall BC, Mayer-Hamblett N, et al. Azithromycin in patients with cystic fibrosis chronically infected with *Pseudomonas aeruginosa*: a randomized controlled trial. JAMA. 2003;290(13):1749–56.
19. Wolter J, Seeney S, Bell S, Bowler S, Masel P, McCormack J. Effect of long term treatment with azithromycin on disease parameters in cystic fibrosis: a randomised trial. Thorax. 2002;57(3):212–6.
20. Balfour-Lynn IM, Lees B, Hall P, et al. Multicenter randomized controlled trial of withdrawal of inhaled corticosteroids in cystic fibrosis. Am J Respir Crit Care Med. 2006;173(12):1356–62.
21. Regelmann WE, Elliott GR, Warwick WJ, Clawson CC. Reduction of sputum *Pseudomonas aeruginosa* density by antibiotics improves lung function in cystic fibrosis more than do bronchodilators and chest physiotherapy alone. Am Rev Respir Dis. 1990;141:914–21.
22. Hodson ME, Gallagher CG, Govan JRW. A randomised clinical trial of nebulised tobramycin or colistin in cystic fibrosis. Eur Respir J. 2002;20:658–66.
23. Oermann CM, Retsch-Bogart GZ, Quittner AL, et al. An 18-month study of the safety and efficacy of repeated courses of inhaled aztreonam lysine in cystic fibrosis. Pediatr Pulmonol. 2010;45(11):1121–34.
24. Ramsey BW, Pepe MS, Quan JM, et al. Cystic Fibrosis Inhaled Tobramycin Study Group. Intermittent administration of inhaled tobramycin in patients with cystic fibrosis. N Engl J Med. 1999;340:23–30.
25. Borowitz D, Baker R, Stallings V. Consensus report on nutrition for pediatric patients with cystic fibrosis. J Pediatr Gastroenterol Nutr. 2002;35:246–59.
26. Eisenberg DM, Davis RB, Ettner SL, et al. Trends in alternative medicine use in the United States, 1990–1997: results of a follow-up national survey. JAMA. 1998;280(18):1569–75.
27. What is complementary and alternative medicine (CAM)? National Center for Complementary and Alternative Medicine [online] 2004; http://nccam.nih.gov/health/whatiscam.
28. Stern RC, Canda ER, Doershuk CF. Use of nonmedical treatment by cystic fibrosis patients. J Adolesc Health. 1992;13(7):612–5.
29. Tanase A, Zanni R. The use of complementary and alternative medicine among pediatric cystic fibrosis patients. J Altern Complement Med. 2008;14(10):1271–3.
30. Samdup DZ, Smith RG, Il Song S. The use of complementary and alternative medicine in children with chronic medical conditions Am J Phys Med Rehabil. 2006;85(10):842–6.
31. Burrows JA, Bajramovic J, Bell SC. Prevalence of complementary and alternative medicine use by adults with cystic fibrosis. J Pharm Pract Res. 2002;32(4):320–3.
32. Chung Y, Dumont RC. Complementary and alternative therapies: use in pediatric pulmonary medicine. Pediatr Pulmonol. 2011;46(6):530–44.
33. Ravilly S, Robinson W, Suresh S, Wohl M, Berde C. Chronic pain in cystic fibrosis. Pediatrics. 1996;98(4):741–7.

34. Festini F, Ballarin S, Codamo T, Doro R, Laganes C. Prevalence of pain in adults with cystic fibrosis. J Cyst Fibros. 2004;3:51–7.
35. Hernandez-Reif M, Field T, Krasnegor J, Martinez E, Schwartzman M, Mavunda K. Children with cystic fibrosis benefit from massage therapy. J Pediatr Psychol. 1999;24(2):175–81.
36. Lee A, Holdsworth M, Holland A, Button B. The immediate effect of musculoskeletal physiotherapy techniques and massage on pain and ease of breathing in adults with cystic fibrosis. J Cyst Fibros. 2009;8(1):79–81.
37. Coulter ID, Hurwitz EL, Adams AH, Genovese BJ, Hays R, Shekelle PG. Patients using chiropractors in North America: who are they, and why are they in chiropractic care? Spine. 2002;27:291–6.
38. Paccou J, Zeboulon N, Combescure C, Gossec L, Cortet B. The prevalence of osteoporosis, osteopenia, and fractures among adults with cystic fibrosis: a systematic literature review with meta-analysis. Calcif Tissue Int. 2010;86:1–7.
39. White A. A cumulative review of the range and incidence of significant adverse events associated with acupuncture. Acupunct Med. 2004;22:122–33.
40. Lin YC, Ly H, Golianu B. Acupuncture pain management for patients with cystic fibrosis: a pilot study. Am J Chin Med. 2005;33(1):151–6.
41. Scott E. Acupuncture for the relief of pain in cystic fibrosis. Cystic Fibrosis Worldwide Newsletter. 22 May 2011. p. 11.
42. Rustøen T, Wahl AK, Hanestad BR, Gjengedal E, Moum T. Expressions of hope in cystic fibrosis patients: a comparison with the general population. Heart Lung. 2004;33:111–8.
43. Pfeffer PE, Pfeffer JM, Hodson ME. The psychosocial and psychiatric side of cystic fibrosis in adolescents and adults. J Cyst Fibros. 2003;2:61–8.
44. Goldbeck L, Besier T, Hinz A, Singer S, Quittner AL, Group T. Prevalence of symptoms of anxiety and depression in German patients with cystic fibrosis. Chest. 2010;138(4):929–36.
45. Szyndler JE, Towns SJ, van Asperen PP, McKay KO. Psychological and family functioning and quality of life in adolescents with cystic fibrosis. J Cyst Fibros. 2005;4:125–44.
46. Napolitano MA, Babyak MA, Palmer S, et al. Effects of a telephone-based psychosocial intervention for patients awaiting lung transplantation. Chest. 2002;122:1176–84.
47. Delk KK, Gevirtz R, Hicks DA, Carden F, Rucker R. The effects of biofeedback assisted breathing retraining on lung functions in patients with cystic fibrosis. Chest. 1994;105:23–8.
48. Glasscoe CA, Quittner AL. Psychological interventions for people with cystic fibrosis and their families. Cochrane Database Syst Rev. 2008;16(3):CD003148.
49. Belsky J, Khanna P. The effects of self-hypnosis for children with cystic fibrosis: a pilot study. Am J Clin Hypn. 1994;36:282–92.
50. Anbar RD. Self-hypnosis for patients with cystic fibrosis. Pediatr Pulmonol. 2000;30:461–5.
51. Grasso M, Button BM, Allison DJ, Sawyer SM. Benefits of music therapy as an adjunct to chest physiotherapy in infants and toddlers with cystic fibrosis. Pediatr Pulmonol. 2000;29:371–81.
52. Wiens ME, Reimer MA, Guyn HL. Music therapy as a treatment method for improving respiratory muscle strength in patients with advanced multiple sclerosis. A pilot study. Rehabil Nurs. 1999;24(2):74–80.
53. Collyer S, Kenny DT, Archer M. The effect of abdominal directives on breathing patterns in female classical singing. Logoped Phoniatr Vocol. 2009;34(3):100–10.
54. Irons JY, Kenny DT, Chang AB. Singing for children and adults with cystic fibrosis. Cochrane Database Syst Rev. 2010;12(5):CD008036.
55. Hurley MN, Forrester DL, Smyth AR. Antibiotic adjuvant therapy for pulmonary infection in cystic fibrosis. Cochrane Database Syst Rev. 2010;6(10):CD008037.
56. Cheng K, Smyth RL, Govan JRW, et al. Spread of beta-lactam-resistant *Pseudomonas aeruginosa* in a cystic fibrosis clinic. Lancet. 1996;348:639–42.
57. Alhede M, Bjarnsholt T, Jensen PØ, et al. *Pseudomonas aeruginosa* recognizes and responds aggressively to the presence of polymorphonuclear leukocytes. Microbiology. 2009;155 (Pt 11):3500–8.
58. Rasmussen TB, Bjarnsholt T, Skindersoe ME, et al. Screening for quorum-sensing inhibitors (QSI) by use of a novel genetic system, the QSI selector. J Bacteriol. 2005;187:1799–814.

59. Bjarnsholt T, Jensen PO, Rasmussen TB, et al. Garlic blocks quorum sensing and promotes rapid clearing of pulmonary *Pseudomonas aeruginosa* infections. Microbiology. 2005;151:3873–80.
60. Hurley MN, Crusz SA, Symonds ME, et al. A commercial garlic preparation exerts global inhibition of the quorum sensing (QS) system and virulence factor production of laboratory and clinical strains of *Pseudomomas aeruginosa*. J Cyst Fibros. 2011;10 Suppl 1:S24.
61. Smyth AR, Cifelli PM, Ortori CA, et al. Garlic as an inhibitor of *Pseudomonas aeruginosa* quorum sensing in cystic fibrosis—a pilot randomized controlled trial. Pediatr Pulmonol. 2010;45(4):356–62.
62. O'Hara M, Kiefer D, Farrell K, Kemper K. A review of 12 commonly used medicinal herbs. Arch Fam Med. 1998;7:523–36.
63. Song Z, Johansen HK, Faber V, et al. Ginseng treatment reduces bacterial load and lung pathology in chronic *Pseudomonas aeruginosa* pneumonia in rats. Antimicrob Agents Chemother. 1997;41:961–4.
64. Song Z, Kharazmi A, Wu H, Johansen HK, Faber V, Høiby N. Immunomodulatory properties of ginseng—effects on *Pseudomonas aeruginosa* lung infection. Clin Microbiol Infect. 1999;5:S37–8.
65. Song Z, Konga KF, Wub H, et al. Panax ginseng has anti-infective activity against opportunistic pathogen *Pseudomonas aeruginosa* by inhibiting quorum sensing, a bacterial communication process critical for establishing infection. Phytomedicine. 2010;17:1040–6.
66. Egan ME, Pearson M, Weiner SA, et al. Curcumin, a major constituent of turmeric, corrects cystic fibrosis defects. Science. 2004;304(5670):600–2.
67. Wang W, Bernard K, Li G, Kirk KL. Curcumin opens cystic fibrosis transmembrane conductance regulator channels by a novel mechanism that requires neither ATP binding nor dimerization of the nucleotide-binding domains. J Biol Chem. 2007;16:4533–44.
68. Harada K, Okiyoneda T, Hashimoto Y, et al. Curcumin enhances cystic fibrosis transmembrane regulator expression by down-regulating calreticulin. Biochem Biophys Res Commun. 2007;353:351–6.
69. Song Y, Sonawane ND, Salinas D, et al. Evidence against the rescue of defective DeltaF508-CFTR cellular processing by curcumin in cell culture and mouse models. J Biol Chem. 2004;279(39):40629–33.
70. Yu YC, Miki H, Nakamura Y, et al. Curcumin and genistein additively potentiate G551D-CFTR. J Cyst Fibros. 2011;10(4):243–52.
71. Brown RK, Wyatt H, Price JF, Kelly FJ. Pulmonary dysfunction in cystic fibrosis is associated with oxidative stress. Eur Respir J. 1996;9(2):334–9.
72. Back EI, Frindt C, Nohr D, et al. Antioxidant deficiency in cystic fibrosis: when is the right time to take action? Am J Clin Nutr. 2004;80(2):374–84.
73. Lancellotti L, D'Orazio C, Mastella G, Mazzi G, Lippi U. Deficiency of vitamins E and A in cystic fibrosis is independent of pancreatic function and current enzyme and vitamin supplementation. Eur J Pediatr. 1996;155:281–5.
74. Shamseer L, Adams D, Brown N, Johnson JA, Vohra S. Antioxidant micronutrients for lung disease in cystic fibrosis. Cochrane Database Syst Rev. 2010;12:CD007020.
75. Olveira G, Olveira C, Acosta E, et al. Fatty acid supplements improve respiratory, inflammatory and nutritional parameters in adults with cystic fibrosis. Arch Bronconeumol. 2010;46:70–7.
76. McKarney C, Everard M, N'Diaye T. Omega-3 fatty acids (from fish oils) for cystic fibrosis. Cochrane Database Syst Rev. 2007;17:CD002201.
77. Bruzzese E, Raia V, Spagnuolo MI, et al. Effect of Lactobacillus GG supplementation on pulmonary exacerbations in patients with cystic fibrosis: a pilot study. Clin Nutr. 2007;26:322–8.
78. Bruzzese E, Raia V, Gaudiello G, et al. Intestinal inflammation is a frequent feature of cystic fibrosis and is reduced by probiotic administration. Aliment Pharmacol Ther. 2004;20:813–9.
79. Weiss B, Bujanover Y, Yahav Y, Vilozni D, Fireman E, Efrati O. Probiotic supplementation affects pulmonary exacerbations in patients with cystic fibrosis: a pilot study. Pediatr Pulmonol. 2010;45:536–40.

Chapter 7
Integrative Therapies for People with Lung Cancer

Karen K. Swenson and Alice C. Shapiro

Abstract Lung cancer is a serious illness with a myriad of harmful effects due to both the disease itself and its treatments. Many patients with lung cancer use both complementary and alternative therapies to alleviate symptoms and sometimes for treatment. It is important for healthcare practitioners to be aware of the prevalence and use of these therapies by their patients because of their potential biological effects, which may interact with current therapies including chemotherapy, biological therapy, and radiation treatments. Practitioners must help patients distinguish between "complementary" and "alternative" therapies in oncology care because complementary care incorporates the use of nonpharmacological interventions in addition to evidence-based medicine, while alternative care is often given in place of traditional medicine with little or no existing information regarding safety and efficacy. Recognizing patients' interest in both complementary and alternative options and the importance of having a patient-centered approach to cancer care, the use of complementary therapies has gradually been incorporated into the oncology care in the United States through integrative therapy programs. Research on both complementary and alternative therapies in oncology is in the infancy stage due to difficulty designing high-quality randomized clinical trials, lack of funding, and use of these interventions by patients without scientific evidence of their efficacy. Therefore, more rigorous research is needed to determine the safety, efficacy, and long-term outcomes of these modalities. This chapter summarizes the current research on complementary therapies that are available to patients with lung cancer.

Keywords Cancer • Integrative medicine • Complementary therapy • Mind–body practices • Energy medicine • Botanicals

---

K.K. Swenson, PhD (✉) • A.C. Shapiro, PhD, RD, LN
Department of Oncology Research, Park Nicollet Health Services,
St. Louis Park, MN 55426, USA
e-mail: Karen.Swenson@parknicollet.com

L. Chlan and M.I. Hertz (eds.), *Integrative Therapies in Lung Health and Sleep*,
Respiratory Medicine 4, DOI 10.1007/978-1-61779-579-4_7,

Overview and Introduction

Lung cancer is one of the leading causes of mortality in the world. In the United States, lung cancer is diagnosed in over 222,000 people each year and is the leading cause of cancer-related deaths in both men and women—estimated to have caused over 160,000 deaths in 2010 [1]. Among patients with a cancer diagnosis, complementary and/or alternative practices are in widespread use; it is estimated that 36–88% of patients use some form of these therapies [2–5]. Because of the poor prognosis of lung cancer with current treatments and care, patients may be particularly vulnerable to alternative care practices that falsely promote unproven claims of cure [6]. Integrative therapy provides a seamless approach of complementary care with traditional lung cancer therapy with a goal of guiding patients toward appropriate sources of care.

In the 2002 National Health Interview Survey (NHIS), cancer patients reported significantly more use of complementary and alternative cancer therapies in the previous year than people without a cancer history [7]. In surveys of lung cancer patients in Sweden and Germany, over half of the patients use some form of dietary supplement and natural remedy [8, 9]. Some studies include the use of religious practices such as intercessory prayer and faith-based healing when reporting on complementary modalities [10]. In addition, chaplain services are typically offered in hospitals and clinics for oncology patients who are dealing with spiritual issues. It is important that researchers identify which practices are included in their analyses in order to accurately estimate the prevalence rates of complementary therapy use in oncology patients [11].

Despite the very serious prognosis of lung cancer, some patients with early-stage disease are cured, and patients may live for months or years with a lung cancer diagnosis. Both the treatment and the disease itself can cause significant morbidity, and patients may seek complementary and/or alternative therapies to cope with disease and treatment-related side effects to improve their quality of life and to do something positive to control their disease and affect their overall health [12, 13]. As might be expected, patients who are symptomatic and who have a poorer prognosis appear to be more likely to use these therapies [14, 15].

Recognizing patients' interests and the importance of having a patient-centered approach to cancer care, certain therapies have been gradually incorporated into the conventional medical system in the United States through integrative therapy programs. These programs empower patients to be more involved in managing their cancer care. Many integrative therapy programs also conduct clinical research to test promising modalities and provide evidence-based information about complementary therapies when it is available [16]. An example is the Mayo Clinic Complementary and Integrative Medicine Program, which has an extensive research program to test complementary modalities for patient care and provide reliable scientific information [17].

Practice-based guidelines are available for professionals and oncology patients through the Society for Integrative Oncology, a nonprofit, multidisciplinary organization committed to the study and application of complementary and botanicals for cancer therapy [18]. The American Cancer Society also provides a comprehensive review of complementary and alternative cancer therapies that can be used by patients and clinicians to evaluate the current research on commonly used therapies [19]. In 2007, the World Cancer Research Fund (WCRF) reported on effects of foods and nutrients on cancer risk, including a review of 32 case-controlled studies, 25 cohort studies, and 3 randomized clinical trials [20, 21]. In March of 2011, a conference on integrative cancer care was held in Amsterdam, and reports from this conference will provide another resource for patients and providers [22].

Regardless of the addition of supplemental treatments, smoking and tobacco products cause 85–90% of lung cancer cases, and recent trends in smoking cessation and prevention are the most effective method of reducing lung cancer incidence and mortality [23]. Therefore, integrative cancer therapy programs should include smoking cessation programs as an integral component of the program for lung cancer treatment, prevention, and risk reduction.

Palliative care programs also play an important role in comprehensive management of symptoms experienced by patients with lung cancer. A recent study found that patients with metastatic lung cancer who were randomized to an outpatient palliative care program vs. usual care had significant improvements in quality of life, mood states, and survival time if they received palliative care [24]. Palliative care programs emphasize the team approach and employ integrated services from many disciplines to address the complex needs of lung cancer patients and their family members. These include professionals from medicine, nursing, social work, chaplaincy, nutrition, rehabilitation, and pharmacy [25].

Integrative Therapies to Treat or Manage Lung Cancer

Mind–Body Practices

Mind–body practices focus on the interactions between the mind, body, and behavior with the intent to use the mind's capacity to influence bodily functions and symptoms [26]. Mind–body interventions include yoga, meditation, acupuncture/acupressure, guided imagery, qigong, deep breathing techniques, and hypnosis. These modalities are frequently used by lung cancer patients to control physical and psychological symptoms that are related to their disease and its treatment. Lung cancer patients may frequently experience a cluster of symptoms including coughing, breathlessness, and pain related to their disease and nausea, fatigue, and neuropathy related to their treatment. Some of the mind–body interventions are effective in helping to control symptoms of disease and treatment [27].

Yoga

Yoga is an ancient mind–body practice that combines physical posture, breathing techniques, and visual imagery, meditation, or relaxation. It has been practiced for millennia in Eastern cultures from India, China, and Japan. There are many different types of yoga, and programs can vary greatly depending on the instructor and philosophy of the program. Yoga has been studied in patients with cancer, primarily breast cancer survivors, and it has been shown to improve mental health, vitality, bodily pain, anxiety, positive affect, and overall quality of life [28–32]. A randomized study comparing yoga to a wait-list group in breast cancer patients showed that although the yoga group reported significantly better general health perceptions and physical functioning scores, there were no differences between the groups in fatigue, depression, or sleep scores [33]. One study measured the diurnal salivary cortisol levels (which correlates with anxiety and depression scores) and found improvements in the early morning salivary cortisol levels in a group of breast cancer patients who practiced yoga [34]. A recent evidence-based review was conducted to determine the effects of yoga on psychological adjustment among cancer patients; although positive findings were noted, study variability and methodological issues limit the extent to which yoga can be deemed effective for managing cancer and treatment-related symptoms [35].

Meditation and Mindfulness-Based Therapies

Meditation techniques include psychological exercises that focus patients' attention on being present in the moment. Patients are asked to pay close attention to bodily sensations, thoughts, and emotions and to learn possible ways to handle stresses through meditative exercises with deep breathing techniques. Although no meditative studies have been conducted specifically with lung cancer patients, most of the meditation programs employed with oncology patients use the mindfulness-based stress reduction approach developed by Kabat-Zinn [36, 37]. This technique is taught to participants through weekly sessions for 2–2.5 h for 8–10 weeks, culminating in an all-day, intensive practice session. In addition, participants are asked to practice the technique daily for approximately 45 min per day. Mindfulness-based programs have been shown to decrease distress, tension, depression, and anxiety and to improve quality of life [38–42]. In a heterogeneous group of oncology patients, Carlson and colleagues found significant improvements in sleep, mood states, and fatigue among participants in a mindfulness-based program [43]. A meta-analysis of mindfulness-based stress reduction studies for cancer patients found that these techniques may be useful for mental health, but more research is needed to show evidence of effectiveness for physical health outcomes [44]. Most studies of mindfulness-based therapy have lacked sufficient scientific rigor to make definitive conclusions because they use no or nonrandomized controls, have short follow-up periods, and do not use intent-to-treat analyses. Certain meditation techniques require extensive training and practice, which makes these programs impractical for many oncology patients. However, programs offering meditation are often accessible and in the community and can readily be incorporated into oncology care.

Acupuncture/Acupressure

Acupuncture is a procedure used in traditional Chinese medicine, which stimulates anatomical locations on the body using thin, metallic needles to penetrate the skin along hypothesized channels or "meridians." The manual manipulation and/or electrical stimulation at these anatomical points have been shown to have therapeutic effects. Acupressure is derived from acupuncture but uses physical pressure applied by the hands, elbows, or devices instead of needles to acupuncture points to stimulate the same meridians to produce similar effects. Acupuncture, and acupressure to a lesser extent, has been widely used to help control symptoms in oncology patients.

Acupuncture has been shown to be beneficial for the treatment of chemotherapy-induced nausea and vomiting in several randomized clinical trials [45–48]. The most effective acupuncture point to prevent nausea is at pericardium-6 (PC-6) on the palmar aspect of the forearm, just above the wrist. Acupressure bands (wrist bands placed at the PC-6 area) have reduced the need for antiemetics and provided relief for nausea in patients with high levels of expected nausea [49, 50]. Acupuncture using needles placed along the major salivary glands has been shown to be effective for the treatment of radiation-induced xerostomia (dry mouth) [51, 52]. Acupuncture has also been found to be effective for the treatment of postchemotherapy fatigue and cancer-related pain [53, 57].

A comprehensive review found that acupressure was effective in reducing chemotherapy-induced nausea and vomiting; however, more rigorous studies are needed to evaluate the effectiveness of acupuncture and acupressure on managing other oncology-related symptoms [58]. When choosing acupuncture services, recommendations are given to identify a safe and effective acupuncturist: (1) a licensed practitioner, (2) general medical training, (3) hospital system experience, (4) good communication skills, and (5) previous experience with treating oncology patients [59].

Qigong

Qigong is a type of traditional Chinese medicine that combines movement, meditation, and controlled breathing exercises with the intent of improving blood flow through the flow of qi (vital energy) and the practice of yi (consciousness or intention). A randomized controlled trial comparing usual medical care to usual care plus qigong found that qigong improved overall quality of life, fatigue, and mood disturbances in cancer patients [60]. One small study designed to determine whether qigong could shrink breast cancer and improve quality of life prior to surgery found that it was ineffective for both [61]. Further studies are needed to evaluate qigong therapy because the evidence of effectiveness for cancer care is currently inadequate based on a systematic review of controlled studies [62].

Tai Chi

Tai chi is a form of traditional Chinese martial art that combines meditative practice and aerobic exercises. A series of postures or movements are performed in a slow, deliberate manner with each posture flowing into the next with the body in constant motion. One small study of breast cancer survivors found beneficial effects of tai chi on health-related quality of life and self-esteem [63]. However, very few studies have been done using tai chi for oncology patients, and the existing evidence does not show definitively that tai chi is beneficial for supportive cancer care; [64] several additional studies are under way [65].

Vitamin, Mineral, and Herbal Supplements

Substances found in foods and herbs such as micronutrients (vitamins and minerals) and phytochemicals (plant chemicals) are widely used by oncology patients as cancer treatment or to alleviate the side effects of treatment. These products are often perceived as safe and efficacious because they are "natural" and easily obtained over the counter. However, many of these products contain active compounds that can interact and/or interfere with chemotherapy and other cancer therapies. An example of this is St. John's wort, an herbal product commonly used to treat depression, anxiety, and sleep disorders. It is metabolized by the cytochrome P450 pathway, which is also responsible for metabolism of several chemotherapy drugs. Therefore, synchronous use of St. John's wort with chemotherapy may decrease the plasma levels of the chemotherapy drugs, thus diminishing potential efficacy [66]. Because herbal therapies and other dietary supplements are not regulated by federal agencies, the dose of the active ingredients as listed on the product label may be variable and these products may contain pesticides or heavy metals, as well as other contaminants including hormones and commonly prescribed medicines [67].

The relationships between diet, cancer prevention, and cancer recurrence have been studied in large cohort studies. Certain food groups in the diet appear to have an impact on lung cancer rates in population-based studies [68]. However, the results from randomized trials of nutritional supplements taken in addition to the diet, such as alpha-tocopherol (vitamin E), beta-carotene (a precursor of vitamin A), and other supplements, have been disappointing [69–71]. In a notable example, increased risk of lung cancer has been found for supplements in cancer prevention trials [69, 70]. Randomized, controlled trials have shown that beta-carotene supplements increased lung cancer risk; a prospective cohort study showed a small increase in incident lung cancer with supplemental vitamin E [72]. In general, dietary supplements are not helpful and in some cases have shown to be harmful in lung cancer prevention studies.

Diet: Fruit and Vegetable Consumption

The 2007 WCRF reported a 20% increased risk for incident lung cancer in those in the lowest quintile of fruit intake. Observational studies have found beneficial effects of fruits and vegetable consumption on reduced rates of lung cancer, particularly among tobacco users [73]. In the European Prospective Investigation into Cancer and Nutrition (EPIC) study, a significant inverse association was found between dietary consumption of fruits and vegetables and lung cancer risk [68]. A pooled analysis of cohort studies also found a protective effect of fruit and vegetable consumption on the risk of lung cancer [74]. The positive effects of fruit consumption in lung cancer prevention and in possibly reducing recurrences are most likely from the effects of micronutrient composition as well as the phytochemical composition of the foods themselves.

Alpha-Tocopherol (Vitamin E)

Favorable observational studies of the protective effects of fruit and vegetable intake on lung cancer risk prompted randomized clinical trials to evaluate alpha-tocopherol in the supplement form. The Alpha-Tocopherol, Beta-Carotene Cancer Prevention Trial (ATBC) examined whether alpha-tocopherol 50 mg po daily vs. placebo would prevent lung cancer in a group of nearly 30,000 male smokers [69]. They found that alpha-tocopherol supplements had no effect on the lung cancer incidence or overall mortality. However, in the Diet, Cancer, and Health Study in Denmark, a large observational study of a cohort of 55,557 participants found that higher levels of dietary vitamin E had significant protective effects against lung cancer development [71].

Beta-Carotene (Vitamin A Precursor)

Randomized clinical trials have also evaluated the effects of beta-carotene (a precursor of vitamin A) on lung cancer incidence and mortality. The ATBC examined whether beta-carotene 20 mg po taken daily vs. placebo would prevent lung cancer in a group of nearly 30,000 male smokers [69]. The results were surprising in that the patients who took beta-carotene had an increased incidence of lung cancer and overall mortality. Similar results were found in the Beta-Carotene and Retinol Efficacy Trial (CARET), which examined the use of 30 mg of beta-carotene daily along with 25,000 IU of retinyl palmitate (vitamin A) compared to placebo taken daily in a study group of over 18,000 men and women at high risk of developing lung cancer [70]. The Diet, Cancer, and Health Study in Denmark also found a higher lung cancer risk with supplemental beta-carotene [71]. Thus, beta-carotene supplementation is not recommended for lung cancer prevention or as a complementary therapy during lung cancer treatment.

Vitamin D

Vitamin D is a steroid hormone that plays an important role in calcium absorption and bone mineralization. Research interest in vitamin D and its possible role in the development of lung cancer are due to its role as a nuclear transcription factor that regulates cell growth, differentiation, and apoptosis [75]. Circulating 25-hydroxy vitamin D levels have been associated with improved survival in early-stage non–small cell lung cancer (NSCLC) [76]. Higher nuclear vitamin D receptor expression has also been associated with better overall survival in NSCLC patients [77]. The results from these reports are intriguing and warrant further study to determine whether vitamin D may be useful as a supplement or as a prognostic marker in lung cancer.

Green Tea

Green tea has several properties that are being investigated for potential chemopreventive effects against lung cancer. It contains epigallocatechin-3-gallate (EGCG), epigallocatechin (EGC), epicatechin-3-gallate (ECG), and epicatechin (EC), which may have potential molecular targets against cancer through inhibition of cell growth and induction of apoptosis [78, 79]. While epidemiological and animal models have yielded promising results [80], a negative Phase II study was published in hormone-refractory prostate cancer [81]. Future studies will be necessary to determine if there is a synergistic role of green tea with anticancer drugs for lung cancer [79].

Toona sinensis

Toona sinensis (TS) is a traditional Chinese herb leaf extract which possesses antitumor properties against lung cancer adenocarcinoma cells in animal models. These effects appear to be mediated by producing G1 phase arrest through downregulation of cyclin-D1 protein and inducing apoptosis by antioxidation [82]. Clinical studies will be necessary to validate antiproliferative effects in humans.

Valerian

Valeriana officinalis (Valerian) is a perennial herb containing essential oils, which provide active ingredients promoted as helping with sleep, restlessness, and anxiety. It was studied in a randomized, placebo-controlled trial and had no effect on quality of sleep but did show positive effects on fatigue and drowsiness [83].

Ginseng

The potential mechanisms of cancer prevention with ginseng are not well known, but ginseng may activate nuclear factor kappa B and extracellular kinase, inhibit cell proliferation, and induce apoptosis [84]. A randomized, prospective study was performed to determine the anticarcinogenic effects of red ginseng (*Panax ginseng*) extracts compared to placebo in 643 participants with chronic atrophic gastritis who were followed for cancer incidence over 11 years. During the follow-up period, 24 cancers were detected, with 6 lung cancers in the placebo group and 2 lung cancers in the red ginseng group (RR = 0.54; 95% CI 0.23–1.28; $P = 0.13$) [84]. A pilot study was conducted of American ginseng (*Panax quinquefolius*) to evaluate the effect of three different dose levels on cancer-related fatigue when compared to placebo. This pilot study of diverse cancer patients showed reduced cancer-related fatigue (as measured by the Brief Fatigue Inventory) and tolerable toxicity; further studies will be needed to confirm results [85].

Manipulative and Body-Based Practices

Manipulative and body-based practices focus on interventions that affect the body systems including the bones, soft tissues, and circulatory and lymphatic systems. Interventions include chiropractic medicine, massage, and reflexology. Chiropractors use their hands and other devices to apply controlled force to a joint, moving it beyond the usual range of motion. Chiropractic medicine is commonly used for low back pain in a healthy population but is not advised for lung cancer patients who have bone metastases because of vulnerability to fracture and spinal cord injury. Massage is a more common intervention offered in integrative therapy clinics because of its ability to increase patients' relaxation and improve overall quality of life.

Massage

Massage is the manipulation of muscles and other soft tissues of the body with the practitioner's hands or fingers. Massage is used primarily to relieve pain, reduce stress, increase relaxation, and improve general well-being. In patients with cancer, massage has been found to reduce stress, pain, fatigue, depression, and anxiety [86–92]. However, most of these studies were not specifically conducted in patients with lung cancer.

Reflexology

Reflexology is the practice of applying pressure to the feet and hands based on a system of zones and reflex areas that reflect an image of the entire body, with a premise that such work effects a physical change in specific areas of the body. This intervention has been found to significantly reduce pain intensity and anxiety in patients who have metastatic cancer [93].

Energy Medicine

Energy medicine involves manipulation of energy fields to improve health. These modalities are collectively termed by NCCAM as "biofield therapies" and include the practices of therapeutic touch (TT), healing touch, and Reiki. Although many of these practices have been used since ancient times for the purpose of healing physical disorders, there has been a recent resurgence of interest in these modalities in the clinical and hospital setting. Studies testing biofield therapies are sparse, in part due to a lack of research funding to conduct large-scale randomized controlled trials in this area. However, integrative therapy clinics may offer therapeutic touch as one of the complementary therapies because of perceived safety of the intervention with conventional therapy as well as frequent requests by patients [94].

Therapeutic Touch

Therapeutic touch (TT) (also called "healing touch") is a biofield therapy that promotes healing and reduces pain and anxiety. Practitioners place their hands on or near the patient in order to "manipulate" the patient's energy field. Aghabaite et al. found that pain, as measured by the Visual Analogue Scale (VAS), and fatigue, as measured with the Rhoten Fatigue Scale, were reduced with daily use of TT as compared to a control group in patients undergoing chemotherapy [95]. Post-White et al. found that healing touch and massage, when compared to presence alone or standard care, lowered total mood disturbance, fatigue, and pain in patients receiving chemotherapy [96]. However, other studies have found that TT did not significantly impact pain or fatigue in oncology patients [97, 98]. TT interventions lost some credibility when a 9-year-old girl, Emily Rosa, decided for her science project to investigate in a blinded study whether TT practitioners were able to actually perceive a human energy field; she found that experienced practitioners were not able to correctly identify the patient's energy field [99].

Reiki

Reiki is a spiritual practice developed in 1922 by Japanese Buddhist Mikao Usui. It uses a technique commonly called "palm healing" as a form of biofield therapy—practitioners claim to transfer healing energy in the form of *ki* through the palms. A small randomized clinical trial examined the effects of Reiki vs. a control group for patients with advanced cancer and found a positive outcome on pain for the Reiki group [100]. Another pilot, crossover Reiki study in a diverse group of oncology patients found reductions in pain over a 2-week intervention period; however, these reductions were not significantly better than the control group [101].

A recent review by Jain and Mills found evidence for positive effects of biofield therapies on acute cancer pain. However, there is conflicting evidence for long-term pain, fatigue, quality of life, and physiologic effects. There have been very few studies conducted in this area, especially in light of the high utilization of these modalities by cancer patients. Further studies are necessary to evaluate their efficacy for common symptoms in cancer [102].

Implications of the Evidence and Science for Practice

Although the practice of complementary therapies is very common in patients with lung cancer, there are relatively few clinical studies that have been conducted to validate the safety and efficacy of these therapies. Practice-based guidelines are available for professionals and oncology patients through the Society for Integrative Oncology, a nonprofit, multidisciplinary organization committed to the study and application of complementary and botanicals for cancer therapy [18]. The American Cancer Society provides a comprehensive review of complementary and alternative cancer therapies that can be used by patients and clinicians to evaluate the current research on commonly used therapies [19]. In 2007, the WCRF reported on the effects of foods and nutrients on cancer risk, including a review of 32 case-controlled studies, 25 cohort studies, and 3 randomized clinical trials [20, 21]. These sources should be used to guide physicians in their recommendations to patients.

Mind–body practices are useful in reducing common cancer-associated side effects including fatigue, distress, mood disturbance, nausea, and vomiting and have been shown to improve some aspects of quality of life. However, there is limited information pertaining specifically to the lung cancer population and little data to show the impact of these practices on prevention, treatment, and survival.

Physicians should provide patients who are interested in *biologically based therapies* with a framework for safely pursuing these therapies:

- Advise patients to check with a pharmacist, physician, registered nurse, or dietician about possible drug interactions with nutritional supplements.
- Provide reliable sources of information regarding complementary modalities (i.e., American Cancer Society, NCCAM, or WCRF).
- Advise patients to get most of their nutritional intake from foods rather than supplements. Eat a diet with a variety of fruits, vegetables, and whole grains to obtain phytochemical and minerals that might influence lung cancer incidence and recurrence.
- Advise patients to obtain consultation from a registered oncology dietitian to assist with questions about safety and efficacy of supplements during lung cancer therapy.
- Include documentation of intake of supplements and vitamins in patients' medication records.

Manipulative and body-based therapies such as massage are used to relieve pain, reduce stress, increase relaxation, and improve general well-being. In patients with cancer, massage reduces stress, pain, fatigue, depression, and anxiety.

Positive effects have been found for *energy medicine* on acute cancer pain. However, there is conflicting evidence for chronic pain, fatigue, and quality of life. There have been very few studies conducted in this area relative to the high utilization of these modalities by cancer patients. Further studies are necessary to evaluate their efficacy for common symptoms in cancer.

General recommendations for practitioners who are providing care for lung cancer patients interested in complementary therapies are to:

- Assess patients' use of complementary therapies and respect their choices about using complementary or alternative therapies but inform them of the possible risks vs. benefits so that they can make informed decisions.
- Refer patients to reputable and evidence-based integrative therapy programs where available.

Directions for Future Research

More rigorous research is needed to determine the safety, efficacy, and long-term outcomes of these modalities. Research effort should be made to conduct well-designed randomized controlled trials to evaluate the efficacy and safety of complementary therapies before widespread adoption in integrative therapy programs. Supplements and natural compounds are often perceived of as safe and efficacious because they are easily obtained over the counter. However, many of these products contain active compounds that can interact and/or interfere with chemotherapy and other cancer therapies. Therefore, conduct of research should include evaluation of safety measures such as pharmacokinetic studies to determine effects on proven lung cancer therapies.

Summary and Conclusions

Research on both complementary and alternative therapies in oncology is in the infancy stage due to difficulty designing high-quality randomized clinical trials, lack of funding, and the high rate of use of these interventions by patients prior to scientific evidence of their efficacy.

References

1. Jemal A, Siegel R, Xu J, Ward E. Cancer Statistics, 2010. CA Cancer J Clin. 2010;60: 277–300.
2. Barnes PM, Powell-Griner E, McFann K, Nahin RL. Complementary and alternative medicine use among adults: United States, 2002. Adv Data. 2004;343:1–19.

3. Richardson M, Sanders T, Palmer J, et al. Complementary/alternative medicine use in a comprehensive cancer center and the implications for oncology. J Clin Oncol. 2000;18: 2505–14.
4. Trinkaus M, Burman D, Barmala N, et al. Spirituality and use of complementary therapies for cure in advanced cancer [published online ahead of print May 19, 2010]. Psychooncology. 2010. PMID: 20878865.
5. Lo CB, Desmond RA, Meleth S. Inclusion of complementary and alternative medicine in US state comprehensive cancer control plans: baseline data. J Cancer Educ. 2009;24(4):249–53.
6. Cassileth BM, Deng GE, Gomez JE, Johnstone PA, Kumar N, Vickers AJ, American College of Chest Physicians. Complementary therapies and integrative oncology in lung cancer: ACCO evidence-based clinical practice guidelines (2nd edition). Chest. 2007; 132(Suppl 3):340S–54S. PMID: 17873179.
7. Mao JJ, Farrar JT, Xie SX, Bowman MA, Armstrong K. Use of complementary and alternative medicine and prayer among a national sample of cancer survivors compared to other populations without cancer. Complement Ther Med. 2007;15(1):21–9.
8. Lovgren M, Wilde-Larsson B, Hok J, Levealahti H, Tishelman C. Push or pull? Relationships between lung cancer patients' perceptions of quality of care and use of complementary and alternative medicine [published online ahead of print November 17, 2010]. Eur J Oncol Nurs.2010. PMID: 21093373.
9. Micke O, Buntzel J, Kisters K, Schafer U, Micke P, Mucke R. Complementary and alternative medicine in lung cancer patients: a neglected phenomenon? In: Heide J, Schmittel A, Kaiser D, Hinkelbein W, editors. Controversies in the treatment of lung cancer. Basel: Karger; 2010. p. 198–205.
10. Wells M, Sarna L, Cooley ME, et al. Use of complementary and alternative medicine therapies to control symptoms in women living with lung cancer. Cancer Nurs. 2007;30(1): 45–55.
11. Crammer C, Kaw C, Gansler T, Stein KD. Cancer survivors' spiritual well-being and use of complementary methods: a report from the American Cancer Society's studies of cancer survivors. J Relig Health. 2011;50(1):92–107.
12. Eisenberg DM, Kessler RC, Van Rompay MI, et al. Perceptions about complementary therapies relative to conventional therapies among adults who use both: results from a national survey. Ann Intern Med. 2001;135(5):344–51.
13. Richardson MA, Masse LC, Nanny K, Sanders C. Discrepant views of oncologists and cancer patients on complementary/alternative medicine. Support Care Cancer. 2004;12(11):797–804.
14. Fouladbakhsh JM, Stommel M. Gender, symptom experience, and use of complementary and alternative medicine practices among cancer survivors in the U.S. cancer population. Oncol Nurs Forum. 2010;37(1):E7–15.
15. Krisstoffersen AE, Fonnebo V, Norheim AJ. Do cancer patients with a poor prognosis use complementary and alternative medicine more often than others? J Altern Complement Med. 2009;15(1):35–40.
16. Frenkel M, Cohen L, Peterson N, Palmer JL, Swint K, Bruera E. Integrative medicine consultation service in a comprehensive cancer center: findings and outcomes. Integr Cancer Ther. 2010;9(3):276–83.
17. Barton DL, Bauer BA, Loprinzi CL. Integrative oncology at Mayo Clinic. In: Cohen L, Markman M, editors. Integrative oncology: incorporating complementary medicine into conventional cancer care. Totowa, NJ: Humana; 2008. p. 123–35.
18. Deng GE, Frenkel M, Cohen L, et al. Evidence-based clinical practice guidelines for integrative oncology: complementary therapies and botanicals. J Soc Integr Oncol. 2009;7(3): 85–120.
19. American Cancer Society. Complete Guide to Complementary and Alternative Cancer Therapies. 2nd ed. Atlanta, GA: American Cancer Society; 2009.
20. World Cancer Research Fund, American Institute for Cancer Research. Food, nutrition, physical activity, and the prevention of cancer: a global perspective. Washington, DC: American Institute for Cancer Research; 2007.

21. American Institute for Cancer Research. The Expert Report http://www.aicr.org/site/PageServer?pagename=research_science_expert_report. Accessed 28 March 2011.
22. Integrative Care for the Future Web Site. http://www.integrativecareftfuture.org. Accessed 30 March 2011.
23. Jemal A, Thun MJ, Ries LAG, et al. Annual report to the nation on the status of cancer, 1975–2005, featuring trends in lung cancer, tobacco use, and tobacco control. J Natl Cancer Inst. 2008;100:1672–94.
24. Temel JS, Greer JA, Muzikansky A, et al. Early palliative care for patients with metastatic non-small cell lung cancer. N Engl J Med. 2010;363(8):733–42.
25. Kelley AS, Meier DE. Palliative care—a shifting paradigm. N Engl J Med. 2010;363(8):781–2.
26. National Center for Complementary and Alternative Medicine. What is complementary and alternative medicine? National Institute of Health Web site. http://nccam.nih.gov/health/whatiscam. Accessed 5 February 2011.
27. Kwekkeboom KL, Cherwin CH, Lee JW, Wanta B. Mind-body treatments for the pain fatigue sleep disturbance symptom cluster in persons with cancer. J Pain Symptom Manage. 2010;39(1):126–38.
28. Danhauer SC, Mihalko SL, Russell GB, et al. Restorative yoga for women with breast cancer: findings from a randomized pilot study. Psychooncology. 2009;18(4):360–8.
29. Duncan MD, Taylor-Brown JW. Impact and outcomes in an iyengar yoga program in a cancer centre. Curr Oncol. 2008;15(Suppl 2):S109.Es72–8. PMID: 18769575.
30. Speed-Andrews AE, Stevinson C, Belanger LJ, Mirus JJ, Courneya KS. Pilot evaluation of an iyengar yoga program for breast cancer survivors. Cancer Nurs. 2010;33(5):369–81.
31. Ulger O, Yagli NV. Effects of yoga on the quality of life in cancer patients. Complement Ther Clin Pract. 2010;16(2):60–3.
32. Vadiraja HS, Rao MR, Nagarathna R, et al. Effects of yoga program on quality of life and affect in early breast cancer patients undergoing adjuvant radiotherapy: a randomized controlled trial. Complement Ther Med. 2009;17(5–6):274–80.
33. Chandwani KD, Thornton B, Perkins GH, et al. Yoga improves quality of life and benefit finding in women undergoing radiotherapy for breast cancer. J Soc Integr Oncol. 2010;8(2):43–55.
34. Vadiraja HS, Raghavendra RM, Nagarathna R, et al. Effects of a yoga program on cortisol rhythm and mood states in early breast cancer patients undergoing adjuvant radiotherapy: a randomized controlled trial. Integr Cancer Ther. 2009;8(1):37–46. Erratum in: Integr Cancer Ther. 2009;8(2):195. PMID: 19190034
35. Smith KB, Pukall CF. An evidence-based review of yoga as a complementary intervention for patients with cancer. Psychooncology. 2009;18(5):465–75.
36. Kabat-Zinn J, Lipworth L, Burney R. The clinical use of mindfulness meditation for the self-regulation of chronic pain. J Behav Med. 1985;8:163–89.
37. Kabat-Zinn J. Full catastrophe living: using the wisdom of your body and mind to face stress, pain, and illness. New York: Delacourt; 1990.
38. Ando M, Morita T, Akechi T, et al. The efficacy of mindfulness-based meditation therapy on anxiety, depression, and spirituality in Japanese patients with cancer. J Palliat Med. 2009;12(12):1091–4.
39. Branstrom R, Kvillemo P, Brandberg Y, Moskowitz JT. Self-report mindfulness as a mediator of psychological well-being in a stress reduction intervention for cancer patients-A randomized study. Ann Behav Med. 2010;39:151–61.
40. Foley E, Baillie A, Huxter M, Price M, Sinclair E. Mindfulness-based cognitive therapy for individuals whose lives have been affected by cancer: a randomized controlled trial. J Consult Clin Psychol. 2010;78(1):72–9.
41. Kieviet-Stijnen A, Visser A, Garssen B, Hudig W. Mindfulness-based stress reduction training for oncology patients: patients' appraisal and changes in well-being. Patient Educ Couns. 2008;72:436–42. PMID 18657376.

42. Kvillemo P, Branstrom R. Experiences of a mindfulness-based stress-reduction intervention among patients with cancer. Cancer Nurs. 2011;34(1):24–31.
43. Carlson LE, Garland SN. Impact of mindfulness-based stress reduction (MBSR) on sleep, mood, stress and fatigue symptoms in cancer outpatients. Int J Behav Med. 2005;12(4): 278–85.
44. Ledesma D, Kumano H. Mindfulness-based stress reduction and cancer: a meta-analysis. Psychooncology. 2009;18(6):571–9.
45. Boa T. Use of acupuncture in the control of chemotherapy-induced nausea and vomiting. J Natl Compr Canc Netw. 2009;7(5):606–12.
46. Acupuncture. NIH Consens Statement. 1997;15(5):1–34. PMID: 10228456.
47. Nystrom E, Ridderstrom G, Leffler AS. Manual acupuncture as an adjunctive treatment of nausea in patients with cancer in palliative care—a prospective, observational pilot study. Acupunct Med. 2008;26(1):27–32.
48. Shen J, Wenger N, Glaspy J, et al. Electroacupuncture for control of myeloablative chemotherapy-induced emesis: a randomized controlled trial. JAMA. 2000;284:2755–61.
49. Roscoe JA, O'Neill M, Jean-Pierre P, et al. An exploratory study on the effects of an expectancy manipulation on chemotherapy-related nausea. J Pain Symptom Manage. 2010;40(3): 379–90.
50. Lee J, Dibble S, Dodd M, Abrams D, Burns B. The relationship of chemotherapy-induced nausea to the frequency of pericardium 6 digital acupressure. Oncol Nurs Forum. 2010;37(6): E419–25.
51. Wong RK, Jones GW, Sagar SM, Babjak AF, Whelan T. A phase I-II study in the use of acupuncture-like transcutaneous nerve stimulation in the treatment of radiation-induced xerostomia in head-and-neck cancer patients treated with radical radiotherapy. Int J Radiat Oncol Biol Phys. 2003;57:472–80.
52. Johnstone PA, Pneg YP, May BC, Inouye WS, Niemtzow RC. Acupuncture for pilocarpine-resistant xerostomia following radiotherapy for head and neck malignancies. Int J Radiat Oncol Biol Phys. 2001;50:353–7.
53. Alimi D, Rubino C, Pichard-Leandri E, Fermand-Brule S, Dubreuil-Lemaire ML, Hill C. Analgesic effects of auricular acupuncture for cancer pain: a randomized, blinded, controlled trial. J Clin Oncol. 2003;21:4120–6.
54. Balk J, Day R, Rosenzweig M, Beriwal S. Pilot, randomized, modified, double-blind, placebo-controlled trial of acupuncture for cancer-related fatigue. J Soc Integr Oncol. 2009; 7(1):4–11.
55. Mao JJ, Styles T, Cheville A, Wolf J, Fernandes S, Farrar JT. Acupuncture for nonpalliative radiation therapy-related fatigue: feasibility study. J Soc Integr Oncol. 2009;7(2):52–8.
56. Vickers AJ, Straus DJ, Fearon B, Cassileth BR. Acupuncture for post chemotherapy fatigue: a phase II study. J Clin Oncol. 2004;22:1731–5.
57. Zick SM, Alrawi S, Merel G, Burris B, Sen A, Litzinger A, Harris RE. Relaxation acupressure reduces persistent cancer-related fatigue [published online ahead of print Sept 2 2010]. Evid Based Complement Alternat Med. 2011;pii:142913. PMID: 20924499.
58. Chao LF, Zhang AL, Liu HE, Cheng MH, Lam HB, Lo SK. The efficacy of acupoint stimulation for the management of therapy-related adverse events in patients with breast cancer: a systematic review. Breast Cancer Res Treat. 2009;118(2):255–67.
59. Lu W, Dean-Clower E, Doherty-Gilman A, Rosenthal DS. Acupuncture in cancer care at Dana-Farber Cancer Institute: an integrative medical practice. In: Cohen L, Markman M, editors. Integrative oncology: incorporating complementary medicine into conventional cancer care. Totowa, NJ: Humana; 2008. p. 181–99.
60. Oh B, Butow P, Mullan B, et al. Impact of medical qigong on quality of life, fatigue, mood and inflammation in cancer patients: a randomized controlled trial. Ann Oncol. 2010;21(3): 608–14.
61. Cohen L, Zhen C, Arun B, et al. External qigong therapy for women with breast cancer prior to surgery. Integr Cancer Ther. 2010;9(4):348–53.

62. Lee MS, Chen KW, Sancier KM, Ernst E. Qigong for cancer treatment: a systematic review of controlled clinical trials. Acta Oncol. 2007;46(6):717–22.
63. Mustian KM, Katuloa JA, Gill DL, Roscoe JA, Lang D, Murphy K. Tai Chi Chuan, health-related quality of life and self-esteem: a randomized trial with breast cancer survivors. Support Care Cancer. 2004;12(12):871–6.
64. Lee MS, Choi TY, Ernst E. Tai chi for breast cancer patients: a systematic review. Breast Cancer Res Treat. 2010;120(2):309–16.
65. Lee EO, Chae YR, Song R, Eom A, Lam P, Heitkemper M. Feasibility and effects of a Tai Chi self-help education program for Korean gastric cancer survivors. Oncol Nurs Forum. 2010;37(1):E1–6.
66. He SM, Yang AK, Li XT, Du YM, Zhou SF. Effects of herbal products on the metabolism and transport of anticancer agents. Expert Opin Drug Metab Toxicol. 2010;6(10):1195–213.
67. National Center for Complementary and Alternative Medicine. Using dietary supplements wisely. National Institutes of Health Web site. http://nccam.nih.gov/health/supplements/wiseuse.htm. Accessed 6 March 2011.
68. Gonzalez C, Riboli E. Diet and cancer prevention: contributions from the European Prospective Investigation into Cancer and Nutrition (EPIC) study. Eur J Cancer. 2010;46:2555–62.
69. Albanes D, Heinonen OP, Taylor PR, et al. Alpha-tocopherol and beta-carotene supplements and lung cancer incidence in the alpha-tocopherol, beta-carotene cancer prevention study: effects of baseline characteristics and study compliance. J Natl Cancer Inst. 1996;88(21):1560–70.
70. Omenn GS, Goodman GE, Thornquist MD, et al. Risk factors for lung cancer and for intervention effects in CARET, the beta-carotene and retinol efficacy trial. J Natl Cancer Inst. 1996;88(21):1550–9.
71. Roswall N, Olsen A, Christensen J, Dragsted LO, Overvad K, Tjonneland A. Source-specific effects of micronutrients in lung cancer prevention. Lung Cancer. 2010;67:275–81.
72. Slatore CG, Littman AJ, Au DH, Satia JA, White E. Long-term use of supplemental multivitamins, vitamin C, vitamin E, and folate does not reduce the risk of lung cancer. Am J Respir Crit Care Med. 2008;177:524–30.
73. Block G, Patterson B, Subar A. Fruit, vegetables, and cancer prevention: a review of the epidemiological evidence. Nutr Cancer. 1992;18:1–29.
74. Smith-Warner SA, Spiegelman D, Yaun SS, et al. Fruits, vegetables and lung cancer: a pooled analysis of cohort studies. Int J Cancer. 2003;107:1001–11.
75. Ingraham BA, Bragdon B, Nohe A. Molecular basis of the potential of vitamin D to prevent cancer. Curr Med Res Opin. 2008;24(1):139–49.
76. Zhou W, Heist RS, Liu G, Asomaning K, Neuberg DS, Hollis BW. Circulating 25-hydroxyvitamin D levels predict survival in early-stage non-small-cell lung cancer patients. J Clin Oncol. 2007;25:479–85.
77. Srinivasan M, Parwani AV, Hershberger PA, Lenzner DE, Weissfeld JL. Nuclear vitamin D receptor expression is associated with improved survival in non-small cell lung cancer. J Steroid Biochem Mol Biol. 2011;123:30–6.
78. Gullett NP, Ruhul Amin ARM, Bayraktar S,et al. Cancer prevention with natural compounds. Semin Oncol. 2010;37(3):258–81. PMID: 20709209.
79. Suganuma M, Saha A, Fjuiki H. New cancer treatment strategy using combination of green tea catechins and anticancer drugs. Cancer Sci. 2011;102(2):317–23.
80. Bushman JL. Green tea and cancer in humans: a review of the literature. Nutr Cancer. 1998;31(3):151–9.
81. Jatoi A, Ellison N, Burch PA, et al. A phase II trial of green tea in the treatment of patients with androgen independent metastatic prostate carcinoma. Cancer. 2003;97:1442–6.
82. Yang CJ, Huang YJ, Wang CY, et al. Antiproliferative effects of *Toona sinensis* leaf extract on non-small cell lung cancer. Transl Res. 2010;155(6):305–14.
83. Barton DL, Atherton PJ, Bauer BA, et al. The use of *Valeriana officinalis* (Valerian) in improving sleep in patients who are undergoing treatment for cancer: a phase III randomized, placebo-controlled, double-blind study (NCCTG Trial, N01C5). J Support Oncol. 2011;9: 24–31.

84. Yun TK, Zheng S, Choi SY, et al. Non-organ-specific preventive effects of long-term administration of Korean red ginseng extract on incidence of human cancers. J Med Food. 2010; 13(3):489–94.
85. Barton DL, Soori GS, Bauer BA, et al. Pilot study of *Panax quinquefolius* (American ginseng) to improve cancer-related fatigue: a randomized, double-blind, dose-finding evaluation: NCCTG trial N03CA. Support Care Cancer. 2010;18:179–87.
86. Jane SW, Wilkie DJ, Gallucci BB, Beaton RD, Huang HY. Effects of a full-body massage on pain intensity, anxiety, and physiological relaxation in Taiwanese patients with metastatic bone pain: a pilot study. J Pain Symptom Manage. 2009;37(4):754–63.
87. Keir ST. Effect of massage therapy on stress levels and quality of life in brain tumor patients-observations from a pilot study [published online ahead of print November 3, 2010]. Support Care Cancer. 2010. PMID: 21046417.
88. Krohn M, Listing M, Tjahjono G, et al. Depression, mood, stress, and Th1/Th2 immune balance in primary breast cancer patients undergoing classical massage therapy [published online ahead of print July 20, 2010]. Support Care Cancer. 2010. PMID: 20644965.
89. Listing M, Krohn M, Liezmann C, et al. The efficacy of classical massage on stress perception and cortisol following primary treatment of breast cancer. Arch Women's Ment Health. 2010;13(2):165–73.
90. Listing M, Reisshauer A, Krohn M, et al. Massage therapy reduces physical discomfort and improves mood disturbances in women with breast cancer. Psychooncology. 2009;18(12): 1290–9.
91. Sharp DM, Walker MB, Chaturvedi A, et al. A randomized, controlled trial of the psychological effects of reflexology in early breast cancer. Eur J Cancer. 2010;46(2):312–22.
92. Sturgeon M, Wetta-Hall R, Hart T, Good M, Dakhil S. Effects of therapeutic massage on the quality of life among patients with breast cancer during treatment. J Altern Complement Med. 2009;15(4):373–80.
93. Stephenson NL, Swanson M, Dalton J, Keefe FJ, Engelke M. Partner-delivered reflexology: effects on cancer pain and anxiety. Oncol Nurs Forum. 2007;34(1):127–32.
94. Pierce B. The use of biofield therapies in cancer care. Clin J Oncol Nurs. 2007;11(2):253–8.
95. Aghabati N, Mohammadi E, Pour Esmaiel Z. The effect of Therapeutic Touch on pain and fatigue of cancer patients undergoing chemotherapy [published online ahead of print February 2, 2008]. Evid Based Complement Alternat Med. 2008. PMID: 18955319.
96. Post-White J, Kinney ME, Savik K, Gau JB, Wilcox C, Lerner I. Therapeutic massage and healing touch improve symptoms in cancer. Integr Cancer Ther. 2003;2(4):332–44.
97. Frank LS, Frank JL, March D, Makari-Judson G, Barham RB, Mertens WC. Does therapeutic touch ease the discomfort or distress of patients undergoing stereotactic core breast biopsy? A randomized clinical trial. Pain Med. 2007;8(5):419–24.
98. Sood A, Barton DL, Bauer BA, Loprinzi CL. A critical review of complementary therapies for cancer-related fatigue. Integr Cancer Ther. 2007;6(1):8–13.
99. Rosa L, Rosa E, Sarner L, Barrett S. A close look at therapeutic touch. JAMA. 1998;279(13): 1005–10.
100. Olson K, Hanson J, Michaud M. A phase II trial of Reiki for the management of pain in advanced cancer patients. J Pain Symptom Manage. 2003;26(5):990–7.
101. Tsang K, Carlson L, Olson K. Pilot crossover trial of Reiki versus rest for treating cancer-related fatigue. Integr Cancer Ther. 2007;6(1):25–35.
102. Jain S, Mills PJ. Biofield therapies: helpful or full of hype? A best evidence synthesis. Int J Behav Med. 2010;17(1):1–16. PMCID: PMC2816237.

Chapter 8
Integrative Therapies for Lung Transplantation Recipients

Annette DeVito Dabbs, Mi-Kyung Song, and Sheila D. Switzer

Abstract The prevalence of integrative therapy usage after lung transplantation is high. The interest in seeking integrative therapies for better symptoms management and health maintenance is likely to grow given the overall symptom burden and psychological distress and complications after lung transplantation. However, empirical evidence regarding the effects and safety of particular integrated therapy practices in lung transplant populations is seriously lacking. Also unknown are the interactions between complementary and alternative therapies and the conventional medical therapies prescribed for lung transplantation. In this chapter, we present what little evidence exists to guide clinicians in advising lung transplant recipients regarding the safety and efficacy of integrative therapy usage. Nonetheless, the success of integrative therapies in other settings and populations demand that more attention be paid to this important area in the future.

Keywords Lung transplantation • Symptom management • Integrative therapy • Complementary and alternative therapies • Mind–body practices

Overview and Introduction

Lung and heart-lung transplantations offer individuals with end-stage cardiopulmonary disease a chance for prolonged survival and improved quality of life [1]. Accordingly, the rate of lung transplantation procedures performed in the United States and

A.D. Dabbs, PhD, RN, FAAN (✉)
School of Nursing, University of Pittsburgh, Pittsburgh, PA, USA
e-mail: ajdst42@pitt.edu

M.-K. Song, PhD, RN
School of Nursing, University of North Carolina at Chapel Hill, Chapel Hill, NC, USA

S.D. Switzer, BSN
University of Pittsburgh School of Nursing, Camp Hill, PA, USA

L. Chlan and M.I. Hertz (eds.), *Integrative Therapies in Lung Health and Sleep*, Respiratory Medicine 4, DOI 10.1007/978-1-61779-579-4_8,

worldwide has increased markedly during the last decade [2–4]. As of June 2009, more than 36,000 lung transplants had been performed worldwide, with nearly 3,000 procedures performed annually [2]. This increase in lung transplantation has coincided with improvements in post-transplant survival. Unadjusted survival rates at 1, 3, 5, and 10 years post-transplant are currently 79, 63, 52, and 29%, respectively. Since the implementation of refined organ allocations systems internationally, including the Lung Allocation Score (LAS) System in the United States [5–7], reductions in the size of waiting lists, waiting time, and wait list mortality have also been realized [8]. Chronic obstructive pulmonary disease (36%), interstitial pulmonary fibrosis (22%), cystic fibrosis (16%), and α_1-antitrypsin deficiency emphysema (7%) were the major indications for lung transplantation during the period from January 1995 through June 2009 [2]. Graft failure and non-cytomegalovirus (CMV) infections account for most early mortality, while deaths after the first year are primarily due to chronic rejection, also known as bronchiolitis obliterans syndrome (BOS), and non-CMV infections. Malignancies account for approximately 12% of deaths between 5 and 10 years post-transplantation.

Most lung recipients experience relief of symptoms from their underlying condition, yet the typical course of illness after transplantation is punctuated by complications, secondary illnesses, and side effects of the requisite life-long immunosuppression. Chronic comorbidities such as hypertension, diabetes mellitus, dyslipidemia, and renal dysfunction are common [9]. Few recipients escape acute rejection during the first year [10], and the development of BOS is common with as many as half of recipients developing BOS by year 5 [2]. From the onset of chronic rejection until death, lung transplant recipients experience frequent emergency department visits, rehospitalizations, and intensive care unit (ICU) admissions to manage symptoms and organ dysfunction associated with chronic rejection and its treatment [11, 12]. Complications are rarely avoided and often undermine the health-related quality of life and survival benefits expected after transplantation [13].

While the majority of recipients report significant symptomatic improvements from pre- to post-transplantation [14], quality of life remains significantly lower than the normative mean in the physical and functional domains [15]. Furthermore, for a large proportion of lung and heart-lung recipients, the prevalence of symptoms is high relative to normative rates reported by healthy adults and exceeds levels reported by recipients of other solid organ transplants [16]. In the most comprehensive assessment of symptom reports after lung transplantation to date [17], 120 recipients returning for routine transplant evaluations between 1 and 100 months post-transplant, reported, on average, 10.5+6.7 symptoms. They frequently described new physical and psychological symptoms, arising primarily from side effects of prolonged immunosuppression, complications such as infection and rejection, as well as the emotional demands of managing health and medical uncertainty post-lung transplantation [18].

The success of lung transplantation at prolonging life demands that control of associated symptoms receive careful attention. This is imperative because relief of patient reported outcomes are themselves critical indicators of the utility and success

Table 8.1 Most frequently reported symptoms after lung transplantation (listed alphabetically) [16, 17, 22–24]

Anxiety symptoms
Cough
Depressive symptoms
Diarrhea
Fatigue
Headache
Heartburn
Leg cramps
Nausea
Pain, incisional
Pain, lower back
Shortness of breath
Sleep problems
Sputum
Weakness

of lung transplantation [19, 20]. Furthermore, there are implications of uncontrolled symptoms beyond their impact on quality of life. Thoracic transplant recipients who experience symptoms and side effects are at increased risk for persistent medication nonadherence [21]. Table 8.1 presents the most frequently endorsed symptoms compiled from multiple empirical studies of symptoms after lung transplantation [16, 17, 22–24].

State of the Evidence on Integrative Therapies in Lung Transplantation

Poor symptom management and uncontrolled medication side effects are among the primary reasons persons with chronic illnesses seek integrative therapies [25–30]. Yet in spite of the high symptom burden reported by lung transplant recipients, little is known about the extent to which lung transplant recipients use complementary and alternative therapies. In fact, there is extremely limited evidence related to the use of integrative therapies to treat or manage symptoms, illness, or conditions after lung transplantation. After an exhaustive literature search, only three studies [31–33] were found regarding the frequency of integrative therapy usage among organ transplant recipients in the United States, and all were single-center-based surveys. Another publication reported on a survey of 356 renal transplant recipients' use of such therapies in Switzerland [34]. Finally, there have been two published guidelines for over-the-counter medication use: one for solid organ transplant recipients [35] was published nearly two decades ago, and therefore, contents are likely out of date; the other was limited to cardiac transplant recipients [36]. Only two studies examined the effectiveness of mind–body practices among solid organ recipients, including lung recipients [37, 38]. No studies were identified that evaluated the impact of any other integrative therapies, including biologically based practices, manipulative and body-based practices, or energy medicine practices.

The prevalence of integrative therapy usage, particularly herbal medicines and food supplements, among solid organ transplant patients was first reported by Crone and colleagues in 1997 [31]. Both pre- and post-transplant patients ($N = 323$) participated in the survey, including 79 cardiothoracic patients (24.4% of the total), only four of whom were lung transplant patients. In this study, 20% of the sample reported using some type of integrative therapy. However, the specific modalities used, for what symptoms or conditions, and data regarding their effectiveness and safety were not reported.

The only study of the frequency of integrative therapy usage among lung transplant recipients was conducted by Matthees and colleagues [32]. This mail survey included 99 lung transplant recipients: the median age of the sample was 52.1 years, 58% were women, 99% were white, 64% completed at least some college education, and months since transplant ranged from 9 months to 10.3 years. In this study, 89% of the sample reported using at least one integrative therapy modality: 68.7% used prayer, 43.4% used support groups, 43.4% used a mind–body therapy (e.g., relaxation techniques, meditation), 23.2% used a manipulative therapy (e.g., massage, chiropractic), 41.4% used a biologically based therapy (e.g., herbals, megavitamins), and 17.2% used other (e.g., energy, acupuncture, homeotherapy). Of these users, 63.4% reported their use to their healthcare provider. The primary reasons for using integrative therapies were to relieve anxiety and other symptoms and to maintain overall health. Nearly 70% of integrated therapy users reported benefits ranging from "quite effective" to "extremely effective." Similar to the findings of the most recent National Health Interview Survey on the Use of Complementary and Alternative Medicine Use in the United States conducted by the National Centers for Disease Control and Prevention [27], lung transplant recipients who used integrative therapies were more likely to be female and college-educated. No significant difference was found between integrative therapy users and nonusers in their level of adherence to the medical regimen (e.g., immunosuppressive medications) or health-related quality of life. A limitation of this study is that data regarding targeted symptoms, effectiveness, and safety for particular integrative therapy practices among lung transplant recipients were not reported.

In comparison, a survey of integrative therapy use in 32 liver transplant recipients [33] reported that 34.4% used a form of integrative therapy, and among those who used integrative therapies, 45% were using herbal products for improving liver function. A survey of renal transplant recipients in Switzerland [34] reported that of 356 respondents, 11.8% used integrative therapies, and the most frequently used types were homeopathy (42.9%) and Chinese medicine (23.8%). Although these surveys shed light on the frequency of integrative therapy use among transplant populations, systematic evaluations are lacking regarding the prevalence of specific practices, their effectiveness and safety.

Mind–body practices. Mindfulness meditation was the only mind–body practice evaluated in any solid organ transplant population [37–39]. Using a pre- and post-test design, Gross and colleagues [37] examined the preliminary effects of a mindfulness-based stress reduction (MBSR) intervention on self-reported depression, anxiety, sleep, illness-intrusiveness, and transplant-related stress in a pilot sample of 20 organ transplant recipients (only two of whom were lung transplant recipients). The intervention included group training in types of meditation and gentle hatha yoga for 2.5-h sessions for 8 weeks. Participants were instructed to practice the program 5 days per week for 45 min per day using audiotapes and were assessed at the completion of the intervention and at 3 and 6 months post-intervention. Compared to baseline, depressive symptoms (Center for Epidemiologic Studies Depression Scale, CES-D) improved significantly at the completion of the intervention (mean score from 12.95 to 7.47, $p<0.01$). State-Trait Anxiety Inventory (STAI) scores significantly improved at 3 months post-intervention only (mean score from 33.16 to 29.18, $p<0.05$). Sleep quality (Pittsburgh Sleep Quality Index, PSQI) improved statistically significantly at all time points; however, mean scores remained at > score 5, indicating "poor sleep." The illness–intrusiveness rating scores did not change after intervention. The overall transplant-related stress scores only marginally improved at 6 months post-intervention (from 25.79 to 22.05, $p<0.05$).

The same MBSR intervention was further evaluated in a full-scale trial for its long-term effects on primary outcomes of self-reported anxiety (STAI), depression (CES-D), and sleep quality (PSQ), and secondary outcomes of health-related quality of life (mental and physical summary scores of the Short-Form 12 version of the Health Survey and Bodily Pain and Vitality subscales of the Short Form 36 Version of the Health Survey) and visual analogue scales of perceived health, quality of life, and global health state [38, 39]. The sample included 26 lung or heart, 26 liver, and 98 kidney and/or pancreas transplant recipients in an intent-to-treat, controlled trial with a two-staged randomization. Recipients were stratified by use of medications for anxiety, depression, or sleep disturbances in the past year and initially randomized equally within strata to three groups: MBSR, health education, or delayed intervention (waitlist) control. Recipients who were randomized to the waitlist were randomized again after 6 months to either MBSR or health education. MBSR and health education classes were held in parallel. Both interventions were composed of 8 weekly, 2.5-h training sessions. The outcomes were assessed at baseline, 8 weeks, 6 months, and 1 year. Outcome analyses included all randomized recipients ($n=122$) who completed one or more follow-up evaluations after final assignment to MBSR ($n=67$) or health education ($n=60$). Demographic characteristics and baseline scores for outcomes of interest were equivalent between the three groups. Of note, baseline anxiety, depression, and sleep disturbances exceeded clinically meaningful levels in 39, 38, and 42% of recipients, respectively. Results revealed that the MBSR group reported fewer symptoms of anxiety ($F[1, 108]=5.21$, $P=0.02$) and sleep problems ($F[1,106]=5.28$, $P=0.02$) than health education and waitlist groups over time with medium treatment effects. These reductions were detected as early as 8 weeks and sustained through 1 year after the intervention. Symptom reductions in the health education group were smaller and not sustained. Depressive symptoms at

1 year remained significantly lower than baseline levels in the MBSR group; however, the difference in depressive symptoms between MBSR and health education groups did not reach statistical significance (effect size = 0.41, $P = 0.08$). Both groups reported improvements in secondary outcomes, but benefits were more durable within the MBSR group. Improvements in vitality were significantly higher in MSBR group at 1 year (effect size = 0.59, $P < 0.01$). Correlations between better adherence to MBSR (participation in >5 training sessions and more home practice time) and changes in sleep, depression, and mental dimensions of quality of life were in the expected direction; however, adherence was only significantly correlated with reduced anxiety and increased vitality (coefficients = 0.3–0.4, $P < 0.01$). Comparisons to the waitlist group confirmed the impact of MBSR on both symptoms and quality of life, whereas health education improvements were limited to quality-of-life ratings. The authors concluded that MBSR reduced distressing symptoms of anxiety, depression, and poor sleep and improved quality of life with benefits sustained over 1 year. The health education program provided fewer benefits, and effects were not as durable. MBSR is a relatively inexpensive, safe, and effective community-based intervention.

Biologically based practices. No reports regarding the effectiveness and/or safety of any biologically based practices for lung transplant recipients or any other solid organ transplant populations were identified.

Manipulative and body-based practices. There are no reports regarding the effectiveness and/or safety of any manipulative and body-based practices for lung transplant recipients or any other solid organ transplant populations.

Energy medicine. There are no reports regarding the effectiveness and/or safety of any energy medicine practices for lung transplant recipients or any other solid organ transplant populations.

Implications of the Evidence and Science for Practice

Overall symptom burden, psychological distress, and complication rates are high after lung transplantation, as is the reported use of integrative therapies among lung transplant recipients. Yet, only one type of integrative therapy, MBSR, has been systematically evaluated and found to be successful in reducing anxiety, depression, and sleep disturbances in solid–organ transplant recipients, including lung transplant recipients. While many mind–body, manipulative and body-based, and energy medicine practices have been proven to be safe and effective for a wide variety of symptoms and conditions in other settings and populations, and therefore likely to be safe for use after lung transplant, empirical studies in lung transplant recipients are lacking. However, there is too little evidence to guide clinicians in advising lung transplant recipients regarding the type, dose, duration, interactions, and contraindications of specific biologically based therapies (e.g., herbals and dietary supplements). Therefore, the need for empirical trials of the effects and safety of additional integrated therapy practices after solid organ transplantation and in lung transplant recipients in particular is paramount.

Most clinicians report concerns about the impact of complementary and alternative therapy usage on recipients' adherence to prescribed therapies and the potential or unknown interactions between biologically based therapies (e.g., herbals and dietary supplements) and conventional medications. However, as Matthees and colleagues suggested [32], most post-lung transplant recipients who use integrative therapies are likely to use them as complementary to managing symptoms and conditions rather than using integrative therapies as a substitute for their prescribed medical regimens. Therefore, there is a need for clinicians to keep the dialogue open, assess potential usage, and explore potential interactions and application of integrative therapies as adjuvant and complementary to the traditional medical regimen.

Directions for Future Research

The burden of symptoms is high after lung transplantation, arising primarily from side effects of prolonged immunosuppression, complications such as infection and rejection, as well as the emotional demands of managing health and the uncertain prognosis for continued organ function [16–18, 22–24]. The literature also indicates that subclinical psychological symptoms and distress improve little over time and that episodes of mood and anxiety disorders in lung transplant recipients are often severe but tend to be undertreated [40]. Furthermore, when the impact of concurrent medical complications was controlled, lung and heart-lung recipients with elevated psychological distress remained significantly more likely to report more physical symptoms and physical impairment [16]. Since many integrative therapies are known to safely reduce symptoms of anxiety, depression, and general psychological distress in a wide variety of populations, future research regarding which specific integrative therapies are most likely to be safe and effective in reducing psychological distress among lung recipients appears to have the most promise for improving the quality of life for lung transplant recipients.

Summary and Conclusions

Integrative therapy usage after lung transplantation is high, and interest in seeking integrative therapies for better symptom management and health maintenance is likely to grow. However, empirical evidence of the effects and safety of particular integrative therapy practices in lung transplant populations is seriously lacking. Also unknown are the interactions between integrative and conventional medical therapies. Currently, there is too little evidence to guide clinicians in advising lung transplant recipients regarding integrative therapy usage. Yet, the success of integrative therapies in other settings and populations, particularly in reducing symptoms of psychological distress, coupled with the overall symptom burden, psychological distress, and complication rates after lung transplantation, demand that more attention be paid to this important area in the future.

References

1. McCurry KR, Shearon TH, Edwards LB, Chan KM, Sweet SC, Valapour M, Yusen R, Murray S. Lung transplantation in the United States, 1998–2007. Am J Transplant. 2009;9(Part 2):942–58.
2. Christie JD, Edwards LB, Kucheryavaya AY, Aurora P, Dobbels F, Kirk R, Rahmel AO, Stehlik J, Hertz MI. The Registry of the International Society for Heart and Lung Transplantation: twenty-seventh official adult lung and heart-lung transplant report—2010. J Heart Lung Transplant. 2010;29(10):1104–18.
3. U.S. Organ Procurement and Transplantation Network and the Scientific Registry of Transplant Recipients. 2009 Annual Report, Transplant Data 1999–2008. Richmond: United Network for Organ Sharing; 2006. http://optn.transplant.hrsa.gov/ar2009/. Accessed December 20, 2010.
4. Eurotransplant International Foundation. Annual report 2009. Leiden: Eurotransplant International Foundation.
5. Department of Health & Human Services. Organ procurement and transplantation network: final rule. Federal Register 1999;42 CFR:56649–61.
6. Egan TM, Murray S, Bustami RT, et al. Development of the new lung allocations system in the United States. Am J Transplant. 2006;6:1212–27.
7. Organ Procurement and Transplantation Network (OPTN). Policies. Revision to policy 3.7.6.1. 2010. http://www.optn.org/PoliciesandBylaws2/policies/pdfs/policy_9.pdf. Accessed December 19, 2010.
8. Levine GN, McCullough KP, Rodgers AM, Dickinson DM, Ashby VB, Schaubel DE. Analytical methods and database design: implications for transplant researchers. Am J Transplant. 2005;6(Part 2):1128–242.
9. DeVito Dabbs AJ, Song MK. Risk profile for cardiovascular morbidity and mortality after lung transplantation. Nurs Clin North Am. 2008;43:37–53.
10. DeVito Dabbs AJ, Hoffman LA, Iacono AT, Wells CL, Grgurich W, Zullo TG, McCurry KR, dauber JH. Pattern and predictors of early rejection after lung transplantation. Am J Crit Care. 2003;12(6):497–507.
11. Song MK, De Vito Dabbs AJ. Advance care planning after lung transplantation: a case of missed opportunities. Prog Transplant. 2006;16(3):222–5.
12. Song MK, De Vito Dabbs A, Studer SM, Zangle SE. Course of illness after the onset of chronic rejection in lung transplant recipients. Am J Crit Care. 2008;17(3):246–53.
13. Dew MA, Switzer GE, Goycoolea JM, Allen AS, DiMartini A, Kormos RL, Griffith BP. Does transplantation produce quality of life benefits? A quantitative analysis of the literature. Transplantation. 1997;64(9):1261–73.
14. Lanuza DM, Lefaiver CA, Farcas GA. Research on the quality of life of lung transplant candidates and recipients: an integrative review. Heart Lung. 2000;29:180.
15. Myaskovsky L, Dew MA, McNulty ML, Switzer GE, DiMartini AF, Kormos RL, McCurry KR. Trajectories of change in quality of life in 12-month survivors of lung or heart transplant. Am J Transplant. 2006;6(8):1939–47.
16. DeVito Dabbs AJ, Dew MA, Stilley CS, Manzetti J, Zullo T, McCurry KR, Kormos RL, Iacono A. Psychosocial vulnerability, physical symptoms and physical impairment after lung and heart-lung transplantation. J Heart Lung Transplant. 2003;22:1268–75.
17. DeVito Dabbs AJ, Hoffman LA, Lacono AT, Zullo TG, Mc Curry KR, Dauber JH. Are symptom reports useful for differentiating between acute rejection and pulmonary infection after lung transplantation? Heart Lung. 2004;33(6):372–80.

18. Cupples S, Dew MA, Grady KL, DeGeest S, Dobbels F, Lanuza D, Paris W. Report of the Psychosocial Outcomes Workgroup of the Nursing and Social Sciences Council of the International Society for Heart and Lung Transplantation: present status of research on psychosocial outcomes in cardiothoracic transplantation: review and recommendations for the field. J Heart Lung Transplant. 2006;25(6):716–25.
19. Krakauer H, Beiley RC, Lin MJ. Beyond survival: the burden of disease in decision making in organ transplantation. Am J Transplant. 2004;4:1555–61.
20. Rothman ML, Beltran P, Cappelleri JC, Lipscomb J, Teschendorf B; Mayo/FDA Patient-Reported Outcomes Consensus Meeting Group. Patient-reported outcome: conceptual issues. Value Health. 2007;10 Suppl 2:S66–75.
21. Dew MA, DiMartini AF, DeVito Dabbs A, Zomak R, De Geest S, Dobbels F, Myaskovsky L, Switzer GE, Unruh M, Steel JL, Kormos RL, McCurry KR. Adherence to the medical regimen during the first two years after lung transplantation. Transplantation. 2008;85(2):193–202.
22. DeVito Dabbs AJ, Johnson B, Wardzinski WT, Iacono A, Studer S. Development and evaluation of the electronic version of the Questionnaire for Lung Transplant Patients (e-QLTP). Prog Transplant. 2007;17(1):29–35.
23. Lanuza DL, McCabe M. Care before and after lung transplant and quality of life research. AACN Clin Issues. 2001;12:186–201.
24. Stilley CS, Dew MA, Stukas AA, et al. Psychological symptom levels and their correlates in lung and heart-lung transplant recipients. Psychosomatics. 1999;40:503–9.
25. Astin JA. Why patients use alternative medicine: results of a national survey. JAMA. 1998;279(19):1548–53.
26. Astin JA, Pelleiter KR, Marie A, Haskell WL. Complementary and alternative medicine use among elderly persons: one year analysis of a Blue Shield Medicare supplement. Gerontol A Biol Sci Med Sci. 2000;55(1):M4–9.
27. Barnes PM, Bloom BL, Nahin RL. Complementary and alternative medicine use among adults and children: United States, 2007. National Health Statistics Reports: no. 12. Hyattsville. National Center for Health Statistics; 2008.
28. Humpel N, Jones SC. Gaining insight into the what, why, and where of complementary and alternative medicine use by cancer patients and survivors. Eur J Cancer Care. 2006; 15(4):362–8.
29. Shen J, Andersen R, Albert PS, Wenger N, Glaspy J, Cole M, Shekelle P. Use of complementary/alternative therapies by women with advanced-stage breast cancer. BMC Complement Altern Med. 2002;2:8.
30. Wolsko PM, Eisenberg DM, Davis RB, Ettner SL, Phillips RS. Insurance coverage, medical conditions and visits to alternative medicine providers: results of a national survey. Arch Intern Med. 2002;162(3):281–7.
31. Crone CC, Wise TN. Survey of alternative medicine use among organ transplant recipients. J Transpl Coord. 1997;7:123–30.
32. Matthees BJ, Anantachoti P, Kreitzer MJ, Savik K, Hertz MI, Gross CR. Use of complementary therapies, adherence, and quality of life in lung transplant recipients. Heart Lung. 2001;30(4):258–68.
33. Tinkerhoof L, Wagener MM, Cacciarelli T, Singh N. Alternative therapy in liver transplant recipients. Prog Transplant. 2006;16(3):226–31.
34. Hess S, DeGeest S, Hatler K, Dickenmann M, Denhaerynck K. Prevalence and correlates of selected alternative and complementary medicine in adult renal transplant patients. Clin Transplant. 2009;23:56–62.
35. Lake KD, Nolen JG, Slaker RA, Reutzel TJ, Milfred SK, Solbrack D, Hoffman FM. Over-the-counter medications in cardiac transplant recipients: guidelines for use. Ann Pharmacother. 1992;26(12):1566–75.
36. Ellingson T, Wipke-Tevis D, Messina C, Livesay T. The use of over-the-counter medications by transplant recipients: a guideline. J Transpl Coord. 1999;9(1):17–24.
37. Gross CR, Kreitzer MJ, Russas V. Mindfulness meditation to reduce symptoms after organ transplant: a pilot study. Altern Ther Health Med. 2004;10(3):58–66.

38. Gross CR, Kreitzer MJ, Thomas W, Reilly-Spong M, Cramer-Bornemann M, Nyman JA, Frazier P, Ibrahim HN. Mindfulness-based stress reduction for solid organ transplant recipients: a randomized controlled trial. Altern Ther Health Med. 2010;16(5):30–8.
39. Gross CR, Kreitzer MJ, Reilly-Spong M, Winbush NY, Schomaker EK, Thomas W. Mindfulness meditation training to reduce symptom distress in transplant patients: rationale, design, and experience with a recycled waitlist. Clin Trials. 2009;6:76–89.
40. Dew MA, DiMartini AF. Psychological disorders and distress after adult cardiothoracic transplantation. J Cardiovasc Nurs. 2005;20:S51–66.

Part III
Integrative Therapies in Critical Care and Sleep Disorders

Chapter 9
Integrative Therapies in the Management of Critically Ill Patients

Mary Fran Tracy

Abstract The intensive care unit (ICU) is a highly technical environment where providers gravitate toward cutting-edge equipment to cure patients. It is becoming increasingly evident, however, that integrative therapies may be important adjunctive therapies to maximize care and healing of the critically ill patient. With approximately 55,000 patients in the ICU on any given day in the United States, use of integrative therapies is an area that has potential to have significant impact on both outcomes and satisfaction of ICU patients. This chapter will provide a general overview of the four main categories of integrative therapies and a more in-depth review of four selected integrative therapies that are currently in use or being explored in critical care. These therapies include music therapy, early mobility in mechanically ventilated patients, animal-assisted therapy, and the use of probiotics in the prevention of ventilator-associated pneumonia.

Keywords Integrative therapies • Critical care • Mechanical ventilation • Music therapy • Animal-assisted therapy • Early mobility • Probiotics

Introduction

The intensive care unit (ICU) is a highly technical environment in which providers can lose sight of the person in the bed given the amount of technology that surrounds them. Intensive care providers gravitate toward technical, cutting-edge therapies to cure patients. However, it is becoming increasingly evident that integrative therapies may be important adjunctive therapies to maximize care and promote healing of the critically ill patient.

M.F. Tracy, PhD, RN (✉)
University of Minnesota Medical Center,
500 Harvard Street SE, Minneapolis, MN 55455, USA
e-mail: mtracy1@fairview.org

L. Chlan and M.I. Hertz (eds.), *Integrative Therapies in Lung Health and Sleep*,
Respiratory Medicine 4, DOI 10.1007/978-1-61779-579-4_9,

Use of complementary and alternative medicine (CAM)—also known as integrative therapies—is increasing in the United States [1]. The National Center for Complementary and Alternative Medicine (NCCAM) continues to use the term CAM, while there is increasing use of the term "integrative therapies." (These two terms will be considered interchangeable for the purposes of this chapter.) CAM is defined as a diverse array of healthcare products and practices that are generally not considered part of mainstream, traditional Western medicine [2]. Typically, four main categories of CAM are identified: mind–body practices, biologically based practices, manipulative and body-based practices, and energy-based practices. Though there is scientific evidence available for some of these therapies, in general, there is a dearth of rigorous research that clearly answers questions about safety and efficacy for most of these therapies and even less research evidence in the population of critically ill patients.

The 2007, National Health Interview Survey showed that 38% of American adults used some form of CAM the preceding 12 months [1]. This translates into 83 million adults who spent $33.9 billion on CAM therapies out of pocket. More than 11% of total out-of-pocket spending for health care is used for CAM. Approximately 354 million visits were reportedly made to CAM practitioners in those 12 preceding months, costing $11.9 billion. Types of therapies used vary over time. For example, use of nonvitamin, nonmineral natural products, deep breathing exercises, and yoga increased between 2002 and 2007, while therapies for head and chest colds decreased during that same period. Women, those with higher incomes, and those with more education were more likely to report use of CAM therapies. In addition, many Americans are using CAM to treat conditions such as back, neck, and joint pain—conditions that can easily continue or be exacerbated during a critical illness [1]. This survey demonstrates that patients and families are increasing their use of integrative therapies in daily life. It can be presumptuous of critical care providers to believe that just because patients cross the threshold of the hospital does not mean they will not want to use these therapies in the hospital.

The Critical Care Environment

More than five million patients are admitted annually to the nearly 6,000 ICUs in the United States [3, 4]. The approximately 55,000 patients in an ICU on any given day are admitted for a variety of reasons but primarily for respiratory insufficiency/failure, postoperative management, ischemic heart disease, sepsis, and heart failure [3, 4]. There is increasing pressure to transition patients through their hospital course, including their ICU stay, as expeditiously as possible. Longer lengths of stay translate into higher health costs as well as increasing the risk for patients to acquire a nosocomial complication. In addition, health-care facilities are emphasizing focus on patient and family satisfaction with their hospital stay and care. It behooves health-care providers to explore all options for maximizing healing and outcomes for critically ill patients for all the above reasons.

Use of integrative therapies is an area that has potential to impact both outcomes and satisfaction of ICU patients. The critical care environment may be especially suitable for exploration of the impact of integrative therapies on improving the critically ill patient's course of illness. Multiple stressors impact the critically ill [5], including noise in the environment from monitor alarms, ventilator noise at the head of the bed, conversations of the multiple care providers that can occur both in the room over the patient as well as in the hallways and at the desk, and the continuous artificial lighting in the ICU with little night/day variation. Critically ill patients frequently experience discomfort and pain from procedures and invasive equipment [5].

Intersection of the Stress Response and Integrative Therapies

With the most frequent ICU admission diagnosis being respiratory insufficiency/failure as noted above, many patients are intubated and mechanically ventilated at some point in their ICU stay. While any patient in an ICU can experience unpleasant sensations and potential for increased anxiety, patients who are mechanically ventilated (MV) are particularly at risk for experiencing stress. Mechanical ventilation can be a painful, uncomfortable, terrifying experience. Patients who are MV report stressors such as discomfort from the endotracheal tube, fear, anxiety, immobility, isolation, lack of control, loneliness, lack of sleep, spells of terror, loss of control, and stress at the inability to communicate with others [6–9].

The physiologic response to stress activates the sympathetic nervous system releasing adrenaline from the adrenal medulla. This results in an increase in blood pressure, heart rate, respiratory rate, and an increase in anxiety [10]. Unrelieved stress can cause long-term symptoms that can impact patient recovery [11, 12]. Patients often receive sedation to ameliorate the anxiety that can trigger this stress response. Unfortunately, use of sedation in MV patients can have potentially deleterious effects. Oversedation can result in respiratory depression, hypotension, muscle weakness, changes in mental status, and decreased gut motility [6, 11, 13]. Use of continuous sedation can result in prolonged requirement of the ventilator, [14, 15] placing patients at risk for development of ventilator-associated pneumonia and increased costs. The possibility of supplementing or supplanting traditional sedative use with use of integrative therapies is appealing as an opportunity to prevent the risk of nosocomial complications and delay in healing. Integrative therapies provide the possibility to ameliorate the stress response through promotion of relaxation and an opportunity to "escape" from what can seem like an endless barrage of alarms, noises, bright lights, frequent manipulation, and interruptions in the critical care environment. Other integrative therapies may serve as adjuncts that can directly impact physiological status, such as nutritional supplements.

Very few integrative therapies have been rigorously researched in critically ill patients. The critical care environment is a difficult one in which to carry out randomized controlled trials (RCTs) without encountering recruitment challenges such as patients who are able to give consent, changing physiologic stability of subjects, and potential for deviation from the protocol [16]. Integrative therapy researchers may be hesitant to conduct protocols in this challenging environment.

Despite the lack of extensive research evidence for integrative therapies and the relatively new concept of developing integrative therapy programs in ICUs, healthcare providers do show an interest in providing these therapies to patients. In a national survey of critical care nurses, the vast majority were interested or very interested in offering integrative therapies to their patients in ICUs (91.1%) [17]. However, many reported multiple barriers to the use of integrative therapies including lack of knowledge and training, lack of equipment, lack of time, unavailability of credentialed providers, and reluctance on the part of physicians, peers, and themselves [17].

This chapter will provide a general overview of the four main categories of integrative therapies and a more in-depth review of four selected integrative therapies that are currently in use or being explored in critical care—some with a growing body of evidence and some just beginning to have research evidence reported. These therapies include music therapy, early mobility in MV patients, animal-assisted therapy (AAT), and the use of probiotics in the prevention of ventilator-associated pneumonia.

Mind–Body Practices

NCCAM defines mind–body integrative practices as those interventions that promote the connection between the mind, body, and behavior to improve physiologic functioning and health [2]. Examples of mind–body practices include meditation, progressive relaxation, and guided imagery. Mind–body practices can be a challenge for ICU patients if the therapy requires focus on the part of the patient for any length of time. Very few studies of mind–body practices have been carried out in critically ill patients though some research has been done in the cardiovascular population.

Seskevich et al. [18] examined the use of integrative therapies in patients undergoing percutaneous coronary interventions (PCI) and the effects on mood and perceived stress. A sample of 108 patients were randomly assigned to receive one of five interventions—guided imagery, stress management (slowed breathing and repeated mental phrase), healing touch, intercessory prayer, and standard care. There was a significant decrease in self-reported worry (30%) in patients receiving guided imagery, stress management, and healing touch compared to the other two groups. In fact, the reported level of worry actually increased 16% in the standard care patient group as the patients got closer in time to the actual PCI procedure. There was no change in reported level of worry in the intercessory prayer group. There were no significant differences between groups in other of the other mood states measured (happiness, hope, calm, satisfaction, sadness, feeling upset, or shortness of breath).

In a review of integrative therapy studies in cardiac surgical patients, Casida and Lemanski [19] reported that five studies demonstrated a significant decrease in anxiety with use of guided imagery [20–24]. In addition, some of the studies also demonstrated a significant decrease in pain in this population [21, 23, 24] and a decreased length of stay [21, 22, 24]. Even though there is increasing work being done with guided imagery in the cardiac surgery population, the authors acknowledge that the research studies frequently lack statistical power and high-level quality designs [19]. Music therapy and AAT are arguably some of the most studied mind–body practices and will be discussed in more depth.

Music Therapy

Music therapy has some of the most research and evidence of all integrative therapies for use in MV ICU patients. It has been studied in a variety of procedural situations and is starting to be researched more consistently in the MV population. It is believed that music works both physiologically and psychologically to ameliorate the stressors of MV patients. By using music that is between 60 and 80 beats a minute with a flowing rhythm and pleasing harmonies, the body may trend toward entrainment, a synchronization of body rhythms with those of the music [10, 25]. Entrainment of body rhythms can thus diminish the sympathetic nervous system response, resulting in decreases in heart rate, respiratory rate, skeletal muscle tension, and oxygen consumption, and gastric and sweat gland activity [10, 25].

Music is thought to also have an affective component in patient response. Music can have an anxiolytic component, provide distraction from painful procedures and from the stress-invoking environment and situation, and promote relaxation and sleep by approximating a peaceful atmosphere [6, 12]. The consistent flowing rhythm may induce a hypnotic effect [13, 16]. Auditory stimulation with music, rather than the potentially stress-invoking noise of the ICU, can affect the limbic system, reducing the transmission of negative feelings by neurotransmitters [10, 16]. This can thus lead to a relaxation response, as evidenced by decreases in anxiety, heart rate, respiratory rate, and blood pressure.

While research evidence to date is promising for the use of music with MV patients in decreasing anxiety, results have been mixed. Studies have shown a consistent decrease in anxiety [10, 12, 13, 26, 27], heart rates [10, 11, 13, 27, 28], and respiratory rates [10, 12, 13, 27–29]. There have been inconsistent results for systolic and diastolic blood pressures and oxygen saturation [26]. Many of these studies had small sample sizes, had differences between types of music with patients, and may or may not have solicited patient input as to the type of music, were not RCTs, or had varying lengths and numbers of music listening sessions.

Implications for Practice Related to Music Therapy in Critical Care

Despite the lack of rigorous evidence to unequivocally support the use of music therapy, there is enough evidence to support its use in the critical care environment.

Table 9.1 Development of a music therapy program in critical care [16, 26, 30]

• Educate staff about the definition of music therapy
• Develop a wide selection of music that meets criteria for entrainment (60–80 beats/min, predictable dynamics, flowing and regular rhythm, no sudden changes in tempo or dynamics, pleasing harmonies)
• Allow patient to choose music to listen to
• Allow use of patient equipment
• Use headphones to block out background noise and optimize music experience
• Use MP3 players
• Allow for uninterrupted listening time
• Allow patient to choose times to listen but remember to offer music as they may not be able to initiate themselves due to weakness or restrictions from invasive lines, tubes, etc.
• Allow patient to determine length of listening session. Provide for at least 30 min if able

It is a safe and relatively easy therapy to implement and is easy to engage patients and families [10, 25, 26]. Collaboration with a trained music therapist, if at all feasible, is ideal as this can optimize music as an interventional therapy rather than as simply another instance of background noise for patients [26]. Music therapists are skilled at implementing music that incorporates the entrainment criteria while also using music to which a patient prefers to listen. Music therapy can be a relatively inexpensive therapy to implement. The majority of costs are associated with purchase of headphones, MP3 players, and maintaining a music library (see Table 9.1) [16, 26, 30].

Considerations

There are multiple factors that influence responses to music—age, gender, cognitive function, severity of tress, anxiety, distress, pain, training in music, familiarity and preference for music, culture, and personal associations with music. An individual may have a unique imagery experience evoked by a particular piece of music [26].

Having the patient listen to music that is not pleasing can heighten the stress response rather than lessen it. Similarly, if patients are not allowed to choose music they wish to listen to, they may inadvertently listen to music that evokes negative personal connotations or is linked to prior negative experiences.

While promoting relaxation as a goal, music therapy in combination with sedatives, pain medications, and vasoactive medications could result in untoward hemodynamic changes.

Future Research Directions

There is still much research to be done in determining in the extent of music's therapeutic effect in critically ill patients. Areas for future research should include exploring answers to the optimal and minimal "dose" of music that is beneficial, the number of sessions that optimize the relaxation response, carrying out larger RCTs, timing of music listening, exploring the interaction of sedative and pain medications during music intervention, and determining whether there is a cumulative effect to the use of music as an intervention, impact on mechanical ventilation days, and patient/family satisfaction [26]. There are also intriguing questions being posed about music listening having a direct effect on hormone responses and the hypermetabolic response of the critically ill that requires further exploration [25, 31].

Animal-Assisted Therapy and Pet Visitation

The use of animal visitation was recognized as long ago as in Nightingale's era and is another integrative therapy that can promote a healing environment for patients who are critically ill [32]. There are two distinct methods for using animals in this way: through a formal AAT program and visitation by patient-owned pets. AAT is "an intentional healing modality used to achieve therapeutic goals through facilitated interaction between patients and trained animals (as therapist) accompanied by human owners or handlers" [33]. AAT is a formal program where handlers train animals to visit residents of care facilities or hospital in-patients with the specific goal to improve cognitive and physical functioning [34]. Pet visitation is a circumstance where the patient's own pet is allowed to visit the patient while they are in the hospital.

There is very limited research on the impact of AAT or pet visitation on patients' physiological or psychological status. What evidence is available does point to the positive impact that the animal–human bond may have on patient response in both areas. Cole et al. performed an experimental research protocol comparing the impact of visits by volunteer dogs with a group receiving human volunteer visits and a control group of patients hospitalized with heart failure [35]. Visits lasted 12 min as tolerated by patients with significant changes in hemodynamic readings. Patients who had visits by volunteer dogs showed decreases in right atrial pressure, systolic and diastolic pulmonary artery pressures, pulmonary capillary wedge pressures, and epinephrine levels during the visit compared to both the human volunteer visit and the control. In addition, these same patients demonstrated a significant decrease in state anxiety and in norepinephrine levels after the volunteer dog visits compared to the other two groups. Stoffel and Braun [36] documented patient testimonials in a research protocol utilizing AAT canine visits with hospitalized pediatric and adult patients. Patients reported a significant increase in feelings of relaxation, calmness, and peace. Forty-nine percent of subjects reported a reduction in pain during the AAT visit. Also reported were improvements in attitude, an increase in energy, and improvement in temperature [36]. Both research groups recommend AAT as a viable complementary therapy to explore as part of the patient's plan of care.

In addition, Giuliano et al. [37] reported on development of a pet visitation program in critical care. While they report that they had no quantitative research data to formally evaluate the impact of the program, both staff and participant reports were very positive about the success of pet visitations. They report that critically ill patients may experience loneliness, depression, and feelings of lack of emotional support. Pet visitation may be one therapeutic option that can mitigate those psychosocial issues. The American College of Critical Care Medicine has recognized the role pet visitation can play in promoting a patient-centered critical care environment [38]. Their recommendations are that pets that are clean and properly immunized should not be restricted from visiting the ICU and recommend the development of unit guidelines to accommodate that practice. Patients may not be the only ones receiving benefit from either AAT or pet visitation programs. Nurses also reported that animals in the work environment made it a happier and more interesting place and reported that it had no negative impact on the working environment [33].

Implications for Practice Related to Animal Therapy in Critical Care

Implementation of pet visitation program can be initiated through development of a policy and guidelines and education of staff about the process. A plan should be in place for preparatory work prior to the visit. Implementation of an official AAT program can be more complex as a process for animal and handler assessments and ongoing evaluation need to be in place in addition to the policy and guidelines. Implementation of animal visitation can be inexpensive to develop. For pet visitation, the majority of the cost may be associated with the time needed to prepare for and closely monitor the animal during the visit. For an official AAT program, there are some costs associated with screening handlers and animals that will come into the institution to visit patients and maintaining information on continued appropriateness of participants. Typically, handlers and animals are volunteers, providing a cost-effective therapy [34].

Both the Centers for Disease Control and Prevention and the Association for Professionals in Infection Control and Epidemiology (APIC) have published recommendations for allowing animal visitation in hospital inpatient areas [39, 40]. Highlights of the recommendations call for limiting visits to domestic companion animals and prohibiting visits by animals such as primates, reptiles, hamsters, and gerbils; utilizing hand hygiene principles before and after animal contact; and ensuring that animals are appropriately vaccinated, clean, and healthy (see Table 9.2) [34, 38–40]. Refer to APIC Guidelines for more in-depth information about institution of both pet visitation and AAT programs [40].

Considerations

ICUs who allow animal visits should have plans in place for potential risk of animal bites or scratches or for animals which become excitable or out of control. Consider the access routes of animals to and from units to avoid potential inadvertent interactions with the public or other patients. Patient-owned animals should visit only their owner and not other patients [40].

Table 9.2 Basic guidelines in implementing an animal visitation program [34, 38, 39]

Refer to APIC and CDC for more detailed recommendations [39, 40]

- Minimize contact with animal saliva, dander, urine, and feces
- Perform hand hygiene both before and after animal contact
- Allow visits only from domestic companion animals that are pets and avoid visitation from animals such as primates, reptiles, hamsters, gerbils, mice, hedgehogs, and other noncompanion animals
- Ensure animals are fully vaccinated and healthy
- Ensure pets have had veterinarian visit within the past year
- Prior to visit, encourage handler to brush/comb hair and bathe pet if needed
- Provide animal opportunity to urinate and defecate prior to visit
- Place disposable, water-proof barriers between the animal and the bed; if not available, a sheet or towel can be used
- Restrict animals from visiting areas such as dialysis, burn units, operating rooms, neonatal nurseries, and medication or food storage, and preparation areas
- Ensure that handler maintains control of the animal at all times

Future Research

More research is needed regarding the impact of animal visitation, both through AAT programs or patient-owned pets. Areas of exploration should include impact of animal visitation on patient stress response and symptoms, impact on weaning of MV patients, satisfaction levels of patients involved with animal visitation, impact on ICU and hospital length of stay, morbidity, mortality, and quality of life.

Manipulative and Body-Based Practices

NCCAM defines manipulative and body-based integrative therapies as those therapies focused on body structures and systems—for example, joints, soft tissues, bones, and circulatory and lymphatic systems [2]. Spinal manipulation falls into this category but will be rarely used in the critically ill patient. The other common intervention in this category is massage therapy.

Massage had traditionally been a routine component of care provided by nurses but has become infrequently provided despite the research that has shown it to be beneficial to patients [41]. Benefits of massage have been shown to include decreases in heart rate, respiratory rate, muscle tension, and anxiety [42]. Even a 5-min foot massage can decrease blood pressure, heart rate, and respiratory rate during the intervention in critically ill patients [43]. Though the results were transient in the study, patients expressed very positive psychological effects from the intervention. As little as 5–10 min of massage prior to bedtime can improve both the quality and quantity of sleep [44]. Patients receiving massage slept longer, had longer periods of rapid eye movement (REM) sleep, and an improved sleep efficiency. The massage promoted an increase in relaxation and a decrease in perception of pain [44].

Use of massage may have the potential to decrease the need for sedatives and hypnotics [41].

In a descriptive study of hospitalized patients receiving twice-weekly massages, Smith et al. [45] found that 98% of patients reported increased relaxation and more than 87% reported improved sense of well-being and positive mood with the therapy. Other positive reports included improved mobility, energy, and sleep and decreased pain and anxiety.

Research has also been conducted with the use of tactile touch (effleurage) with critically ill patients. Tactile touch performed daily for 5 days in ICU patients resulted in significant decreases in anxiety and diastolic blood pressure, though no differences in systolic blood pressure or heart rate [46].

Clearly, massage has a continuing place in the care of critically ill patients. More research is needed to continue to define optimal timing and length of massage therapy and the effects and contraindications of its use. Protocols have been developed to assist providers in reinstituting massage as a part of nursing care [47]. Another intervention that could be considered a type of body-based practice is early mobility in MV patients. This is an increasing area of research and will be explored here in more depth.

Early Mobility in Mechanically Ventilated Patients

As increasing numbers of critically ill patients survive to be discharged from ICUs and hospitals, increased attention has been paid to the physiological status of these patients on discharge and the potential need for extended rehabilitation. These patients may frequently exhibit neuromuscular weakness related to prolonged immobility and muscle atrophy [48, 49], though the exact cause of this condition is unknown. In some cases, this neuromuscular weakness can last as long as 1–2 years [49].

Development of ICU-acquired weakness can occur quickly, resulting in activity intolerance, particularly for those who are MV [50]. Varied reasons are hypothesized as the cause for this ICU-acquired weakness. Immobility can lead to decreased muscle mass related to both diminished protein synthesis and proteolysis [48, 50]. Muscle atrophy can start to occur as quickly as 3 days in ICU patients who are maintained on bed rest [50]. A proinflammatory state can result in muscle damage from cytokine imbalance and shifting. Additionally, malnutrition may develop in critically ill patients who are unable to maintain adequate caloric intake or patients may arrive in a malnourished state on admission with potential for worsening during their critical care stay [49].

Patients exhibiting neuromuscular weakness can have prolongation of mechanical ventilation and increased lengths of stay [49], leading to a vicious cycle of ongoing immobility. Early mobility and physical therapy may have a positive impact on avoiding the development or mitigating the extent of neuromuscular weakness in MV patients.

There has been an increase in research the past 5 years with a focus on demonstrating the feasibility, safety, and potential impact of early mobility in MV patients. There are currently wide variations in the extent of therapy provided to ICU patients across the United States, ranging from active and early engagement of interdisciplinary team members to those critical care areas waiting to initiate therapy after the patient is discharged from the ICU.

Several studies have demonstrated the feasibility and safety of early therapy and mobility of MV patients [51–54]. These studies utilized a combination of interdisciplinary team members to initiate and maintain early mobility including physical therapy (PT), occupational therapy (OT), respiratory therapy (RT), nursing, and nursing assistants. All studies also utilized standardized protocols that advanced activity from passive range of motion to sitting to standing to walking based on patient alertness, hemodynamic stability, and respiratory status [51–54].

Bailey et al. demonstrated that patients intubated for more than 4 days were able to ambulate >100 ft. at discharge from a respiratory ICU when early mobility with an interdisciplinary team was in place [51]. Morris et al. found an early mobility protocol through use of a Mobility Team was associated with more therapy sessions and a decrease in ICU and hospital length of stay for patients who survived to discharge [52]. While several studies have enrolled patients who have been intubated for several days, Pohlman et al. demonstrated the feasibility of initiating a PT/OT protocol starting immediately after intubation. Even in this newly intubated medical ICU (MICU) population, therapy occurred on 90% of MICU days when patients were on mechanical ventilation [53]. Thomsen et al. demonstrated that when MV patients were transferred from their initial ICU to an ICU with an early mobility culture, they were three times more likely to be ambulating. They postulate that ICUs without an early mobility program may actually be imposing unnecessary immobility constraints on MV ICU patients [54].

A key factor in all the above studies was the concomitant commitment to optimize therapy and mobility sessions when sedation was interrupted. Even intermittent sedative use was associated with a twofold decrease in the likelihood of ambulation [54]. Ensuring that patients are alert and able to engage in their therapy sessions is key to early mobility [51, 55]. Adverse events were uncommon in all of the studies and typically were oxygen desaturations, blood pressure and heart rate changes (which might have been normal response to exercise), and rare dislodgements of tubes such as nasogastric and rectal tubes.

Implications for Practice with Early Mobility

There is increasing evidence that early mobility and initiation of therapy intervention is feasible and safe in MV patients in ICUs [56]. A standardized protocol with clear guidelines about activity progression based on a patient's neurological, cardiovascular, and respiratory status is one component of an early mobility program [55]. Simply having a protocol in place may increase the number and frequency of therapy sessions initiated with MV patients [55].

Table 9.3 Recommendations for implementing an early mobility program for mechanically ventilated patients in the intensive care unit [54, 56]

• Develop interdisciplinary collaborative team
• Promote a culture of early mobility
• Address optimal sedative use
• Develop standardized guidelines for early mobility and activity progression
• Assess for and treat delirium

Optimization of sedative use is a factor that should be closely addressed and aligned with implementation of a successful mobility program [55, 57].

Medical centers that have early mobility programs for MV patients emphasize the fact that a culture that prioritizes mobility must be in place which takes a significant amount of work to develop [49, 51, 55]. The program needs an interdisciplinary team committed to collaboration. Medical centers were able to initiate teams dedicated to early mobility in the ICU without increasing personnel resources [51] or cost [51, 52].

Considerations

The most frequently cited concern in initiating an early mobility program is for the safety of patients related to maintenance of intact tubes, an adequate airway, and hemodynamic stability. Teams can proactively develop clear plans for how to diminish these risk factors, a process for appropriately increasing activity levels, and a plan to quickly respond to adverse events (see Table 9.3) [54, 56]. Studies mentioned above were able to successfully implement these programs with remarkably few adverse events and none that were life-threatening [51–54].

Future Research

An identified weakness of the above studies is that very few are RCTs. Most have focused on the safety and feasibility of initiating an early mobility program with some short-term outcomes reported such as length of stay and cost. Future research should incorporate larger, multicenter samples; randomized controlled methodologies; development of standardized guidelines; identification of patient characteristics for prescription and tailoring of the intervention; and impact of early mobility on long-term outcomes and functional status [49, 51, 54, 58].

Biologically Based Therapies

Biologically based therapies include use of nutrients such as herbal medicines, minerals, vitamins, and dietary supplements. While use of these products is becoming increasingly popular by the public, there can be significant risks associated with their use as they are not regulated by the Food and Drug Administration, and products with similar ingredients can vary widely in concentration and dose. Herbal medicines and megavitamins are rarely used in the critical care population, but there is an increasing focus on the potential for specific nutritional supplements to positively impact the immune system and promote healing.

Perspectives on nutritional supplementation in the critically ill have started to shift toward administering them independently rather than relying on them as incorporated into parenteral or enteral nutrition. It is difficult to maintain adequate parenteral or enteral nutrition in ICU patients, and some key nutrients may require individual titration based on patient needs. Much of the recent focus has been on the effects and benefits of glutamine and selenium replacement, particularly as they relate to the function of the immune system.

A study on the use of "pharmaconutrients" administered separately from enteral nutrition was conducted by Beale et al. [59]. Septic patients received pharmaconutrients (e.g., glutamine, vitamins C and E, beta-carotene, selenium, and zinc among others) daily for 10 days. Plasma levels of nutrients were measured to assess absorption, and organ function was assessed through use of the Sequential Organ Failure Assessment (SOFA) score. Results showed that the nutrients were successfully absorbed and well tolerated with significant increases in key nutrient levels and amino acids by day 3 of administration. The combination of an immune-enhanced enteral formula with the nutrients resulted in significantly faster improvement in organ function, as evidenced by improved SOFA scores. There were no significant differences between groups in lengths of stay or development of secondary infections.

Dechellotte et al. [60] studied the use of parenteral glutamine supplementation in ICU patients receiving parenteral nutrition in a multicenter trial. Findings included decreases in infectious complications (primarily a decrease in pneumonia) and hyperglycemia and fewer patients requiring insulin. There was a trend toward decreased length of time on mechanical ventilation, though this finding was not significant. There were no differences in mortality, hospital length of stay, or ICU length of stay.

There have been conflicting results on the effectiveness of glutamine and selenium use [61]. It is known that levels of these nutrients diminish in critical illness and sepsis. Glutamine has been found to be a safe nutrient to administer, and enough evidence exists that it is recommended to be parenterally supplemented in critically ill patients receiving parenteral nutrition [61]. There is insufficient data to recommend parenteral supplementation in patients receiving enteral nutrition. Selenium, on the other hand, has a risk for toxicity with supplementation due to varying concentrations available with required conutrients. RCTs with selenium have been reported to be of low quality, and so recommendations for its use and dosing are not well developed [61].

It may take years before research on key nutrients gives clear guidance on their use. There are multiple trace elements and amino acids to be evaluated along with their potential interplay. There is also the potential lack of feasibility to titrate each nutrient individually if required. In the meantime, there is also an increasing focus on the use of probiotics in the ICU population which will be explored more here.

Probiotics to Reduce Incidence of Ventilator-Associated Pneumonia

Heighted attention has been directed at the prevention of ventilator-associated pneumonia (VAP) over the past several years to avoid a potentially preventable complication that can prolong mechanical ventilation, increase morbidity and mortality, and lengthen ICU and hospital length of stay [62]. The use of probiotics, prebiotics, and synbiotics has been studied as a method to normalize gut flora in attempts to control diarrhea in ICU patients. Recently, more research has emerged in evaluating the effectiveness of probiotics in preventing VAP.

The gastrointestinal tract is populated with both pathogenic and protective bacteria that, in healthy persons, maintain a homeostatic relationship in the normal functioning gut [62]. When an imbalance in this relationship occurs, the gut can become inflamed and dysfunctional [63]. It is believed that by repopulating protective bacteria in the gut, homeostatic balance can be restored.

Probiotics is a term used to identify a category of normally occurring protective flora, the most commonly recognized probiotic being lactic acid bacteria (LAB) [64]. Prebiotics are substances that act in the gut to promote fermentation and production of nutrients, vitamins, and antioxidants with synbiotics being a combination of both prebiotics and probiotics [64]. The main characteristics of a probiotic are that they should be natural flora of the gut, resist degradation, and remain in the gut through colonization [63]. Probiotics function through various mechanisms including inhibiting growth and adherence of pathogenic bacteria [63], decreasing translocation of gut microbes [63, 64], enhancing function of macrophages, reducing toxins [64], and modulating the immune response [63].

While probiotics have traditionally been studied for use in critically ill patients particularly related to addressing diarrhea and gut function with inconsistent results, there is a growing body of research in the use of probiotics to prevent VAP—in part thought to be caused by aspiration of pathogens residing in the stomach and oropharynx in MV patients [65].

Siempos et al. performed a meta-analysis of RCTs in the use of probiotics to decrease incidence of VAP [65]. The meta-analysis included five RCTs which used either a single LAB or a combination LAB probiotic in conjunction with a fiber prebiotic [66–70]. Four of the five RCTs administered the LAB via naso/orogastic tubes [66, 67, 69, 70], while the fifth study applied the probiotic to the oral cavity [68]. Findings of the meta-analysis included a significant reduction in VAP in the experimental groups compared to controls, decreased ICU length of stay, and fewer patients colonized with *Pseudomonas aeruginosa*. There were no differences between probiotic and control groups in all-cause mortality, mechanical ventilation days, or incidence of diarrhea [65].

Implications for Practice Related to Probiotic Use in Critically Ill Patients

Recent research studies show promise in the use of probiotics to decrease the incidence of VAP. This can be an exciting avenue for exploration for several reasons:

development of resistance to antibiotics is an ever-present concern, driving the need to minimize the development of infections as much as possible; and there is increased scrutiny on ICUs to prevent a nosocomial-acquired complication that can have significant impact on mortality and morbidity. It is unclear, however, whether there is sufficient evidence on safety and efficacy of this intervention to promote widespread implementation.

Considerations

There are significant issues to be considered when exploring use of probiotics for prevention of VAP. Probiotics are not considered medications but rather nutritional supplements and therefore are not regulated with the same level of rigor and oversight as medications [65]. There are multiple formulations of LAB, and careful thought must be used in determining which, if any, should be utilized in any particular situation [71]. There have also been reports of probiotic-induced diseases which can be a significant risk for a critically ill patient who may already have immune response issues [72, 73].

Future Research

If use of probiotics is to be considered as a viable option to reduce the incidence of VAP, it is essential that additional well-designed RCTs be performed [65]. Research needs to support development of guidelines regarding the dosage, administration route, and length of therapy [65]. Different formulas of probiotics need to be evaluated to determine whether single-source formulations or combination products are appropriate for different situations [63]. Trial should also include surveillance of blood cultures to better ascertain the safety of this treatment approach [63].

Energy-Based Therapies

The fourth main category of integrative therapies is energy-based practices. The goal of these interventions is to manipulate energy fields to promote health and includes therapies such as magnet therapy, light therapy, Reiki, healing touch, and Qigong [2]. Very few of these therapies have been researched at all in the critically ill.

Acupressure has been researched in a few pulmonary populations. Use of acupressure has been show to significantly decrease dyspnea when compared to sham acupressure in the pulmonary rehabilitation and chronic obstructive pulmonary disease populations [74, 75]. Tsay et al. [76] studied the use of acupressure in patients receiving longer-term mechanical ventilation (>21 days). Three acupressure points were utilized—two points on the hands bilaterally and one on the ears bilaterally. Acupressure was performed daily for 10 days, with significant reductions in heart rate, respiratory rate, dyspnea, and anxiety.

Energy-based therapy is the least studied of the four integrative therapy categories in the critically ill population at this time. There is no compelling evidence for broad-based implementation without further research. The initial results of acupressure research show promise for continued exploration of this therapy with critically ill patients. Healing touch may also be an energy-based therapy that has had some research in nonhealthy subjects, so further research in the acutely ill may be warranted.

Summary

There is increasing interest in exploring the use of integrative therapies in the critical care environment. It is a challenge to conduct RCTs in critically ill patients in general and can be even more so with therapies that have no baseline "dosages" identified, that are not regulated in the same manner as allopathic medications and interventions, or that impact both physiological and psychological functioning.

It is in the best interest of critically ill patients for health-care providers to be open to the fact that many patients may arrive to our ICUs with a history of integrative therapy use as well as the fact that appropriate use of some therapies may play an important adjunctive role in optimal healing of the critically ill.

There are several steps ICU care providers can take as the foundation of evidence expands. First, health-care providers can ask patients and families about their integrative therapy use on admission to the ICU, keeping in mind that inappropriate use of integrative therapies may actually be the cause of the ICU admission—for example, when excessive or inappropriate use of nutritional supplements leads to severe electrolyte or nutritional imbalances. Health-care providers should be prepared for patients and families to ask to use integrative therapies during their ICU stay. Providers need to keep in mind the influence of cultural diversity in the request for and use of integrative therapies. Lastly, health-care providers can explore opportunities to develop integrative therapy programs in the ICU setting, considering those therapies that require little equipment, minimal training, little time, and expense that are, at minimum, safe interventions.

When offering integrative therapy interventions to patients and families, providers should be cognizant that they may be unfamiliar with the intervention and hesitant to participate. As with any intervention utilized in the ICU, good communication is required with patient/family input and concerns addressed. Finally, offer education to staff and other health-care providers about integrative therapies in general.

There is an increasing amount of research in select integrative therapy modalities, but there is clearly a need for more research across the board in all integrative therapies that indicate clear potential to improve the healing and outcomes of critically ill patients. Continued research in the therapies mentioned in this chapter is certainly warranted. In addition, therapies such as spiritual care, guided imagery, aromatherapy, and acupuncture deserve more exploration regarding their potential place in the critical care environment including use with MV patients.

References

1. Nahin RL, Barnes PM, Stussman BJ, Bloom B. Costs of complementary and alternative medicine (CAM) and frequency of visits to CAM practitioners: United States, 2007. National health statistics reports; no. 18. Hyattsville: National Center for Health Statistics; 2009.
2. National Center for Complementary and Alternative Medicine. 2011. What is CAM? http://nccam.nih.gov/health/whatiscam/. Accessed February 17, 2011.
3. Society of Critical Care Medicine. Critical care statistics in the United States. 2006. http://www.siriusgenomics.com/content/technology/CriticalCareStatistics.pdf Accessed February 17, 2011.
4. Angus DC, Shorr AF, White A, Dremsizov TT, Schmitz RJ, Kelley MA. Critical care delivery in the United States: distribution of services and compliance with Leapfrog recommendations. Crit Care Med. 2006;24(4):1016–24.
5. Thomas LA. Clinical management of stressors perceived by patients on mechanical ventilation. AACN Clin Issues. 2003;14(1):73–81.
6. Austin D. The psychophysiological effects of music therapy in intensive care units. Paediatr Nurs. 2010;22(3):14–20.
7. Chlan L. Description of anxiety levels by individual differences and clinical factors in patients receiving mechanical ventilator support. Heart Lung. 2003;32(4):275–82.
8. Chlan L. A review of the evidence for music intervention to manage anxiety in critically ill patients receiving mechanical ventilator support. Arch Psychiatr Nurs. 2009;23(2):177–9.
9. Rotondi AJ, Chelluri L, Sirio C, et al. Patients' recollections of stressful experiences while receiving prolonged mechanical ventilation in an intensive care unit. Crit Care Med. 2002;30(4):736–52.
10. Lee OKA, Chung YFL, Chan MF, Chan WM. Music and its effect on the physiological responses and anxiety levels of patients receiving mechanical ventilation: a pilot study. J Clin Nurs. 2005;14:609–20.
11. Almerud S, Petersson K. Music therapy—a complementary treatment for mechanically ventilated intensive care patients. Intensive Crit Care Nurs. 2003;19:21–30.
12. Wong HLC, Lopez-Nahas V, Molassiotis A. Effects of music therapy on anxiety in ventilator-dependent patients. Heart Lung. 2001;30(5):376–87.
13. Chlan L. Effectiveness of a music therapy intervention on relaxation and anxiety for patients receiving ventilator assistance. Heart Lung. 1998;27(3):169–76.
14. Kollef MH, Ley NT, Ahren TS, Schaiff R, Prentice D, Sherman G. The use of continuous IV sedation is associated with prolongation of mechanical ventilation. Chest. 1998;114:541–8.
15. Seneff MG, Wagner D, Thompson D, Honeycutt C, Silver M. The impact of long-term acute-care facilities on the outcome and cost of care for patients undergoing prolonged mechanical ventilation. Crit Care Med. 2000;28:342–50.
16. Chlan L, Guttormson J, Tracy MF, Bremer KL. Strategies for overcoming site and recruitment challenges in research studies based in intensive care units. AJCC. 2009;18(5):410–7.
17. Tracy MF, Lindquist R, Savik K. et al; Use of complementary and alternative therapies: a national survey of critical care nurses. AJCC. 2005;14:404–15.
18. Seskevich JE, Crater SW, Lane JD, Krucoff MW. Beneficial effects of noetic therapies on mood before percutaneous intervention for unstable coronary syndromes. Nurs Res. 2004;53(2):116–21.
19. Casida J, Lemanski S. An evidence-based review of guided imagery utilization in adult cardiac surgery. Clin Scholars Rev. 2010;3(1):22–30.
20. Ashton RC, Whitworth GC, Seldomridge JA, Shapiro PA, Michler RE, Smith CR, et al. The effects of self-hypnosis on quality of life following coronary artery bypass surgery: preliminary results of a prospective, randomized trial. J Complement Altern Med. 1995;1(3):288–90.
21. Deisch P, Soukup SM, Adams P, Wild MC. Guided imagery: replication study using coronary artery bypass patients. Nurs Clin North Am. 2000;35(2):417–25.

22. Halpin LS, Speir AM, CapoBianco P, Barnett SD. Guided imagery in cardiac surgery. Outcomes Manag. 2002;6(3):132–7.
23. Kshettry VR, Carole LF, Henly SJ, Sendelbach S, Kummer B. Complementary alternative medical therapies for heart surgery patients: feasibility, safety and impact. Ann Thorac Surg. 2006;81(1):201–5.
24. Tusek DL, Cwynar R, Cosgrove DM. Effect of guided imagery on length of stay, pain and anxiety in cardiac surgery patients. J Cardiovasc Manag. 1999;10(2):22–8.
25. Chlan L, Engeland WC, Anthony A, Guttormson J. Influence of music on the stress response in patients receiving mechanical ventilator support: a pilot study. AJCC. 2007;16(2):141–5.
26. Bradt J, Dileo C, Grocke D. Music interventions for mechanically ventilated patients (Review). The Cochrane Collaboration. 2010;12. http://www.thecochranelibrary.com.
27. Han LH, Sit JWH, Chung L, Jiao ZY, Ma WG. Effects of music intervention on physiological stress response and anxiety level of mechanically ventilated patients in China: a randomized controlled trial. J Clin Nurs. 2010;19:978–87.
28. Chlan L. Psychophysiological responses of mechanically ventilated patients to music: a pilot study. AJCC. 1995;4:233–8.
29. Korhan EA, Khorshid L, Uyar M. The effect of music therapy on physiological signs of anxiety in patients receiving mechanical ventilatory support. J Clin Nurs. 2011; in press.
30. Nelson A, Hartl W, Karl-Walter J, et al. The impact of music on hypermetabolism in critical illness. Curr Opin Clin Nutr Metab Care. 2008;11:790–4.
31. Nightingale F. Notes on nursing. New York: Dover; 1969 (Originally published 1860).
32. Halm M. The healing power of the human-animal connection. AJCC. 2008;17:373–6.
33. DeCourcey M, Russell AC, Keister KJ. Animal-assisted therapy. Evaluation and implementation of a complementary therapy to improve the psychological and physiological health of critically ill patients. Dimens Crit Care Nurs. 2010;29(5):211–4.
34. Cole KM, Gawlinski A, Steers N, Kotlerman J. Animal-assisted therapy in patients hospitalized with heart failure. AJCC. 2007;16:575–85.
35. Stoffel J, Braun C. Animal-assisted therapy: analysis of patient testimonials. J Undergrad Nurs Scholarsh. 2006. http://juns.nursing.arizona.edu/articles/Fall%202006/stoffel.htm. Accessed March 4, 2011.
36. Giuliano KK, Bloniasz E, Bell J. Implementation of a pet visitation program in critical care. Crit Care Nurs. 1999;19(3):43–50.
37. Davidson JE, Powers K, Hedayat K, et al. Clinical practice guidelines for support of the supporting the family in the patient-centered intensive care unit: American College of Critical Care Task Force 2004–2005. Crit Care Med. 2007;35(2):605–22.
38. Centers for Disease Control and Prevention. 2010. Recommendations—animals in health care facilities. http://www.cdc.gov/mmwr/preview/mmwrhtml/rr5210a1.htm Accessed February 17, 2011.
39. Lefebvre SL, Golab GC, Christensen E, et al; For the Writing Panel of the Working Group. Guidelines for animal-assisted interventions in health care facilities. 2008. Association for Professionals in Infection Control and Epidemiology. http://www.apic.org/AM/Template.cfm?Section=Search&section=Consensus_Reports&template=/CM/ContentDisplay.cfm&ContentFileID=11843. Accessed March 4, 2011.
40. Richards K, Nagel C, Markie M, Elwell J, Barone C. Use of complementary and alternative therapies to promote sleep in critically ill patients. Crit Care Nurs Clin North Am. 2003;15(3):329–40.
41. Richards KC, Gibson R, Overton-McCoy AL. Effects of massage in acute and critical care. AACN Clin Issues. 2000;11(1):77–96.
42. Hayes J, Cox C. Immediate effects of a five-minute foot massage on patients in critical care. Intensive Crit Care Nurs. 1999;15:77–82.
43. Richards KC. Effect of a back massage and relaxation intervention on sleep in critically ill patients. Am J Crit Care. 1998;7(4):288–99.
44. Smith MC, Stallings MA, Mariner S, Burrall M. Benefits of massage therapy for hospitalized patients: a descriptive and qualitative evaluation. Altern Ther. 1999;5(4):64–71.

45. Henricson M, Ersson A, Maatta S, Segesten K, Berglund AL. The outcome of tactile touch on stress parameters in intensive care: a randomized controlled trial. Complement Ther Clin Pract. 2008;14:244–54.
46. Richards KC, Benham B, Shannon L, DeClerk L. Promoting sleep in acute and critical care. Aliso Viejo: American Association of Critical-Care Nurses; 1998.
47. Fan E, Zanni JM, Dennison CR, Lepre SJ, Needham DM. Critical illness neuromyopathy and muscle weakness in patients in the intensive care unit. AACN Adv Crit Care. 2009;20(3):243–53.
48. Truong AD, Fan E, Bower RG, Needham DM. Bench-to-bedside review: mobilizing patients in the intensive care unit—from pathophysiology to clinical trials. Crit Care. 2009;13:216. doi:10.1186/cc7885.
49. Winkelman C. Bed rest in health and critical illness. AACN Adv Crit Care. 2009;20(3): 254–66.
50. Bailey P, Thomsen GE, Spuhler VJ, et al. Early activity is feasible and safe in respiratory failure patients. Crit Care Med. 2007;35(1):139–45.
51. Morris PE, Goad A, Thompson C, et al. Early intensive care unit mobility therapy in the treatment of acute respiratory failure. Crit Care Med. 2008;36(8):2238–43.
52. Pohlman MC, Schweikert WD, Pohlman AS, et al. Feasibility of physical and occupational therapy beginning from initiation of mechanical ventilation. Crit Care Med. 2010;38(1):2089–94.
53. Thomsen GE, Snow GL, Rodriguez L, Hopkins RO. Patients with respiratory failure increase ambulation after transfer to an intensive care unit where early activity is a priority. Crit Care Med. 2008;36(4):1119–24.
54. Hopkins RO, Spuhler VJ. Strategies for promoting early activity in critically ill mechanically ventilated patients. AACN Adv Crit Care. 2009;20(3):277–89.
55. Needham DM. Mobilizing patients in the intensive care unit: improving neuromuscular weakness and physical function. JAMA. 2008;300(14):1685–90.
56. Bailey PP, Miller RR, Clemmer TP. Culture of early mobility in mechanically ventilated patients. Crit Care Med. 2009;37(10):S429–35.
57. Gosselink R, Bott J, Johnson M, et al. Physiotherapy for adult patients with critical illness: recommendations of the European Respiratory Society and European Society of Intensive Care Medicine Task Force on physiotherapy for critically ill patients. Intensive Care Med. 2008;34(7):1188–99.
58. Beale RJ, Sherry T, Lei K, Campbell-Stephen L, McCook J, Smith J, et al. Early enteral supplementation with key pharmaconutrients improves Sequential Organ Failure Assessment score in critically ill patients with sepsis: outcome of a randomized, controlled double blind study. Crit Care Med. 2008;36(1):131–44.
59. Dechelotte P, Hasselman M, Cynober L, Allaouchiche B, Coeffier M, Hecketsweller B, et al. L-alanyl-L-glutamine dipeptide-supplemented total parenteral nutrition reduces infectious complications and glucose intolerance in critically ill patients: the French controlled, randomized, double-blind, multicenter study. Crit Care Med. 2006;34(3):598–604.
60. Andrews P. Selenium and glutamine supplements: where are we heading? A critical care perspective. Curr Opin Clin Nutr Metab Care. 2010;13(2):192–7.
61. Safdar N, Dezfulian C, Collard HR, Saint S. Clinical and economic consequences of ventilator-associated pneumonia: a systematic review. Crit Care Med. 2005;33:2184–93.
62. Meier R, Steuerwald M. Place of probiotics. Curr Opin Crit Care. 2005;11:18–325.
63. Bengmark S. Pre-, pro- and synbiotics. Curr Opin Clin Nutr Metab Care. 2001;4:571–9.
64. Siempos II, Ntaidou TK, Falagas ME. Impact of the administration of probiotics on the incidence of ventilator-associated pneumonia: a meta-analysis of randomized controlled trials. Crit Care Med. 2010;38(3):954–62.
65. Knight DJ, Gardiner D, Banks A, et al. Effect of symbiotic therapy on the incidence of ventilator associated pneumonia in critically ill patients: a randomized, double-blind, placebo-controlled trial. Intensive Care Med. 2009;5:854–61.
66. Forestier C, Guelon D, Cluytens V, et al. Oral probiotic and prevention of pseudomonas aeruginosa infections: a randomized, double-blind, placebo controlled pilot study in intensive care unit patients. Crit Care. 2008;12:R669.

67. Klarin B, Molin G, Jeppsson B, et al. Use of the probiotic Lactobacillus plantarum 299 to reduce pathogenic bacteria in the oropharynx of intubated patients: a randomized study in trauma patients. Crit Care. 2008;12:R136.
68. Spindler-Vesel A, Bengmark S, Vovk I, et al. Synbiotics, prebiotics, glutamine, or peptide in early enteral nutrition: a randomized study in trauma patients. J Parenter Enteral Nutr. 2007;31:119–26.
69. Katzampassi K, Giamarellos-Bourboulis EJ, Voudouris A, et al. Benefits of a symbiotic formula (Synbiotic 2000Forte) in critically ill trauma patients: early results of a randomized-controlled trial. World J Surg. 2006;30:1848–55.
70. Bengmark S. Gut microbial ecology in critical illness: is there a role for prebiotics, probiotics, and synbiotics? Curr Opin Crit Care. 2002;8:145–51.
71. Wood GC, Boucher BA, Croce MA, et al. Lactobacillus species as a cause of ventilator-associated pneumonia in a critically ill trauma patient. Pharmacotherapy. 2002;22:1180–2.
72. Snydman DR. The safety of probiotics. Clin Infect Dis. 2008;46(Suppl):S103–11.
73. Maa SH, Gauthier D, Turner M. Acupressure as an adjunct to a pulmonary rehabilitation program. J Cardipulm Rehabil. 1997;17:268–76.
74. Wu HS, Wu SC, Lin JG, Lin LC. Effectiveness of acupressure in improving dyspnoea in chronic obstructive pulmonary disease. J Adv Nurs. 2004;45:252–9.
75. Tsay SL, Wang JC, Lin KC, Chung UL. Effects of acupressure therapy for patients having prolonged mechanical ventilator support. J Adv Nurs. 2005;52(2):142–50.
76. Chlan L, Tracy MF. Music therapy in critical care: indications and guidelines for intervention. Crit Care Nurs. 1999;19(3):35–41.

Chapter 10
Integrative Therapies to Promote Sleep in the Intensive Care Unit

Jessie Casida and LuAnn Nowak

Abstract The prevalence of sleep pattern disturbances (SPDs) in the ICU has been linked to a myriad of factors (e.g., pathologic state, care processes, ICU environment) and unfavorable outcomes such as amplification of stress, immune and inflammatory function in an already altered homeostatic state of critically ill patients resulting in delayed recovery from illness or injury, reduced health-related quality of life and care satisfaction, and among others. Health risk factors and causes of sleep disruptions in patient's sleep/wake pattern in the ICU have been long recognized. However, little effort has been done on promoting sleep among patients in the ICU specifically using nonpharmacologic agents such as integrative therapies. This chapter provides the reader with overview of sleep disturbances the ICU and appraisal of the available knowledge on several integrative therapies that have been investigated and implemented as sleep-promoting interventions in the ICU. Because of the little emphasis on sleep promotion, complexity of patients, difficulty in measuring sleep, and integrating nonpharmacologic sleep interventions in the usual care, strong and high-quality evidence supporting the utilization of integrative therapies is lacking. Implications to clinical practice and research are discussed.

Keywords Sleep pattern • Sleep disturbances • Sleep-promoting therapies • State of the science • Critical care patient symptom management

Introduction

The 2010 Sleep in America Poll showed that 60% of community-dwelling adults reported having a "bad night sleep" every night or almost every night in a given week [1]. Without a doubt, the staggering incidence of sleep deprivation among

---

J. Casida, PhD (✉) • L. Nowak, PhD
College of Nursing, Wayne State University, 5557 Cass Avenue, Detroit, MI 48202, USA
e-mail: jcasida@wayne.edu

L. Chlan and M.I. Hertz (eds.), *Integrative Therapies in Lung Health and Sleep*, Respiratory Medicine 4, DOI 10.1007/978-1-61779-579-4_10,

Table 10.1 Definition of terms [4–6]

Sleep pattern
• *Sleep pattern disturbance* refers to the alterations of the person's nighttime patterns of sleep and daytime awakenings. Sleep–wake pattern is evaluated with self-report questionnaire, sleep diary, wrist actigraphy, and/or polysomnography
• *Sleep latency* refers to the elapsed time between going to bed and the onset of sleep. A normal sleeper has a sleep onset latency of 15 min or less
• *Sleep fragmentation* is the term used to describe sleep disturbances throughout the night characterized by frequent and often lengthy awakenings. Wrist actigraphic data show that normal sleepers have an average sleep fragmentation index of ≤49%
• *Sleep efficiency* is the percentage of time in bed actually spent sleeping (i.e., ratio of total sleep time and the amount of time spent in bed). A normal sleeper has an average sleep efficiency index of ≥85%

adults in the United States can be exaggerated further through hospitalization. Although there is no concrete epidemiologic data on sleep disturbances of patients in the intensive care unit (ICU), healthcare providers have long been concerned of the high prevalence of sleep deprivation and altered circadian rhythm among patients confined in the critical care units [2]. Sleep disturbance, sleep disruption, sleep deprivation, and sleep pattern disturbance (SPD) are the terms interchangeably used to describe symptoms, rather than a "disorder" [3], of the alterations of the patient's nighttime pattern of sleep and daytime awakenings of patients in the ICU (the terms or variables commonly used to describe or measure patient's sleep pattern are summarized in Table 10.1) [4–6]. Difficulty of initiating and maintaining sleep at night and excessive daytime sleepiness are common behavioral characteristics of patients with "disturbed" sleep–wake pattern in the ICU [7]. SPD is a common problem in the ICU primarily due to the patient care delivery practices and the environment in which care is provided. For example, excessive surveillance (e.g., frequent monitoring of vital signs of "stable" patients), providing personal care (e.g., bathing, oral care) at nighttime, diagnostic procedures, treatments, noise level, and lighting practices are among the commonly reported factors causing disturbances in the patient's sleep–wake cycle [2, 8].

In spite of the providers' awareness of the patients' disruptions in their normal sleep–wake/rest-activity pattern in the ICU, many critical care clinicians have the tendency to ignore or do not place a high priority on sleep promotion in planning of care for acutely and/or critically ill patients [8]. Misconceptions and lack of knowledge, combined with nursing unit culture rooted in traditions and ritualistic practices, limit the clinician's motivation to further comprehend the negative consequences of SPD on the patient's healthcare outcomes [9]. Thus, the deficit in competence among the care providers in identifying and designing sleep-promoting interventions may result in longer durations of the patient's recovery from illness or acute injury, fatigue, and psychological distress and diminish health-related quality of life [2, 8]. The purpose of this chapter is to provide the reader with the: (1) state of the science for the utilization of integrative therapies in managing SPD as a symptom, not a disorder or diagnosis, in the ICU and (2) implications of the current science for clinical practice and research.

Overview of Sleep Disturbances in the ICU

A recently published systematic review of the literature revealed that the patient care environment and the underlying pathological processes are the major etiologic factors driving the high prevalence of SPD in the ICU. The common environmental factors that have been identified to cause SPD include noise levels, lighting practices, patient care activities (e.g., vital sign monitoring, medication administration, treatments), diagnostic procedures, and pharmacologic agents such as beta-adrenergic blockers, sedatives, and analgesics. The pathological processes inherent to critical illness, trauma, and/or injury that contribute to, and to some extent cause, SPD include stress, anxiety, hormonal changes, inflammatory response, organ dysfunction, pain, and/or psychosis [8–10]. In addition, standard treatment modalities like mechanical ventilation, hemodialysis machines, and other life-sustaining technological devices have also been known to disrupt the circadian rhythm of these patients [8, 11, 12]. Although much research is still needed to further elucidate the causality among environmental and pathophysiological factors and SPD, the evidence is clear that disturbances in the patients' sleep–wake/rest-activity pattern in the ICU hamper the restitution of their homeostatic state within the biological, physical, and psychological contexts [8, 10]. Consequently, increase in hospitalization days, decrease in care satisfaction, and long-term negative effects on the patients' health, well-being, and overall quality of life prevail [8, 10, 13, 14].

SPD in the ICU is frequently evaluated with objective and/or subjective measurement instruments [8, 10]. Several studies that employed polysomnography (the gold standard for measuring sleep) in measuring sleep architecture and quality have identified common and most significant changes of sleep among medical, surgical, and cardiac ICU patients. A decreased or an absence of rapid eye movement (REM) and the sleep pattern of these critical care populations are often characterized by prolonged sleep latency, increased sleep fragmentation, reduced sleep efficiency, and frequent arousals or awakenings [8, 10].

Despite the sophistication in technology and advancement in critical care knowledge, SPD remains a problem in the ICU. A recently completed unpublished study (2011, March) involving 42 adult cardiac surgery patients showed a significant change in their sleep patterns pre- and postoperatively. An increased sleep latency, fragmentation, and awakenings accompanied by a decrease in total nocturnal sleep time and sleep efficiency on postoperative days 1 through 5 when compared to baseline were found.

Time and again, the ICU patient's sleep becomes severely fragmented and unconsolidated, where it breaks up into small periods and free floats across the 24-h day. As a result, 50% of the ICU patient's "sleep" occurs during the daytime hours to supplement sleep loss [15, 16].The frequent napping (sleep supplementation) occurring during the day disrupts the patient's normal circadian rhythm, which has deleterious effects on the hypothalamic–pituitary function. Thus, amplification of stress, immune, and inflammatory function in an already altered homeostatic state ensues. The ICU patients' sleep characteristics described were corroborated by anecdotal and empirical evidence [10, 17] on the patient's overall hospitalization experience.

For example, one of the most common complaints among hospitalized patients is inability to maintain sleep, which is consistent with the findings that ICU patients perceive their sleep quality as generally poor and their sleep quantity (i.e., total sleep time) as typically shorter than community-dwelling patients [10].

Over the past three decades, critical care investigators have identified the etiology and predisposing factors of sleep disturbances in the ICU. The nature, predictors, consequences, and healthcare outcomes associated with SPD, however, are not clearly established [8, 10]. Likewise, the scientific knowledge on nonpharmacologic sleep-promoting interventions, like complementary and alternative medicine (CAM) or integrative therapies, is still in the formative stage of development. Scientists are constantly faced with methodological as well as measurement challenges in evaluating the effectiveness of any intervention due to the complexity of sleep [18]. Additionally, the physiologic instability of many critically ill patients, time constraints, cost, strong practice traditions, and the speculative attitudes among healthcare providers toward integrative therapies in general are deterrents to the advancement of science supporting the utilization and/or acceptance of integrative therapies in the ICU [8, 18]. Therefore, moving the current knowledge forward requires creative and thoughtful investigations on the efficacy and translation of the evidence to the bedside, paramount for improving patient care quality, satisfaction, and reducing cost.

State of the Science for Utilization of Integrative Therapies as Sleep-Promoting Interventions in the ICU

The latest synthesis of the research literature on the utilization of integrative therapies to promote sleep in the ICU was published in 2003 [13]. The types of therapies reported in the six studies evaluated in the integrated review included the use of music, melatonin, therapeutic touch, massage, and noise reduction (i.e., environmental manipulation) [19–24]. Subjects in these studies consisted of patients from different types of critical care units such as medical/surgical, coronary care, and cardiothoracic ICUs. Sample sizes ranged from 14 to 96 (median = 52.5) subjects, with 6 as smallest and 32 as largest number per group, in studies employing pretest/posttest ($n = 2$) and randomized controlled trial (RCT) designs ($n = 3$). The information of the research design of one study (pilot) is not clear. While the investigator of one study had utilized polysomnography in measuring sleep outcome variables, investigators of the five studies had relied on self-report measures with inconclusive results. The small sample sizes and methodological flaws (e.g., lack of randomization procedures) found in these studies are suggestive of low quality or poor evidence warranting more research.

However, despite the poor evidence on those integrative therapies tested in the ICU for sleep, Richards and colleagues [13], while acknowledging the existing deficit in the scientific merit of these modalities, asserted that such therapeutic modalities can be integrated into the nursing care delivery to improve the sleep quality and quantity outcomes of critically ill patients. The primary bases for their recommendations to implement integrative therapies cited in their review were the lack of adverse effects, and clinical significance, and the meaningful outcomes on patient care demonstrated by high levels of care satisfaction by patients.

Since the 2003 publication and up to this date, the body of knowledge in which the utilization of integrative therapies in the ICU is yet to be established, due in part to disagreement among investigators on the conceptualizations of integrative therapies (i.e., CAM). Also, many of the published intervention studies on the utilization of integrative therapies in the ICU were primarily focused on the reduction of pain and anxiety; less has been focused on sleep as a primary outcome measure. The mechanism by which these therapies (e.g., guided imagery, music, and massage) promote sleep has been attributed as a by-product (i.e., secondary outcome) of psychological supportive interventions [14]. Thus, the scientific advancement has become stagnant in this field, which is reflected in the paucity of published research articles, with the bulk of the publications having been printed in the late 1990s.

Mind–Body Practices

The mind–body therapies commonly cited as sleep-promoting interventions in critical care publications over the past two decades include music, massage, and therapeutic touch. Two RCTs [19, 22] have fairly strong evidence supporting music therapy and massage as safe and effective sleep-promoting interventions. In an RCT involving three groups of postoperative cardiac surgery patients, Zimmerman and colleagues [19] found better sleep scores ($p < 0.05$) reported by those patients who had used video music therapy when compared to (1) patients who had used music only ($n = 32$) and (2) patients who had a 30-min schedule of "undisturbed sleep" (controls, $n = 32$) during the second and third postoperative days.

Biologically Based Practices

Melatonin is secreted by the pineal gland with highest levels of secretion occurring during the dark period of the night. To date, melatonin is the only biologically based therapy that has been used for sleep promotion in the ICU. Decrements in the amount or changes in the timing and rhythm of endogenous melatonin can negatively impact sleep. While research has begun to emerge utilizing exogenous melatonin in small doses to promote sleep, there is paucity in the literature with respect to its use as a sleep-promoting agent in the ICU setting. In one study involving eight critically ill patients, Shilo and colleagues [20] administered melatonin to critically ill patients with chronic obstructive pulmonary disease (COPD). While the investigators found improvements in several parameters of sleep, the evidence is not sufficient to translate into practice due to the small sample size, methodological issues, and lack of clarity in the data as it was reported [20].

Manipulative and Body-Based Practices

Richards [22] tested the effects of effleurage back massage against relaxation techniques and implementation of rest periods (controls) on sleep efficiency, nonrapid and rapid eye movements, total sleep time, sleep latency, and wake after sleep onset in veteran patients with cardiovascular illnesses randomly assigned in one of the three groups in an ICU setting. The findings showed that patients who received the 6-min back massage ($n=24$) had 1 h longer sleep time ($p<0.05$) than patients who received the 7.5-min relaxation technique ($n=28$) and patients who received the 6-min rest period ($n=17$) at bedtime ($p>0.05$).

Energy Medicine

Therapeutic touch is another intervention that has shown potential promise in promoting sleep among ICU patients. Cox and Hayes [21] are the first and only authors that have published the utilization of therapeutic touch as sleep-promoting intervention on 53 subjects in a cardiac care unit (CCU) and ICU settings. Of the 53 patients, 55% ($n=29$) reported having to fall asleep immediately upon initiation or shortly after the session. Clearly, more work is needed to further establish the science underpinning the effectiveness of music, massage, and therapeutic touch on sleep among ICU patients.

It is worth noting that other forms of relaxation techniques like guided imagery (i.e., guided visualization) have gained some attention on its utilization in the ICU, specifically in postoperative cardiac surgical units. A recently published systematic review showed that when guided imagery is used in adult cardiac surgery patients, their anxiety and pain levels were reduced, enabling patients the propensity of falling asleep. Guided imagery with music [13, 14, 18] recorded on a portable device (i.e., MP3 player or iPod®) is a viable option that can be integrated in the routine care of the ICU patient. Guided imagery is defined as a "therapeutic process that facilitates working with the power of the imagination to positively affect the mental attitude and potentiate positive outcomes" [25]. The mechanism by which guided imagery utilization can promote sleep was based on its pain- and anxiety-reducing effects, somewhat similar to music therapy, resulting in a relaxed, positive state. By providing the person with a relaxed state in preparation for sleep, the brain naturally progresses through alpha and delta brain wave states [26, 27], thereby "creating the most conducive overall mind/body state for deep, natural sleep" [28]. However, this known mechanism has not been validated in the ICU setting.

Environmental Manipulation

Although manipulation of the patient care environment is not an integrative therapy per se, the nature of the ICU environment, lighting practices, and high noise levels have been known to significantly disrupt the patient sleep–wake pattern.

Environmental light is the strongest regulator of the circadian rest-activity rhythm. In most hospitals, unit lights are now routinely dimmed during the night hours to assist patients in maintaining regulation of their sleep–wake cycle. For example, Walder and colleagues [23] developed and successfully implemented a protocol designed to have staff dim lights during the night in the ICU. Contrary to what was hypothesized, results showed patients sleep to be more disturbed, with awakenings possibly being triggered by sudden and increased light levels required to conduct nighttime care activities [23]. Another environmental manipulation strategy is the use of "pleasant" sounds to block the noise of the ICU. In this context, a team of investigators [24] implemented a noise reduction protocol for the purposes of facilitating nocturnal sleep among cardiac surgery patients. One group was placed in a room with ocean sounds ($n = 30$) that was played throughout the night, and another group was placed in a room with white noise ($n = 30$) played throughout the night. Patients who listened to ocean sounds had better self-report sleep scores, fewer periods of awakenings, and fell asleep quicker ($p < 0.05$) than those patients who listened to the white noise.

Implications of the Evidence and Science for Practice

Within the limited body of literature that was reviewed and appraised, very few clinical trials have evaluated the feasibility, efficacy, and safety of mind–body, biologically based therapies, and environmental manipulations as sleep-promoting interventions in the ICU. The strength of evidence and quality of these studies are marginally weak and low, respectively [8, 13, 18]. Almost all of the studies were inadequately conceptualized, having small effect and sample sizes, and lack methodological rigor. Notably, the dosage and frequency, procedures employed in reducing the threat to internal validity, and overall fidelity of the interventions were not reported by the authors. Thus, the validity, generalizability, and transferability of the findings to clinical practice remain questionable.

Despite the formative stage of scientific knowledge development in this field, the recommendations by Richards and colleagues [13] should be accepted by the critical care community. Healthcare providers should continue to employ integrative therapies (music therapy, guided imagery, and relaxing massage) that have been shown to be safe and have demonstrated meaningful and clinically significant impact on improving sleep, care satisfaction, overall health, and well-being of the ICU patient. Collectively, these therapies may facilitate patient's sleep by diverting his/her attention to a more tranquil and positive state, thus allowing a patient to drift into a progressive, deep natural sleep [13, 14, 29]. Clearly, well-conceptualized and rigorous studies are needed to advance the science underpinning the utilization of integrative therapies as sleep-promoting interventions in the ICU. Future research must address the issues surrounding the validity of these published studies specifically on the sleep-promoting mechanism and overall treatment fidelity of a particular therapy to promote sleep for ICU patients.

Directions for Future Research

In order to establish a solid and scientific base of a particular integrative therapy, one must develop a clear and explicit conceptual framework for the study. Investigators should conceptualize their studies within the specific, known factors causing SPD in the ICU [2, 8, 10].Whether the intervention is designed to target a single or a set of variables comprising environmental and/or pathophysiological etiologic factors described previously, the proposed mechanisms by which a particular intervention is presumed to take effect must be thoughtfully delineated and tested. Pilot work directed at evaluating the feasibility and acceptability of a particular therapy should be considered essential preliminary groundwork that must be laid prior to undertaking a larger study. Pilot work is crucial to gathering estimates on the proportion of patients who are willing to "try" nontraditional therapies in their treatment plans, determining healthcare providers' nature and level of acceptance, as well as level of institutional support in integrating "integrative therapies" in the customary or standard of care. Through this process, investigators can also identify the appropriate dose (amount, frequency, duration, and timing) and mode of delivery that may confound, mediate, or moderate the outcome of a particular intervention. Finally, investigators can design the treatment fidelity plan, estimate the effect size, and resolve methodological issues essential for the success of a larger scale study. Thus, time, effort, and cost are not wasted. For example, a series of investigations should be implemented in testing the effect of guided imagery (i.e., visualization) on sleep quantity and quality of ICU patients. First, design study with emphasis on testing its mechanism of action on sleep, acceptability, and feasibility of integrating the intervention in the routine care of the patient. Next, a study designed to determine the appropriate dose and frequency of the intervention and critically examine confounders (e.g., pain, noise) prior to implementation of a larger scale research.

Unquestionably, the nature of the critically ill patient and the ICU environment are the two major challenges that any investigator must overcome. Investigators must be creative in navigating this fast-paced, technologically driven, and complex patient care environment to successfully implement a study, regardless of the type and sophistication of the research plan. More so, traditional care deliveries such as administering medications around the clock, ritualistic behaviors that are not supported by science such as the constant, and to some extent, excessive surveillance on monitoring, obtaining, and documenting physiologic parameters (e.g., vital signs and hemodynamic parameters), regardless of the patient's level of acuity, are probably the most significant factors that disrupt the continuity of a patient's sleep.

While there are no data to be used as a basis for changing the way in which patient care activities are delivered in the ICU at night, one should design an intervention study (using mind–body and/or biologically based practices) that can be integrated into the staff routine. One example might be an intervention that can be used to enhance sleep and prevent sleep disruption after midnight through noise and patient care activities. Although there have been reports on clustering patient care activities around wake hours [30], the validity of the results, and the mechanism in which "clustering care" promotes or improves the patient's sleep quality, quantity, efficiency, and sleep–wake/rest-activity pattern in general, are not known. Also, the findings on environmental manipulation such as light and sound regulations are inconclusive due to small sample size and lack of rigorous research methods. Although no study has been published on using earplugs as a noise reduction strategy, it is worth investigating its effect on sleep promotion in the ICU. The findings from a study involving six healthy individuals that were exposed to a simulated ICU noise showed significant reductions in REM latency and increased amounts of REM sleep than nonearplug wearers [31]. Clearly, the function of light and sound regulations, in the context of environmental manipulation, as sleep-promoting interventions in the ICU warrants more investigations.

Several environmental manipulation strategies have been successfully implemented by critical care nurses to reduce the prevalence of SPD in the ICU since 1980s. However, none of the strategies or interventions like noise reduction and light regulation has shown strong and high-quality evidence. Thus, the findings were not sufficient in reaching "policy level" mandating a change in the care delivery processes. While little is known about the effectiveness of these interventions, healthcare providers' frequent interruptions of patients at the peak of their nocturnal sleep are pervasive and remain a major problem [32]. Anecdotal evidence has shown that ICU staff performed these activities because it has been a "routine" and a "hospital policy" to obtain and record vital signs, administer medications during a specific time frame around the clock, turn patients every 2 h, completely bath, and record daily weights before 6:00 am. These ritualistic, scientifically baseless practices must be understood and reconciled first, before any sleep-promoting interventions can be effectively tested and implemented within the ICU.

With the current practices for patient care delivery in the ICU, investigators are confronted with challenges to modify the care delivery routines. However, one can find ways to infuse the intervention with the primary goal of improving patient sleep and allowing patients to have consolidated sleep instead of having their sleep interrupted at night. In this context, investigators should consider pursuing a program of research on integrating melatonin, relaxation techniques, and acupressure [13, 20, 33]. These selected modalities are a few that have shown reasonable acceptability by patients and staff and have potentially strong evidence that requires further investigations to establish a solid scientific ground.

Finally, investigators may also attempt to evaluate some emerging therapies like acupressure, which holds potential promise in improving sleep quantity and quality among diverse groups of non-ICU patients [33]. Acupressure is a viable therapy that may be successfully integrated in the current standard of care in the ICU. It is based on the concept of touch therapy, acupuncture, and traditional Chinese medicine [33, 34]. The same points of the body used in acupuncture are used in acupressure without inserting needles. Rather, the points are stimulated with finger pressure. This allows the brain to modulate the activity of certain chemicals such as serotonin, dopamine, and endogenous opioids that have been known to be sleep-promoting substances particularly in patients with chronic insomnia [33, 34]. However, its effect on "acute" insomnia as a symptom of sleep disruptions in the ICU (i.e., SPD) remains to be explored.

Summary and Conclusion

Over the past three decades, the prevalence of SPD in the ICU has been recognized, and its significant impact on patients' illness, recovery, and overall health had stimulated critical care investigators to study the phenomenon. Unfortunately, all of the integrative therapies that have been tested to promote patient's sleep in the ICU setting have failed to provide a cohesive scientific base. Investigators can facilitate the advancement of the science in this field through development and implementation of strategies outlined in the above "future directions" of research section.

The fact that the science in this field of inquiry has remained idle is due to a myriad of factors including, but not limited to, the complexity of investigating sleep in the ICU setting, strong practices that permeate care delivery processes at night, the skepticisms among healthcare providers in embracing integrative therapies in the ICU, and perhaps funding sources. Moreover, the causative relationships among the environmental, pathophysiological, and SPD with variables that predict, mediate, moderate, or confound the effects of interventions on sleep are not well understood. Therefore, identifying a conceptual framework congruent to the mechanism of action by which a particular intervention or group of interventions can improve ICU patients' sleep outcomes remains a challenging task for many investigators.

Despite these challenges, investigators have the opportunity to craft programs of research based upon well-conceptualized and methodologically rigorous studies, potentially filling the current gap that is now pervasive in the literature for so many of the integrative therapies, particularly those to enhance sleep in the ICU. Ensuring the feasibility, acceptability, practicality, and potentially achievable solid scientific ground is an excellent starting point to consider or develop within the research program. In this context, investigators should reevaluate the function and test the mechanisms of action of music, melatonin, guided imagery, ocean sounds, white noise, and earplugs and design a rigorous clinical trial on each therapy or combinations of two or more therapies.

Several therapies can be integrated in the current standard of care in the ICU; however, the weaknesses in the scientific foundation (e.g., therapeutic touch) [21] and most importantly, the costs associated with the intervention (e.g., massage [13] and acupressure) [33, 34] may add another layer of challenges for research implementation. For example, a trained therapeutic touch practitioner, certified massage therapist, and/or acupressurist are additional direct costs for the hospital, and the scope of practice as well as the legal implications of these emerging practitioners is yet to be delineated and determined in the acute or critical care settings. Finally, in order to adequately test the efficacy and achieve significant improvements in patient sleep outcomes through any type of integrative therapy in the ICU, the reduction or elimination of care interruptions during the peak hours of sleep at night must first be addressed. In conclusion, more work is needed to change nursing unit traditions, rituals, and policies to advance the science of integrating nontraditional therapies as sleep-promoting intervention in the ICU.

References

1. National Sleep Foundation 2010 Sleep in America poll. http://www.sleepfoundation.org/article/sleep-america-polls/2010-sleep-and-ethnicity. Accessed February 1, 2011.
2. Redeker NS. Sleep in acute care settings: an integrative review. J Nurs Scholarsh. 2000;32(1):31–8.
3. Cormier RE. Sleep disturbances. In: Walker HK, Hall WD, Hurst JW, editors. Clinical methods: the history, physical, and laboratory examinations. 3rd ed. Boston: Butterworths; 1990, Chapter 77.
4. Actiware and Actiware CT Software Manual. Bend: Respironics; 2008.
5. Verster JC, Pandi-Perumal SR, Streiner DL. Sleep and quality of life in clinical medicine. Totowa: Humana Press; 2008.
6. Aubert-Tulkens G, Culee C, Hartmant-Van Rijckevorsel K, et al. Ambulatory evaluation of sleep disturbance and therapeutic effects in sleep apnea syndrome by wrist activity monitoring. Am Rev Respir Dis. 1987;136(4):851–6.
7. Casida J, Davis JE, Brewer RM, et al. Sleep and daytime sleepiness of patients with left ventricular assist devices: a longitudinal pilot study. Prog Transplant. 2011; in press.
8. Friese RS. Sleep and recovery from critical illness and injury: a review of theory, current practice, and future directions. Crit Care Med. 2008;36(3):697–705.
9. Tracy MF, Lindquist R, Savik K, et al. Use of complementary and alternative therapies: a national survey of critical care nurses. Am J Crit Care. 2005;14(5):404–14.
10. Redeker NS. Challenges and opportunities associated with studying sleep in critically ill adults. AACN Adv Crit Care. 2008;19(2):178–85.
11. Cooper AB, Thornley KS, Young GB, Slutsky AS, Stewart TE, Hanly PJ. Sleep in critically ill patients requiring mechanical ventilation. Chest. 2000;117:809–18.
12. Parthasarathy S, Tobin MJ. Effect of ventilator mode on sleep quality in critically ill patients. Am J Respir Crit Care Med. 2002;166:1423–9.
13. Richards K, Nagel C, Markie M, Elwell J, Barone C. Use of complementary and alternative therapies to promote sleep in critically ill patients. Crit Care Nurs Clin North Am. 2003;15:329–40.
14. Papathanassoglou E. Psychological support and outcomes for ICU patients. Nurs Crit Care. 2010;15(3):118–28.
15. Rosenberg-Adamsen S, Kehlet H, Dodds C, Rosenberg J. Postoperative sleep Disturbances: mechanisms and clinical implications. Br J Anaesth. 1996;76:552–9.
16. Freedman NS, Gazendam J, Levan L, Pack AI, Schwab RJ. Abnormal sleep/wake cycles and the effect of environmental noise on sleep disruption in the intensive care unit. Am J Respir Crit Care Med. 2001;163:451–7.
17. Flaherty JH. Insomnia among hospitalized older persons. Clin Geriatr Med. 2008;24:51–67.
18. Casida J, Lemanski SA. An evidence-based review on guided imagery utilization in adult cardiac surgery. Clin Scholarsh Rev. 2010;3(1):22–30.
19. Zimmerman L, Nieveen J, Barnason S, Schmaderer M. The effects of music interventions on postoperative pain and sleep in coronary artery bypass graft (CABG) patients. Sch Inq Nurs Pract. 1996;10:153–70.
20. Shilo L, Dagan Y, Smorjik Y, Weinberg U, Dolev S, Komptel B, et al. Effect of melatonin on sleep quality of COPD intensive care patients: a pilot study. Chronobiol Int. 2000;17:71–6.
21. Cox C, Hayes J. Experiences of administering and receiving therapeutic touch in intensive care. Intensive Crit Care Nurs. 1999;15:283–7.
22. Richards KC. Effect of a back massage and relaxation intervention on sleep in critically ill patients. Am J Crit Care. 1998;7:288–99.
23. Walder B, Francioli D, Meyer JJ, Lancon M, Romand JA. Effects of guidelines implementation in a surgical intensive care unit to control nighttime light and noise levels. Crit Care Med. 2000;28:2242–7.

24. Williamson JW. The effects of ocean sounds on sleep after coronary artery bypass surgery. Am J Crit Care. 1992;1:91–7.
25. Ezra S, Reed T. Guided imagery and beyond. Colorado: Outskirts Press; 2008.
26. Reed T. Imagery in the clinical setting: a tool for healing. Nurs Clin North Am. 2007;42:261–77.
27. Restoring sleep through relaxation, guided imagery, and self-hypnosis. 2006. http://www.effective-life-skills.com/sleep/page01.htm. Accessed February 1, 2011.
28. Krieger D. Accepting your power to heal: the personal practice of therapeutic touch. Santa Fe: Bear & Company; 1996.
29. Ackley BJ, Swan BA, Ladwig GB, Tucker SJ. Evidence-based nursing care guidelines: medical-surgical interventions. St. Louis: Mosby; 2007.
30. Olson DM, Borel CO, Laskowitz DT, et al. Quiet time: a nursing intervention to promote sleep in neurocritical care units. Am J Crit Care. 2001;10(2):74–8.
31. Wallace CJ, Robins J, Alvord LS, Walker JM. The effect of earplugs on sleep measures during exposure to simulated intensive care unit noise. Am J Crit Care. 1999;8:210–9.
32. Tamburri LM, DiBrienza R, Zoula R, et al. Nocturnal care interactions with patients in critical care units. Am J Crit Care. 2004;13(2):102–12.
33. Sarris J, Byrne GJ. A systematic review of insomnia and complementary medicine. Sleep Med Rev. 2010. doi:10.1016/j.smrv.2010.04.001
34. Cabyoglu MT, Ergene N, Tan U. The mechanism of acupuncture and clinical applications. Int J Neurosci. 2006;116(2):364–86.

Chapter 11
Future Application of Integrative Therapies for Sepsis: Bench and Experimental Animal Models*

Haichao Wang, Andrew E. Sama, Mary F. Ward, Kathryn L. Miele, and Shu Zhu

Abstract Sepsis refers to a systemic inflammatory response syndrome resulting from a microbial infection and represents the leading cause of death in the intensive care unit. Current therapies for the treatment of sepsis are still largely supportive, with an anticoagulant agent—activated protein C—as the only Food and Drug Administration (FDA)-approved drug for patients with severe sepsis. In animal models of sepsis (induced by cecal ligation and puncture), a nonhistone nucleosomal protein termed "high-mobility group box-1" (HMGB1) has recently been established as a late mediator with a wider therapeutic window than early pro-inflammatory cytokines. The discovery of HMGB1 as a critical mediator of sepsis has initiated a new area of investigation involving the development of experimental therapies. Here, we briefly summarize evidence from bench research and experimental animal models that support integrative strategies, such as vagus nerve stimulation and herbal remedies, as potential therapies for the clinical management of human sepsis. It is important that clinicians be informed about this recent bench and animal research since new clinical interventions will be derived from this new information.

Keywords Experimental animal models • Sepsis • Endotoxemia • HMGB1 • Vagus nerve stimulation • Chinese medicinal herb • Alternative medicine • Innate immune cells

---

*Editor's Note: Xigris [dotrecogin alfa (activated)] was removed from the market on October 25, 2011 after this chapter was completed.

H. Wang, PhD (✉) • A.E. Sama, MD • M.F. Ward, MS, RN
• K.L. Miele, MA • S. Zhu, MD, PhD
Department of Emergency Medicine, North Shore University Hospital,
350 Community Drive, Manhasset, NY 11030, USA
e-mail: hwang@nshs.edu

L. Chlan and M.I. Hertz (eds.), *Integrative Therapies in Lung Health and Sleep*, Respiratory Medicine 4, DOI 10.1007/978-1-61779-579-4_11,

Overview

Following a microbial infection, the innate immune system mounts an immediate inflammatory response in an attempt to remove invading pathogens [1]. If effective, the infection-elicited inflammation resolves normally to restore immunologic homeostasis. Otherwise, exogenous pathogens and/or endogenous immune cell-derived pro-inflammatory mediators can leak into the blood stream, triggering a widespread systemic inflammatory response [1, 2]. Sepsis refers to this systemic inflammatory response syndrome resulting from a microbial infection. As a continuum of increasing clinical severity, sepsis can progress into severe sepsis, leading to the dysfunction of one or multiple organs. The incidence of sepsis is estimated to be on average 3.0 cases per 1,000 population [3], and is expected to increase by 1.5%, annually. If the occurrence of sepsis continues to increase at these rates, by the year 2020, there may be 1,110,000 cases in the USA alone. Despite recent advances in antibiotic therapy and intensive care, the overall mortality rate of sepsis remains high (28.6%) [3], claiming the lives of more than 215,000 people in the USA each year.

The purpose of this chapter is to inform clinicians about recent progress in bench and animal research that aims to develop integrative therapies for future treatment of human sepsis. The content of this chapter will focus on (1) the limitation of current available therapies for sepsis, (2) the experimental animal models employed to search for potential therapeutic targets, and (3) the efficacies of two integrative therapies (vagus nerve stimulation and herbal remedies) in preclinical setting. Possessing a basic understanding of the research on which clinical interventions are founded will help the clinicians to determine the best way to incorporate new therapies into their practice.

Current Therapies for Sepsis

Current therapies for sepsis are still largely supportive and limited to only a few clinical interventions, including broad-spectrum antibiotics, physiological doses of steroidal anti-inflammatory drugs (e.g., hydrocortisone), intensive insulin therapy to regain normoglycemia, early goal-directed therapies (EGDT) to allow for tight control of physiological parameters in order to optimize tissue oxygenation, and adjuvant therapy with an anticoagulant agent (e.g., activated protein C [APC]) (Table 11.1).

Antibiotics

As soon as the infecting agents are identified, appropriate broad-spectrum antibiotics are immediately administered to septic patients to facilitate elimination of invading pathogens [4]. However, antibiotic-mediated microbial disintegration can lead

Table 11.1 Available adjuvant therapies for sepsis

Category	Purpose
Broad-spectrum antibiotics	Antimicrobial
Low-dose steroidal drugs	Regain steroid balance
Insulin	Anti-hyperglycemia
Early goal directed therapy (EGDT)	Tight control of physiological parameters to optimize tissue oxygenation
Activated protein C[a]	Anticoagulant

[a]The only FDA-approved drug for patients with severe sepsis

to the release of microbial toxins (such as endotoxin or CpG-DNA), which may inadvertently amplify a potentially injurious inflammatory response by stimulating innate immune cells to produce more pro-inflammatory cytokines. Thus, other agents capable of attenuating an inflammatory response are needed for the adjuvant therapy of sepsis (Table 11.1).

Low-Dose Steroidal Drugs

At relatively lower doses, steroidal drugs (50 mg hydrocortisone and 50 μg oral fludrocortisone every 6 h for 7 days) have been shown to improve 28-day survival rates of septic patients, particularly those with adrenal insufficiency (i.e., poor endogenous responses to steroid-inducing hormones such as corticotrophin) [5]. However, a recent larger clinical trial did not reproduce the beneficial effect of intravenous hydrocortisone (50 mg every 6 h for 5 days), regardless of the septic patient's response or nonresponse to adrenal stimulation [6]. At higher doses, steroid therapy with methylprednisolone or dexamethasone might even be harmful to septic patients [7]. Thus, it remains unclear whether steroidal drugs are effective adjuvant therapies for sepsis [4].

Insulin

In critically ill patients, hyperglycemia frequently occurs and has long been perceived as a beneficial metabolic response to stress that ensures appropriate glucose supply to insulin-insensitive organs (such as the brain and the immune system) [1]. This notion was challenged by observations in two separate clinical trials in which tight blood glucose control with intensive insulin therapy significantly improved survival in critically ill septic patients [8, 9]. Unfortunately, the zeal for infusing intensive insulin has recently been tempered by the announcement of an unsuccessful multicentered clinical trial [10], which did not increase the 28-day survival rates. In fact, these clinical trials were interrupted early for safety concerns, raising questions about the therapeutic potential of insulin therapy for septic patients.

Early Goal-Directed Therapies

As a therapeutic strategy, EGDT is intended to tightly regulate a number of physiological parameters (such as mean arterial blood pressure, central venous pressure and oxygen saturation, and hematocrit) with discrete, protocol-driven interventions of crystalloid fluid, vasopressors, and blood transfusions. In a prospective clinical trial, it was shown that EGDT, combined with volume resuscitation, catecholamine therapy, and transfusions, reduced the mortality rates (from 46.5 to 30.5%) of patients with septic shock [11]. A large multicenter clinical trial, Protocolized Care for Early Septic Shock (ProCESS), is currently evaluating the therapeutic benefits of EGDT, which is difficult since this labor-intensive approach requires continuous staff commitment [12]. While the medical community waits for these results, there is still debate about the effectiveness of EGDT [13].

Activated Protein C

The systemic inflammatory response is integrally related to intravascular coagulation and endothelial activation. In a clinical study, intravenous infusion of an anticoagulation agent, APC (or drotrecogin alfa, continuously at 24 μg/kg/h for 96 h), reduced 28-day mortality rates from 30.8 to 24.7% [14]. Consequently, APC has become the first FDA-approved intervention for patients with severe sepsis, who are more likely to die if otherwise left untreated. In addition to its antithrombotic and profibrinolytic properties, APC also exhibits anti-inflammatory activities by inhibiting the release of pro-inflammatory mediators (e.g., TNF, MIF, MIP, and nitric oxide) from endotoxin-stimulated macrophages/monocytes [15–18]. Unfortunately, APC therapy is occasionally accompanied by an increased risk of hemorrhagic complication [14].

Experimental Models of Sepsis

Sepsis is routinely simulated in experimental animal models by several techniques, including infusion of exogenous bacterial toxin (endotoxemia), infusion of exogenous bacteria (bacteremia), and disruption of the host epithelial barrier to induce microbial translocation (using cecal ligation and puncture, or CLP). Each of these techniques has particular strengths and weaknesses with respect to their ability to mimic the clinical progression of human sepsis [19], although CLP is widely considered the most clinically relevant model to induce sepsis in animals (Table 11.2). It is important for clinicians to have a basic understanding of the models used to study sepsis so that they can adequately assess the research and the potential for human application.

Table 11.2 Experimental animal models of sepsis

Category	Purpose
Endotoxemia	Septic shock model to study the roles of various cytokines
Bacteremia	Investigating host response to a particular pathogen
Cecal ligation and puncture (CLP)	The most clinically relevant model for sepsis

Endotoxemia

Endotoxemia is induced in animals by infusion of known amounts of bacterial endotoxin such as lipopolysaccharide (LPS). Depending on the doses, LPS can induce transient/nonlethal or persistent/lethal hemodynamic cardiovascular responses. Thus, endotoxemia has generally been considered to be a model of septic shock [19] and is widely used to investigate the roles of various cytokines in lethal systemic inflammation (Table 11.2).

Bacteremia

Infusing an exogenous viable pathogen, typically bacteria, into animals induces bacteremia. Because different bacteria strains may induce distinct cytokine responses, this model is useful to study the host response to a particular pathogen. However, many exogenous bacteria may not colonize or replicate well in the host, and consequently, the doses of bacteria required to induce animal lethality may not mimic the typical host response to infection [19].

Cecal Ligation and Puncture

Sepsis is commonly induced by surgical perforation of the cecum, a technique known as CLP [19]. This procedure allows bacteria spillage and fecal contamination of the peritoneal cavity, mimicking the human clinical conditions of perforated appendicitis or diverticulitis. The severity of sepsis, as reflected by the eventual mortality rates, can be controlled surgically by varying the size of the needle used for cecal puncture. CLP in animals induces biphasic hemodynamic cardiovascular, metabolic, and immunological responses that are similar to those observed during the clinical course of human sepsis. Thus, the CLP model is considered the most clinically relevant model for experimental sepsis.

Pathogenesis of Experimental Sepsis

The pathogenesis of sepsis is complex and remains poorly understood. It is attributable to a dysregulated systemic inflammatory response that is partly mediated by innate immune cells (such as macrophages, monocytes, and neutrophils) (Fig. 11.1).

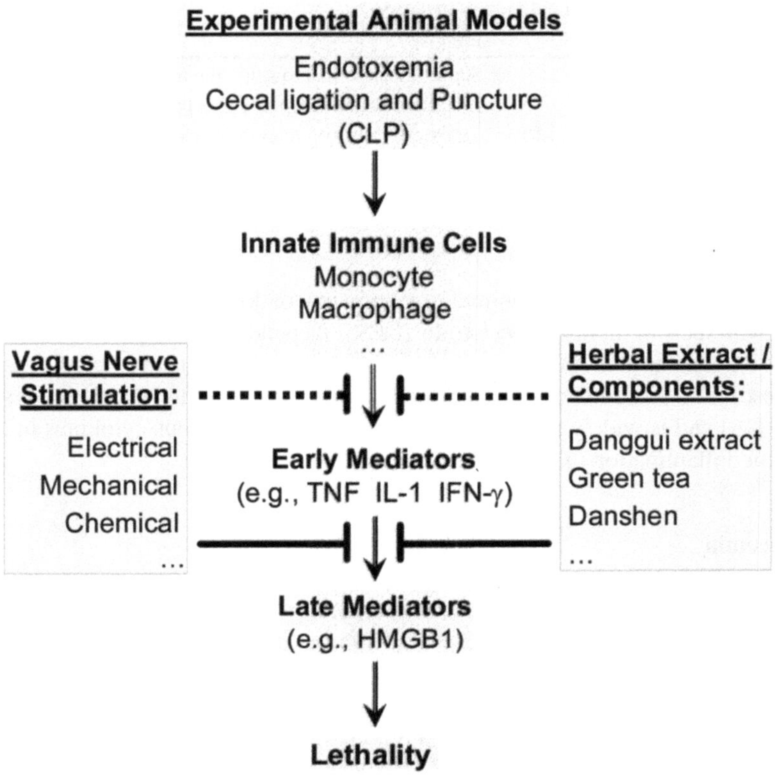

Fig. 11.1 Integrative therapies for sepsis. In response to lethal endotoxemia or sepsis (induced by CLP), innate immune cells sequentially release early and late pro-inflammatory mediators. However, animals typically succumb at latencies of up to 1–3 days, long after early pro-inflammatory cytokines (such as TNF) reach plateau levels in the circulation. In contrast, HMGB1 reaches peak levels in the circulation in a delayed fashion, which parallels with septic lethality, thereby providing HMGB1 with a wider therapeutic window. Although early cytokines may still be protective against experimental sepsis, late-acting pro-inflammatory mediators (such as HMGB1) contribute to the pathogenesis of sepsis by sustaining a rigorous and potentially injurious systemic inflammatory response. Integrative therapies such as vagus nerve stimulation and herbal remedies can be employed strategically in a delayed fashion to attenuate a late inflammatory response, thereby rescuing animals from lethal sepsis

Roles of Early Pro-inflammatory Cytokines

In addition to being able to ingest and eliminate invading pathogens, innate immune cells are also equipped with receptors for recognizing pathogen-associated molecular patterns (PAMPs)—molecules shared by a group of related microbes (such as the toll-like receptor, TLR2, TLR4, and TLR9) [20–22]. Engagement with various PAMPs (such as bacterial peptidoglycan, endotoxin, and CpG-DNA) enables innate immune cells to release a wide array of cytokines and chemokines [23–25].

Although an appropriate inflammatory response is required to defend against infection, uncontrolled systemic inflammation, caused by interaction with PAMPs or other agents, may be injurious to the host. Indeed, excessive accumulation of early pro-inflammatory cytokines, including TNF [26], interleukin (IL)-1 [27], and interferon (IFN)-γ [28], individually or together, contributes to the pathogenesis of lethal systemic inflammation. However, these early cytokines are difficult to target in a clinical setting, prompting a search for other late pro-inflammatory mediators that may offer a wider therapeutic window (Fig. 11.1).

Pathogenic Role of Late Pro-inflammatory Mediators

A decade ago, we and others discovered that a nonhistone nucleosomal protein termed high-mobility group box-1 (HMGB1) is released from activated innate immune cells in response to exogenous microbial products (such as endotoxin or CpG-DNA) [29, 30] or endogenous inflammatory stimuli (e.g., TNF, IFN-γ, or hydrogen peroxide) [29, 31, 32]. In murine models of endotoxemia and sepsis, HMGB1 is first detectable in the circulation 8 h after the onset of diseases, subsequently increasing to plateau levels between 16 and 32 h from the onset [29, 33]. This late appearance of circulating HMGB1 parallels the onset of animal lethality from endotoxemia or sepsis and distinguishes HMGB1 from TNF and other early pro-inflammatory cytokines [34].

Extracellular HMGB1 functions as a pro-inflammatory alarmin signal that stimulates the migration of immune cells (e.g., monocytes, dendritic cells, and neutrophils) [35–38], thereby facilitating recruitment of immune cells to infection sites. In addition, HMGB1 can bind and facilitate innate recognition of various bacterial products (e.g., CpG-DNA or LPS) by innate immune cells to ensure an effective inflammatory response [30, 39, 40]. Lastly, extracellular HMGB1 binds the receptor for advanced glycation end products (RAGE), as well as pattern-recognition receptors such as TLR2 and TLR4 [41, 42], and consequently, HMGB1 activates immune cells to produce pro-inflammatory cytokines, chemokines, and adhesion molecules [41–49].

The pathogenic role of HMGB1 as a late mediator of lethal systemic inflammation was first inferred from an observation that HMGB1-specific neutralizing antibodies conferred dose-dependent protection against lethal endotoxemia [29]. In a clinically relevant animal model of sepsis (induced by CLP), delayed administration of HMGB1-neutralizing antibodies, beginning 24 h *after* CLP, significantly rescued mice from lethality [33, 50]. Notably, the first dose of anti-HMGB1 antibodies was given 24 h after CLP, a time point when mice developed clear signs of sepsis, including lethargy, diarrhea, and piloerection. An increasing number of agents (e.g., ethyl pyruvate, stearoyl lysophosphatidylcholine, and anti-IFN-γ antibodies) have shown efficacy in inhibiting endotoxin-induced HMGB1 release and in protecting animals from lethal endotoxemia [29] and sepsis [33, 51]. Conversely, the administration of exogenous HMGB1 to mice recapitulates many clinical signs of sepsis, including fever [52], derangement of intestinal barrier function [53], and tissue injury [54–57].

Collectively, these experimental data establish extracellular HMGB1 as a critical late mediator of experimental sepsis with a wider therapeutic window than early pro-inflammatory cytokines (Fig. 11.1) [34, 58]. Thus, although early pro-inflammatory cytokines (such as TNF) may still be protective against infection [59], a dysregulated inflammatory response sustained by late-acting mediators (such as HMGB1) contributes to the pathogenesis of lethal sepsis [1, 2]. Therefore, agents capable of selectively attenuating systemic HMGB1 accumulation may hold potential in the treatment of sepsis.

Experimental Evidence for Integrative Therapies for Sepsis

The discovery of late-acting mediators has initiated a new area of investigation involving the development of integrative therapies for experimental sepsis. The following is a review of emerging evidence generated from using experimental models of sepsis in support of integrative strategies (such as vagus nerve stimulation and herbal remedies) as potential therapies for sepsis (Fig. 11.1).

Nerve Stimulation

Traditionally, electrotherapy is a strategy where electricity is used to stimulate muscles and nerves to release endogenous chemicals that cause the relief of pain and other inflammatory ailments. For instance, Benjamin Franklin successfully used electrotherapy to relieve his neighbor's intense shoulder pain in the 1700s [60]. Contemporary electrotherapy includes electroacupuncture (EA) and transcutaneous electrical nerve stimulation (TENS). EA is applied to the skin (at acupoints) through a pair of acupuncture needles attached to an electronic device that generates continuous electric pulses. TENS is applied via surface electrodes embedded in pads coated with electroconductive gel. Both are connected to a source of continuous electric pulses that cause an electrical current to travel towards the brain along specific nerve pathways.

In a rat model of CLP-induced sepsis, acupuncture at several acupoints (e.g., space between the vertebrate, surface of the ear tip, midline between anus and tail, and lumbosacral space) significantly elevated peritoneal neutrophil counts and reduced peritoneal bacterial load [61]. In animal models of carrageenan-induced joint edema, TENS attenuated inflammation-elicited musculoskeletal pain by activating endogenous opioid receptors [62, 63].

Originating in the brain, the vagus nerve travels through the body to major organs, including the heart, spleen, lungs, kidneys, liver, and digestive organs [64]. Recently, Dr. Kevin J. Tracey et al. discovered that the vagus nerve is instrumental to the central nervous system's modulation of a peripheral inflammatory response [65]. For instance, electrical stimulation of the vagus nerve prevented TNF release in animal

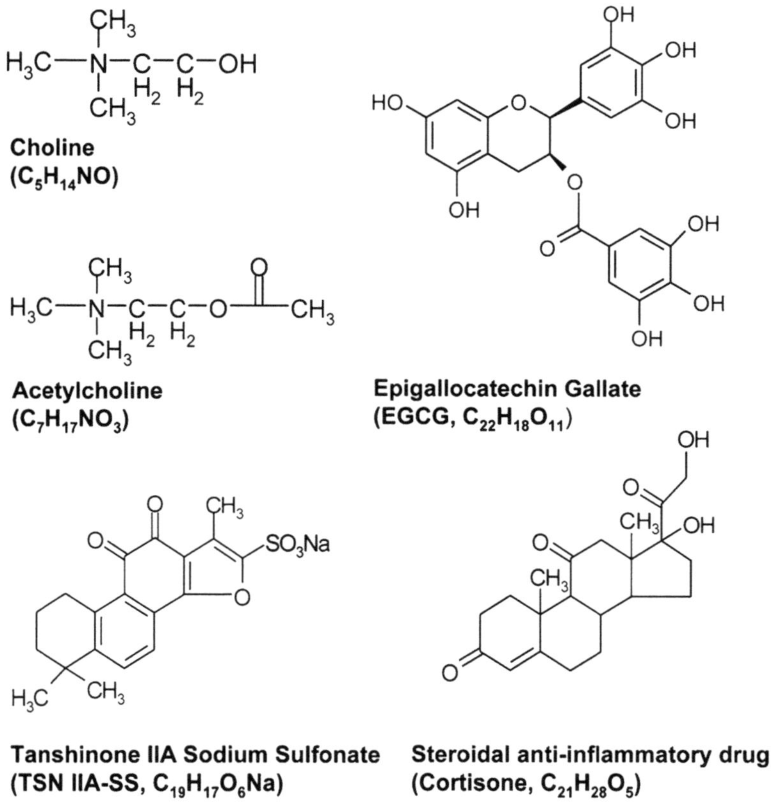

Fig. 11.2 Chemical structure of anti-inflammatory molecules. Acetylcholine is a neurotransmitter of both the central and peripheral nervous system, including the vagus nerve. EGCG is a major catechin of green tea, whereas TSNIIA is a major pigment of Danshen. Note that tanshinone IIA-SS is composed of four fused rings, and structurally similar to steroidal anti-inflammatory drugs, including cortisone

models of endotoxemia, whereas surgical vagotomy (e.g., resection of part of the vagus nerve) abolished electrical stimulation-mediated protective effects [65]. It is possible that electrical stimulation of the vagus nerve triggers release of a neurotransmitter called acetylcholine (Fig. 11.2), which binds to the alpha-7 nicotinic acetylcholine receptor (alpha-7 nAChR), thereby inhibiting cytokine release from activated macrophages [66]. Indeed, disruption of alpha-7 nAChR expression abolished acetylcholine-mediated cytokine inhibition and impaired electrical stimulation-mediated protection against lethal endotoxemia [66].

The vagus nerve can be stimulated by transcutaneous mechanical massage using a cotton-tipped applicator to apply alternating direct pressure perpendicularly and directly adjacent to the border of the trachea [67]. Intriguingly, this stimulation reduced serum HMGB1 levels and consequently improved survival in animal models of sepsis [67]. In addition to physical stimulation, a number of cholinergic chemical agonists have also been tested in experimental animal models of sepsis. Similarly, these cholinergic agonists (including nicotine, choline, GTS-21, and PHA568487) conferred protection against lethal endotoxemia, bacteremia, and sepsis, partly by attenuating systemic HMGB1 accumulation [51, 68–70].

Medicinal Herbal Therapies

Along with electrotherapy, traditional herbal medicine is the basis of folk remedies for various inflammatory ailments. The use of willow bark extract to reduce pain and fever was documented by a Greek physician (Hippocrates) in the fifth century BC; the subsequent discovery of salicylic acid as the pain/fever-relief active component gave rise to the first synthetic nonsteroidal anti-inflammatory drug (NSAID), aspirin. For many centuries, traditional Chinese herbal medicine has been used to treat various inflammatory diseases. To assess their therapeutic potential, the Feinstein Institute for Medical Research Laboratory of Emergency Medicine has screened a few dozen medicinal herbs for HMGB1-inhibiting properties in bench and animal models of sepsis. Among them, the aqueous extracts of Danggui (*Angelica sinensis*), Green tea (*Camellia sinensis*), and Danshen (*Saliva miltorrhiza*) efficiently inhibited endotoxin-induced HMGB1 release and protected animals against lethal endotoxemia and sepsis (Fig. 11.1) [71–74].

Danggui

Danggui (*A. sinensis*) has been regarded as the "ginseng" for women and, as such, is traditionally used to treat gynecological disorders including dysmenorrhea and hot flashes. After extracting Danggui root in hot water (85°C) for 4 h, the water-soluble fraction was fractionated by ultrafiltration using a Centriprep YM-10 Centrifugal Filter (with a defined molecular weight cutoff of 10 kDa). The low (<10 kDa) molecular weight fraction dose-dependently attenuated endotoxin-induced HMGB1 release in macrophage cultures [71]. In animal models of lethal endotoxemia, prophylactic administration of Danggui extract significantly attenuated systemic HMGB1 accumulation and increased the animal survival rate from 30 to 90% [71]. Furthermore, the delayed administration of herbal extract, beginning 24 h after CLP, significantly rescued mice from lethal sepsis.

Green Tea

Brewed from the leaves of *C. sinensis*, tea has been the most popular beverage for almost fifty centuries. Its popular consumption has been associated with health benefits enabling protection, to some degree, from oxidative stress [75], atherosclerosis [75], cancer [76], and cardiovascular diseases [77]. These healing properties are attributed to Green tea's abundance of polyphenolic catechins, such as

(−)-epigallocatechin-3-gallate (EGCG) (Fig. 11.2), (−)-epicatechin-3-gallate (EG), (−)-epigallocatechin (EGC), and (−)-epicatechin (EC). Among them, EGCG accounts for 50–80% of all of the catechins in a serving, which is approximately 50 mg in a single cup (100 mL) of green tea [78]. We and others found that EGCG effectively inhibited endotoxin-induced HMGB1 release in murine macrophages, with an estimated half maximal inhibitory concentration (IC_{50}) < 1.0 μM. Similarly, in primary cultures of human peripheral blood mononuclear cells, EGCG (15 μM) effectively abolished LPS-induced HMGB1 release, but only partly attenuated LPS-induced TNF secretion.

Prophylactic administration of EGCG in animal models of lethal endotoxemia led to a dose-dependent reduction of circulating HMGB1 levels and an increase in survival rates [73]. Since EGCG also inhibits LPS-induced TNF secretion [79], EGCG was strategically administered, thereby preserving a potentially beneficial early TNF response. Delayed administration of EGCG beginning 24 h post-CLP did not affect circulating levels of TNF but significantly attenuated systemic accumulation of HMGB1, as well as IL-6 and KC—two surrogate markers of lethal sepsis [73]. At a clinically feasible dose (4.0 mg/kg), EGCG significantly rescued animals from lethal sepsis, increasing animal survival rates from 53 to 82%.

Danshen

Among hundreds of Chinese medicinal herbs, only a few have been entitled "Shen," meaning medicinal herb (e.g., Ren Shen (*ginseng*) and Danshen (*S. miltiorrhiza*)). Danshen contains a substance of premier medicinal value (termed "Dan" or cinnabar) and has been widely used in China for patients with cardiovascular disorders [80, 81]. Its beneficial effects can be attributed to several red pigments, including tanshinone I, II, and IV, and cryptotanshinone [82], which exhibit anti-inflammatory properties by effectively inhibiting LPS-induced HMGB1 release (IC_{50}<25 μM). However, due to poor solubility and limited bioavailability, these tanshinones (12 mg/kg) failed to rescue mice from lethal sepsis, even after repeated administration at 24, 48, 72, and 96 h post the onset of sepsis, forcing the exploration of other water-soluble derivatives as potential therapeutic agents [72].

A water-soluble tanshinone IIA derivative, tanshinone IIA sodium sulfonate (TSNIIA-SS) (Fig. 11.2), dose-dependently inhibited endotoxin-induced HMGB1 release in macrophage/monocyte cultures. At the concentrations (e.g., 100 μM) that completely abrogated LPS-induced HMGB1 release, TSNIIA-SS merely partially blocked LPS-induced release of nitric oxide or TNF and yet still did not affect the secretion of most cytokines (such as IL-6, IL-12p40/p70, KC, MCP-1, MIP-1s, MIP-2, or TNF). This indicates the relative selectivity of TSNIIA-SS in the inhibition of HMGB1 over most other cytokines. Even when TSNIIA-SS was given several hours after LPS stimulation, HMGB1 release was still effectively blocked, which distinguishes TSNIIA-SS from other HMGB1 inhibitors (such as ethyl pyruvate, nicotine, and stearoyl lysophosphatidylcholine). These unique properties enable the strategic administration of TSNIIA-SS in a delayed fashion, which selectively attenuated systemic HMGB1 accumulation at a late stage of sepsis. Indeed, administration of TSNIIA-SS (15 mg/kg), beginning at +24 h post the onset of sepsis, rescued mice from lethal sepsis, significantly increasing animal survival rates from 33 to 73% [72]. Meanwhile, administration of TSNIIA-SS dose-dependently attenuated circulating HMGB1 levels [72], suggesting that TSNIIA-SS confers protection partly by inhibiting systemic HMGB1 accumulation.

TSNIIA-SS is approved in China as a drug for patients with cardiovascular disorders (such as heart attack), which encouraged the evaluation of whether it improves cardiovascular function in septic animals. In animal model of sepsis, rodents developed early hyperdynamic (around 5 h post-CLP) and late hypodynamic (between 20 and 24 h post-CLP) cardiovascular responses [83]. Notably, TSNIIA-SS dramatically reduced total peripheral vascular resistance, but significantly increased cardiac stroke volume and output in septic animals [72]. Taken together, these data indicate that TSNIIA-SS confers protection against sepsis-induced cardiovascular dysfunction and lethality in animal models of sepsis.

Other Herbs

A number of other herbs have also been tested in animal models of sepsis. For instance, a component of *Magnolia officinalis* called magnolol, promoted protection against lethal sepsis when given 6 h post onset of sepsis [84]. Similarly, a component of Cortex lycii, Kukoamine B (KB), attenuated LPS- and CpG-DNA-elicited activation of NF-kappa B in macrophages and conferred significant protection against lethal bacteremia [85]. Thus, the continued screening of medicinal herbs may lead to the discovery of potential integrative therapies for sepsis.

Implications of the Evidence and Science for Practice

At the bench, several animal models of sepsis have been employed to understand the pathogenesis of sepsis and to develop potential novel therapies. The clinical relevance of these models remains a subject of debate because it has been difficult to translate successful animal studies into clinical applications for sepsis [1]. For instance, although neutralizing antibodies against early cytokines (e.g., TNF) were protective in animal models of bacteremia/endotoxemia [26, 86], these agents all failed in clinical trials of sepsis [87–89]. This failure reflects partly on the complexity of the underlying pathogenic mechanisms of sepsis and partly on the heterogeneity of the patient population [4, 90]. In addition, the difficulty applying findings from animal models to clinical scenarios may also be attributable to pitfalls in the selection of feasible therapeutic targets or drugs, optimal doses and timing of drugs, and nonrealistic clinical outcome measures (such as mortality rates) [1].

However, the recent discovery of several HMGB1-targeting integrative therapies has potential implications for treating human sepsis. For instance, vagus nerve stimulation has been safely performed on patients with epilepsy and is expected to be beneficial for septic patients [67]. The stimulator used is designed to prevent seizures by sending regular, mild pulses of electrical energy to the brain via the vagus nerve and is known as a "pacemaker for the brain" [67]. It is placed under the skin on the chest wall and connected to the vagus nerve in the neck by an electrical wire [67]. Similarly, several herbal extracts and components, including Danggui, Green tea, and Danshen, may also hold potential as therapies for human sepsis. The doses of Danggui used in animal models of sepsis are comparable with the daily dosages (3–15 g/person) recommended for elderly people as a nutrient supplement [71]. Although the doses of EGCG given to septic mice (4 mg/kg, i.e., 10 μM) are higher than those readily available in a cup of green tea [91], purified EGCG is commercially available. Thus, an individual does not need to drink multiple cups of tea to enjoy the health benefits that green tea confers. Finally, TSNIIA-SS, a clinically approved drug for cardiovascular patients in China, also restored cardiovascular functions of septic animals by reducing total peripheral vascular resistance, while also significantly increasing both cardiac volume and cardiac output [72]. The dual effects of TSNIIA-SS in attenuating late inflammatory response and improving cardiovascular function make it a promising therapeutic agent for human sepsis.

Directions for Future Research

Extensive preclinical animal studies have established HMGB1 as an important mediator of experimental sepsis with a wider therapeutic window for future clinical intervention [29, 58, 92]. Recently, a number of integrative strategies (e.g., vagus nerve stimulation and herbal remedies) have been developed to attenuate late-acting pro-inflammatory mediators, resulting in animals being rescued from lethal sepsis. Important directions for future research include:

- Continuous animal studies to determine whether these integrative strategies, taken individually or in combination, influence the outcome of sepsis if given via clinically feasible (intravenous or oral) routes.
- Bench and animal studies to elucidate the mechanisms by which integrative strategies modulate host inflammatory response and protect animals from lethal sepsis.
- Clinical trials of selected integrative strategies to learn more about their efficacy in improving patient survival and to compare therapies.

A new formula of particular interest, termed "Xuebijing," which contains five Chinese herbs (including Danggui, Danshen, Honghua, Chuanxiong, and Chishao), is currently being tested in China as a potential therapy for human sepsis. The investigation of mechanisms underlying the pathogenesis of sepsis, as well as the mechanisms whereby integrative strategies improve animal survival, will likely lead to the discovery of novel integrative therapies for the clinical management of human sepsis.

Summary and Conclusions

The recent explosion of knowledge regarding the molecular pathogenesis of sepsis has led to the identification of late-acting pro-inflammatory mediators (such as HMGB1) of experimental sepsis that may offer a wide therapeutic window for future clinical intervention. This has led to the development of potential integrative therapies, ranging from vagus nerve stimulation to medicinal herbs, which rescued animals from lethal sepsis, even when these therapies were given in a delayed fashion. It is thus critically important to further elucidate the intricate mechanisms underlying the integrative therapy-mediated protection and to investigate their therapeutic potential of integrative therapies in future clinical studies.

Conflict of Interest

AES and HW are coinventors of patent applications related to HMGB1 inhibitors as potential therapeutic agents for sepsis.

Acknowledgments We thank Arvin Jundoria and Dr. Qiuping Zhou for critical reading of the manuscript. Work in authors' laboratory was supported by grants from the National Institutes of Health, National Institute of General Medical Science (R01GM063075), and the National Center of Complementary and Alternative Medicine (R01AT05076).

References

1. Wang H, Zhu S, Zhou R, et al. Therapeutic potential of HMGB1-targeting agents in sepsis. Expert Rev Mol Med. 2008;10:e32.
2. Wang H, Ward MF, Sama AE. Novel HMGB1-inhibiting therapeutic agents for experimental sepsis. Shock. 2009;32:348–57.
3. Angus DC, Linde-Zwirble WT, Lidicker J, et al. Epidemiology of severe sepsis in the United States: analysis of incidence, outcome, and associated costs of care. Crit Care Med. 2001; 29:1303–10.
4. Dellinger RP, Levy MM, Carlet JM, et al. Surviving sepsis campaign: international guidelines for management of severe sepsis and septic shock: 2008. Crit Care Med. 2008;36:296–327.
5. Annane D, Sebille V, Charpentier C, et al. Effect of treatment with low doses of hydrocortisone and fludrocortisone on mortality in patients with septic shock. JAMA. 2002;288:862–71.
6. Sprung CL, Annane D, Keh D, et al. Hydrocortisone therapy for patients with septic shock. N Engl J Med. 2008;358:111–24.
7. Lefering R, Neugebauer EA. Steroid controversy in sepsis and septic shock: a meta-analysis. Crit Care Med. 1995;23:1294–303.
8. Van den BG, Wouters P, Weekers F, et al. Intensive insulin therapy in the critically ill patients. N Engl J Med. 2001;345:1359–67.
9. Van den BG, Wilmer A, Hermans G, et al. Intensive insulin therapy in the medical ICU. N Engl J Med. 2006;354:449–61.
10. Brunkhorst FM, Engel C, Bloos F, et al. Intensive insulin therapy and pentastarch resuscitation in severe sepsis. N Engl J Med. 2008;358:125–39.
11. Rivers E, Nguyen B, Havstad S, et al. Early goal-directed therapy in the treatment of severe sepsis and septic shock. N Engl J Med. 2001;345:1368–77.
12. Sama AE, D'Amore J, Ward MF, et al. Bench to bedside: HMGB1-a novel proinflammatory cytokine and potential therapeutic target for septic patients in the emergency department. Acad Emerg Med. 2004;11:867–73.

13. Russell JA, Walley KR, Singer J, et al. Vasopressin versus norepinephrine infusion in patients with septic shock. N Engl J Med. 2008;358:877–87.
14. Bernard GR, Vincent JL, Laterre PF, et al. Efficacy and safety of recombinant human activated protein C for severe sepsis. N Engl J Med. 2001;344:699–709.
15. Schmidt-Supprian M, Murphy C, While B, et al. Activated protein C inhibits tumor necrosis factor and macrophage migration inhibitory factor production in monocytes. Eur Cytokine Netw. 2000;11:407–13.
16. Brueckmann M, Hoffmann U, De Rossi L, et al. Activated protein C inhibits the release of macrophage inflammatory protein-1-alpha from THP-1 cells and from human monocytes. Cytokine. 2004;26:106–13.
17. Gupta A, Rhodes GJ, Berg DT, et al. Activated protein C ameliorates LPS-induced acute kidney injury and downregulates renal INOS and angiotensin 2. Am J Physiol Renal Physiol. 2007;293:F245–54.
18. Cao C, Gao Y, Li Y, et al. The efficacy of activated protein C in murine endotoxemia is dependent on integrin CD11b. J Clin Invest. 2010;120:1971–80.
19. Wichterman KA, Baue AE, Chaudry IH. Sepsis and septic shock—a review of laboratory models and a proposal. J Surg Res. 1980;29:189–201.
20. Brightbill HD, Libraty DH, Krutzik SR, et al. Host defense mechanisms triggered by microbial lipoproteins through toll-like receptors. Science. 1999;285:732–6.
21. Poltorak A, He X, Smirnova I, et al. Defective LPS signaling in C3H/HeJ and C57BL/10ScCr mice: mutations in Tlr4 gene. Science. 1998;282:2085–8.
22. Hemmi H, Takeuchi O, Kawai T, et al. A Toll-like receptor recognizes bacterial DNA. Nature. 2000;408:740–5.
23. Akira S, Takeda K. Toll-like receptor signalling. Nat Rev Immunol. 2004;4:499–511.
24. Baggiolini M, Loetscher P. Chemokines in inflammation and immunity. Immunol Today. 2000;21:418–20.
25. Balkwill F. Cytokines—soluble factors in immune responses. Curr Opin Immunol. 1988;1:241–9.
26. Tracey KJ, Fong Y, Hesse DG, et al. Anti-cachectin/TNF monoclonal antibodies prevent septic shock during lethal bacteraemia. Nature. 1987;330:662–4.
27. Dinarello CA, Thompson RC. Blocking IL-1: interleukin 1 receptor antagonist in vivo and in vitro. Immunol Today. 1991;12:404–10.
28. Heinzel FP. The role of IFN-gamma in the pathology of experimental endotoxemia. J Immunol. 1990;145:2920–4.
29. Wang H, Bloom O, Zhang M, et al. HMG-1 as a late mediator of endotoxin lethality in mice. Science. 1999;285:248–51.
30. Ivanov S, Dragoi AM, Wang X, et al. A novel role for HMGB1 in TLR9-mediated inflammatory responses to CpG-DNA. Blood. 2007;110:1970–81.
31. Rendon-Mitchell B, Ochani M, Li J, et al. IFN-gamma induces high mobility group box 1 protein release partly through a TNF-dependent mechanism. J Immunol. 2003;170:3890–7.
32. Tang D, Shi Y, Kang R, et al. Hydrogen peroxide stimulates macrophages and monocytes to actively release HMGB1. J Leukoc Biol. 2007;81:741–7.
33. Yang H, Ochani M, Li J, et al. Reversing established sepsis with antagonists of endogenous high-mobility group box 1. Proc Natl Acad Sci USA. 2004;101:296–301.
34. Wang H, Yang H, Czura CJ, et al. HMGB1 as a late mediator of lethal systemic inflammation. Am J Respir Crit Care Med. 2001;164:1768–73.
35. Rouhiainen A, Kuja-Panula J, Wilkman E, et al. Regulation of monocyte migration by amphoterin (HMGB1). Blood. 2004;104:1174–82.
36. Yang D, Chen Q, Yang H, et al. High mobility group box-1 protein induces the migration and activation of human dendritic cells and acts as an alarmin. J Leukoc Biol. 2007;81:59–66.
37. Dumitriu IE, Bianchi ME, Bacci M, et al. The secretion of HMGB1 is required for the migration of maturing dendritic cells. J Leukoc Biol. 2007;81:84–91.
38. Orlova VV, Choi EY, Xie C, et al. A novel pathway of HMGB1-mediated inflammatory cell recruitment that requires Mac-1-integrin. EMBO J. 2007;26:1129–39.

39. Tian J, Avalos AM, Mao SY, et al. Toll-like receptor 9-dependent activation by DNA-containing immune complexes is mediated by HMGB1 and RAGE. Nat Immunol. 2007;8:487–96.
40. Silva E, Arcaroli J, He Q, et al. HMGB1 and LPS induce distinct patterns of gene expression and activation in neutrophils from patients with sepsis-induced acute lung injury. Intensive Care Med. 2007;33:1829–39.
41. Park JS, Svetkauskaite D, He Q, et al. Involvement of TLR 2 and TLR 4 in cellular activation by high mobility group box 1 protein (HMGB1). J Biol Chem. 2004;279:7370–7.
42. Yu M, Wang H, Ding A, et al. HMGB1 signals through toll-like receptor (TLR) 4 and TLR2. Shock. 2006;26:174–9.
43. Park JS, Gamboni-Robertson F, He Q, et al. High mobility group box 1 protein interacts with multiple toll-like receptors. Am J Physiol Cell Physiol. 2006;290:C917–24.
44. Kokkola R, Andersson A, Mullins G, et al. RAGE is the major receptor for the proinflammatory activity of HMGB1 in rodent macrophages. Scand J Immunol. 2005;61:1–9.
45. Pedrazzi M, Patrone M, Passalacqua M, et al. Selective proinflammatory activation of astrocytes by high-mobility group box 1 protein signaling. J Immunol. 2007;179:8525–32.
46. Yamoah K, Brebene A, Baliram R, et al. High-mobility group box proteins modulate tumor necrosis factor-alpha expression in osteoclastogenesis via a novel deoxyribonucleic acid sequence. Mol Endocrinol. 2008;22:1141–53.
47. Fiuza C, Bustin M, Talwar S, et al. Inflammation-promoting activity of HMGB1 on human microvascular endothelial cells. Blood. 2003;101:2652–60.
48. Treutiger CJ, Mullins GE, Johansson AS, et al. High mobility group 1 B-box mediates activation of human endothelium. J Intern Med. 2003;254:375–85.
49. Lv B, Wang H, Tang Y, et al. High-mobility group box 1 protein induces tissue factor expression in vascular endothelial cells via activation of NF-kappaB and Egr-1. Thromb Haemost. 2009;102:352–9.
50. Qin S, Wang H, Yuan R, et al. Role of HMGB1 in apoptosis-mediated sepsis lethality. J Exp Med. 2006;203:1637–42.
51. Wang H, Liao H, Ochani M, et al. Cholinergic agonists inhibit HMGB1 release and improve survival in experimental sepsis. Nat Med. 2004;10:1216–21.
52. O'Connor KA, Hansen MK, Rachal PC, et al. Further characterization of high mobility group box 1 (HMGB1) as a proinflammatory cytokine: central nervous system effects. Cytokine. 2003;24:254–65.
53. Sappington PL, Yang R, Yang H, et al. HMGB1 B box increases the permeability of Caco-2 enterocytic monolayers and impairs intestinal barrier function in mice. Gastroenterology. 2002;123:790–802.
54. Abraham E, Arcaroli J, Carmody A, et al. HMG-1 as a mediator of acute lung inflammation. J Immunol. 2000;165:2950–4.
55. Ueno H, Matsuda T, Hashimoto S, et al. Contributions of high mobility group box protein in experimental and clinical acute lung injury. Am J Respir Crit Care Med. 2004;170:1310–6.
56. Lin X, Yang H, Sakuragi T, et al. Alpha-chemokine receptor blockade reduces high mobility group box 1 protein-induced lung inflammation and injury and improves survival in sepsis. Am J Physiol Lung Cell Mol Physiol. 2005;289:L583–90.
57. Rowe SM, Jackson PL, Liu G, et al. Potential role of high mobility group box 1 in cystic fibrosis airway disease. Am J Respir Crit Care Med. 2008;178(8):822–31.
58. Wang H, Yang H, Tracey KJ. Extracellular role of HMGB1 in inflammation and sepsis. J Intern Med. 2004;255:320–31.
59. Eskandari MK, Bolgos G, Miller C, et al. Anti-tumor necrosis factor antibody therapy fails to prevent lethality after cecal ligation and puncture or endotoxemia. J Immunol. 1992;148: 2724–30.
60. Kahn J. Principles and practice of electrotherapy. 2nd ed. New York: Churchill Livingstone; 1991.
61. Scognamillo-Szabo MV, Bechara GH, Ferreira SH, et al. Effect of various acupuncture treatment protocols upon sepsis in Wistar rats. Ann N Y Acad Sci. 2004;1026:251–6.

62. Ainsworth L, Budelier K, Clinesmith M, et al. Transcutaneous electrical nerve stimulation (TENS) reduces chronic hyperalgesia induced by muscle inflammation. Pain. 2006;120:182–7.
63. Vance CG, Radhakrishnan R, Skyba DA, et al. Transcutaneous electrical nerve stimulation at both high and low frequencies reduces primary hyperalgesia in rats with joint inflammation in a time-dependent manner. Phys Ther. 2007;87:44–51.
64. Rosas-Ballina M, Ochani M, Parrish WR, et al. Splenic nerve is required for cholinergic anti-inflammatory pathway control of TNF in endotoxemia. Proc Natl Acad Sci USA. 2008;105: 11008–13.
65. Borovikova LV, Ivanova S, Zhang M, et al. Vagus nerve stimulation attenuates the systemic inflammatory response to endotoxin. Nature. 2000;405:458–62.
66. Wang H, Yu M, Ochani M, et al. Nicotinic acetylcholine receptor alpha7 subunit is an essential regulator of inflammation. Nature. 2003;421:384–8.
67. Huston JM, Gallowitsch-Puerta M, Ochani M, et al. Transcutaneous vagus nerve stimulation reduces serum high mobility group box 1 levels and improves survival in murine sepsis. Crit Care Med. 2007;35:2762–8.
68. Pavlov VA, Ochani M, Yang LH, et al. Selective alpha7-nicotinic acetylcholine receptor agonist GTS-21 improves survival in murine endotoxemia and severe sepsis. Crit Care Med. 2007;35:1139–44.
69. Parrish WR, Rosas-Ballina M, Gallowitsch-Puerta M, et al. Modulation of TNF release by choline requires alpha7 subunit nicotinic acetylcholine receptor-mediated signaling. Mol Med. 2008;14:567–74.
70. Su X, Matthay MA, Malik AB. Requisite role of the cholinergic alpha7 nicotinic acetylcholine receptor pathway in suppressing Gram-negative sepsis-induced acute lung inflammatory injury. J Immunol. 2010;184:401–10.
71. Wang H, Li W, Li J, et al. The aqueous extract of a popular herbal nutrient supplement, *Angelica sinensis*, protects mice against lethal endotoxemia and sepsis. J Nutr. 2006;136: 360–5.
72. Li W, Li J, Ashok M, et al. A cardiovascular drug rescues mice from lethal sepsis by selectively attenuating a late-acting proinflammatory mediator, high mobility group box 1. J Immunol. 2007;178:3856–64.
73. Li W, Ashok M, Li J, et al. A major ingredient of green tea rescues mice from lethal sepsis partly by inhibiting HMGB1. PLoS One. 2007;2:e1153.
74. Zhu S, Li W, Li J, et al. Caging a beast in the inflammation arena: use of Chinese medicinal herbs to inhibit a late mediator of lethal sepsis, HMGB1. Int J Clin Exp Med. 2008;1:64–79.
75. Frei B, Higdon JV. Antioxidant activity of tea polyphenols in vivo: evidence from animal studies. J Nutr. 2003;133:3275S–84.
76. Crespy V, Williamson G. A review of the health effects of green tea catechins in in vivo animal models. J Nutr. 2004;134:3431S–40.
77. Vita JA. Tea consumption and cardiovascular disease: effects on endothelial function. J Nutr. 2003;133:3293S–7.
78. Graham HN. Green tea composition, consumption, and polyphenol chemistry. Prev Med. 1992;21:334–50.
79. Wheeler DS, Lahni PM, Hake PW, et al. The green tea polyphenol epigallocatechin-3-gallate improves systemic hemodynamics and survival in rodent models of polymicrobial sepsis. Shock. 2007;28:353–9.
80. Ji XY, Tan BK, Zhu YZ. Salvia miltiorrhiza and ischemic diseases. Acta Pharmacol Sin. 2000;21:1089–94.
81. Cheng TO. Cardiovascular effects of Danshen. Int J Cardiol. 2007;121:9–22.
82. Wu TW, Zeng LH, Fung KP, et al. Effect of sodium tanshinone IIA sulfonate in the rabbit myocardium and on human cardiomyocytes and vascular endothelial cells. Biochem Pharmacol. 1993;46:2327–32.
83. Yang S, Chung CS, Ayala A, et al. Differential alterations in cardiovascular responses during the progression of polymicrobial sepsis in the mouse. Shock. 2002;17:55–60.

84. Kong CW, Tsai K, Chin JH, et al. Magnolol attenuates peroxidative damage and improves survival of rats with sepsis. Shock. 2000;13:24–8.
85. Liu X, Zheng X, Long Y, et al. Dual targets guided screening and isolation of Kukoamine B as a novel natural anti-sepsis agent from traditional Chinese herb *Cortex lycii*. Int Immunopharmacol. 2011;11(1):110–20.
86. Beutler B, Milsark IW, Cerami AC. Passive immunization against cachectin/tumor necrosis factor protects mice from lethal effect of endotoxin. Science. 1985;229:869–71.
87. Ziegler EJ, Fisher Jr CJ, Sprung CL, et al. Treatment of gram-negative bacteremia and septic shock with HA-1A human monoclonal antibody against endotoxin. A randomized, double-blind, placebo-controlled trial. The HA-1A Sepsis Study Group. N Engl J Med. 1991;324: 429–36.
88. Ziegler EJ, McCutchan JA, Fierer J, et al. Treatment of gram-negative bacteremia and shock with human antiserum to a mutant *Escherichia coli*. N Engl J Med. 1982;307:1225–30.
89. Abraham E, Wunderink R, Silverman H, et al. Efficacy and safety of monoclonal antibody to human tumor necrosis factor alpha in patients with sepsis syndrome. A randomized, controlled, double-blind, multicenter clinical trial. TNF-alpha MAb Sepsis Study Group. JAMA. 1995;273:934–41.
90. Cohen J. Adjunctive therapy in sepsis: a critical analysis of the clinical trial programme. Br Med Bull. 1999;55:212–25.
91. Yang CS, Chen L, Lee MJ, et al. Blood and urine levels of tea catechins after ingestion of different amounts of green tea by human volunteers. Cancer Epidemiol Biomarkers Prev. 1998;7:351–4.
92. Mantell LL, Parrish WR, Ulloa L. Hmgb-1 as a therapeutic target for infectious and inflammatory disorders. Shock. 2006;25:4–11.

Chapter 12
Integrative Therapies to Manage Acute and Chronic Sleep Disorders

Margaret-Ann Carno

Abstract Integrative therapies have been used in treatment of sleep disorders though some of the evidence is lacking. This chapter will first briefly discuss what sleep is. Impact of sleep on daily life and discussion of reports of the number of sleep complaints will then be presented. The most common sleep disorder treated with integrative therapies, insomnia, will then be discussed in detail. Following the discussion on insomnia, different types of integrative therapies such as mind–body practices, herbal supplements, and manipulative practices will be presented along with supporting evidence of use. Finally, the chapter will move to sections on implications of the evidence and science for practice and directions for future research.

Keywords Sleep • Sleep disorders • Insomnia • Sleep complaints • Integrative therapies in sleep medicine

Introduction

Sleep

Sleep is a necessary biological process that has a restorative function. During sleep, certain hormones are produced and released to assist in cellular repair. Also during sleep, memory is consolidated and memories are moved from "short-term" to "long-term" storage. There are two basic stages of sleep: nonrapid eye movement sleep (NREM) and rapid eye movement (REM) sleep. During NREM sleep, the body is

M.-A. Carno, PhD, MBA, CPNP, DABSM, FNAP (✉)
School of Nursing, University of Rochester, 601 Elmwood Ave., Box 5ON, Rochester, NY 14642, USA
e-mail: margaret_carno@urmc.rochester.edu

L. Chlan and M.I. Hertz (eds.), *Integrative Therapies in Lung Health and Sleep*, Respiratory Medicine 4, DOI 10.1007/978-1-61779-579-4_12,

Table 12.1 Common sleep terms used in research and clinical practice

Sleep term	Definition
Sleep latency	How long it takes a person to fall asleep
Sleep onset	The time that sleep begins
Sleep offset	The time that sleep ends
Sleep efficiency	The percentage of time that the person slept while in bed
Wake after sleep onset (WASO)	The amount of time that the person is awake after the person falls asleep

in a state of repair and growth. During REM, it is thought that memories (both emotional and learning) are moved from short- to long-term storage in the brain.

Sleep can be measured in a number of different ways. Objective measures of sleep include polysomnography which uses electroencephalography and actigraphy which is a small watch-like device that is worn on the body and measures rest and activity. Sleep can also be assessed through sleep diaries/logs where the person writes down what time he or she fell asleep and awoke and standardized sleep questionnaires. Table 12.1 lists commonly used terms in sleep research and clinical practice.

This chapter will primarily focus on the sleep diagnosis of insomnia as this is the diagnosis with the most evidence of use of integrative therapies. There are very limited reports using different integrative therapies for restless leg syndrome. Finally, the use of integrative therapies is so sparse in obstructive sleep apnea (OSA) that there is only one study examining the use of integrative therapies for OSA.

Insomnia

The most common sleep complaint where integrative therapies are used is in the treatment of insomnia. Insomnia is classified by the DSM-IV as the complaint of difficulty falling asleep, frequent or prolonged awakenings, inadequate sleep quality, or short overall sleep duration in an individual who has adequate time available for sleep. Insomnia is not defined by polysomnography or a specific sleep duration. Because insomnia occurs only when there is adequate opportunity for sleep, it must be distinguished from sleep deprivation, in which the individual has relatively normal sleep ability but inadequate opportunity for sleep [1]. Within the classification of insomnia, there are different subtypes. Acute (short-term) insomnia is defined as insomnia that lasts for only a few weeks, and the cause is usually known [2]. Chronic insomnia is defined as occurring for 30 days or more of the symptoms [3]. Insomnia can be classified by either its specific symptoms (sleep onset difficulties or sleep maintenance difficulties) or by the duration of the symptoms (acute vs. chronic) [7]. Both classifications are seen in the literature and in some research studies are not distinguished. Insomnia is usually diagnosed by patient report (general and the use of sleep diaries) along with the objective measure of actigraphy. Actigraphy provides objective information about rest and activity which then can be extrapolated into sleep/wake cycles.

Sleep complaints are one of the leading healthcare concerns across the globe today. In 2005, the National Sleep Foundation published results from a pool of Americans which demonstrated that 75% of those surveyed reported at least one sleep problem a few nights a week or more. Fifty-four percent reported at least one symptom of insomnia at least a few nights a week (primarily awakening unrefreshed; 21% report problems falling asleep at least a few nights a week). Thirty-two percent responded that they snore at least three nights a week, and 15% responded that they have unpleasant sensations in their legs at least three nights a week; in 65% of those that have unpleasant sensations in their legs, it is worse during the night than during the daytime [4].

Some patients find integrative therapies hold relief from these different sleep complaints. According to 2007 National Health Interview Survey (NHIS), 1.4% of the participant stated that they used integrative therapies to assist with sleep [5]. The 2002 data from the NHIS demonstrated that 17.4% of all participants stated that they had trouble sleeping in the past 12 months, and of those participants with insomnia, 4.5% used some form of integrative therapy to treat their symptoms. This number is a staggering 1.6 million adults [6]. 64.8% primarily used biological/herbal therapies, and 39.1% used mind/body relaxation therapies. Most reported that they found these therapies useful [6]. The reasons expressed as why those who were surveyed used integrative therapies were conventional treatments were not helpful (40.7%), conventional therapies were too expensive (24.8%), combined with conventional treatments (63.8%), conventional medical professional suggested (35.2%), and thought it would be interesting to try (66.6%) [7]. (Since the respondents could select more than one reason, the total percentages add up to more than 100%.) Unfortunately, the science behind these therapies has not kept up with the number of people who use them. The purpose of this chapter is to discuss the evidence behind currently used integrative therapies in the treatment of selected sleep disorders commonly experienced by adults and children.

State of the Science/Evidence on Integrative Therapies to Treat or Manage Sleep Issues

To locate available evidence (literature) related to integrative therapies and sleep, PubMed, Ovid, and CINHAL were searched from years 1999 to early 2011. The terms included were sleep, integrative therapies, and complementary and alternative medicine and were limited to the English language. From there, the search was limited to research/humans. Also a Google Scholar search was conducted as a double check to assess the completeness of the search.

Mind–Body Practices

One of the common findings in patients with insomnia is higher states of arousal and higher perceived stress levels. Mindfulness-based stress reduction is one way to decrease stress levels and states of arousals with the goal of improving sleep. Mindfulness-based stress reduction is a formalized intervention based on Buddhist philosophy and developed at the University of Massachusetts Medical Center [8]. It is a psychoeducational, skills-based program that is usually run over 8 weeks. Different meditation techniques are presented and practiced including body-scan medication, sitting meditation, walking meditation, and mindful Hatha yoga [8]. This mind–body practice has been the intervention in a few research studies where the goal was to decrease insomnia and improve sleep in the participants. The most scientifically rigorous of these studies from a sleep prospective was published in 2006. Sixteen subjects were enrolled from a clinical sleep medicine practice in an uncontrolled clinical trial pre-post test design. The study consisted of 8 weekly sessions of 120 min each that provided the subjects with information and practice time on such topics as sitting meditation, "body scan," and walking meditation as well as cognitive treatment elements for insomnia. Participants were to practice at home, but amount of time was not specified. The subjects reported a significant increase in total sleep time of 64 min and a decrease in sleep onset of 4 min along with decreased worry and stress [9].

Very little data is available concerning the use of yoga as a therapy for insomnia in a healthy population. One published study examined sleep quality using the Pittsburgh Sleep Quality Index (PSQI) in practitioners of yoga. There were 16 subjects in the group who practiced long-term yoga (practicing regularly for at least 3 years) and were compared to a control group of ten subjects recruited from the community. There were no statistical differences between groups. Neither group reported sleep disturbances, but those who practiced yoga on a regular basis had a significantly lower (meaning better) sleep quality than the control group [10].

Yoga has been used in a pilot treatment program for chronic insomnia. Twenty subjects completed an either week intervention protocol and were instructed in a series of yoga breathing patterns and simple positions to be done at home right before bedtime. Two weeks of pretreatment sleep diaries were collected and during the 8-week treatment phase. Total sleep time and sleep efficiency significantly improved ($p<0.05$), and sleep latency onset and wake after sleep onset all significantly decreased ($p<0.05$) after the either week intervention. There were no reports of difficulties, but the original sample had a 33% dropout rate (13 out of 40 subjects) with the majority of dropouts related to time commitment [11].

Music therapy has little information as a treatment for sleep disturbances. Harmat et al. reported that listening to classical music improved sleep quality as measured on the PSQI in students with self-reported poor sleep when compared to students who listened to audiobooks or a control group. Ninety-six participants were randomized to one of the three conditions and then followed for 3 weeks. The PSQI was completed at baseline (before randomization) and then once a week for the 3 weeks. The music and the audiobooks were selected in advance by the researchers, and the subjects were asked to listen for 45 min before going to bed. The control group was asked not to listen to music before going to bed and was not given any other specific instructions. Listening to music produced significantly longer sleep duration, better sleep efficiency, and shorter sleep latency when compared to either group. The audiobook group demonstrated no significant differences when compared to the control group [12].

Music for relaxation has also been shown in a small study to improve sleep in older persons with insomnia [13]. Fifteen participants took part in the study; all of whom had long-standing insomnia and seven who were on sleep-inducing medications. All subjects spent the first week without any intervention and only completed required surveys. The subjects were then randomly divided into two groups: music relaxation and progressive muscle relaxation. Those in the music relaxation group were provided a compact disk or cassette tape of slow melody piano music which lasted for 40 min before going to bed. Those in the progressive muscle relaxation group were provided a compact disk or cassette tape with recorded instructions in a male voice for muscle relaxation that had a duration of 40 min and was to be completed before going to bed. There was no music on the progressive muscle relaxation recording. After 1 week of the assigned relaxation technique, all subjects were crossed over into the other respective group (e.g., music group now received the muscle relaxation recording). Measures of sleep included two questionnaires and actigraphy to objectively monitor sleep. Music relaxation was shown to improve sleep efficiency ($p < 0.05$) independent of order of group assignment [13].

While all of these studies seem to indicate that music improves sleep quality, both studies are small in sample size and/or did not have control groups to assess whether the subjects did listen to the intervention. Assessment of sleep was strengthened by the use of an objective measure of sleep (actigraphy). Interestingly, music has not been shown to improve sleep quality and other objective measures of sleep on overnight polysomnography. Lazic and Ogilvie enrolled ten female subjects in a study that examined objective (polysomnography) measures of sleep. The subjects spent a total of four nights in the sleep lab and were presented with the following: no sounds, "soothing music" (not described in article), or soft audio tones from lights out until 5 min of continuous sleep. The subjects reported that the music was significantly more relaxing than the audio tones or no sound at all. There was no statistical difference in sleep latency, sleep efficiency, wake after sleep onset, or the different sleep stages [14]. While there are no side effects and very little cost to the use of music to improve sleep, further research is needed to assess the efficacy of the therapy.

Biologically Based Practices

Integrative therapies that are biologically based have frequently been used to self-manage insomnia. While there are a number of herbs or other biologically based practices that have been used, only a small number of these have been found to be safe, and an even smaller number have demonstrated usefulness as a treatment.

This section will focus only on those biologically based therapies that have been shown to be safe as per published literature which was summarized by the American Academy of Sleep Medicine [15] and put forth in a review article. Thus, hops, lemon balm (no safety data available), kava kava (can induce severe liver toxicity), wild lettuce (hallucinogenic), skull cap (can cause seizure activity), and patrinia root (frequent nausea) will not be discussed as per the American Academy of Sleep Medicine [15].

Melatonin

Melatonin is one of the most commonly used biologically based integrative therapies for sleep issues such as insomnia. In humans, melatonin is produced in the pineal gland driven by input from the suprachiasmatic nuclei which receives input from the retinohypothalamic tract [16]. The major regulator of melatonin production is light/dark cycles that the organism lives in [16]. For humans, melatonin is produced when it is dark. The pineal gland does not store melatonin (*N*-acetyl-5-methoxytryptamine); rather, it is excreted as soon as it is produced [16]. Commercially available melatonin may be isolated from the pineal glands of beef cattle or chemically synthesized [17].

Melatonin acts on its own receptors in the brain. When given before bedtime (about 30 min before), it can induce sleep. Multiple studies across a wide number of patient populations have demonstrated reduced sleep latency, improved sleep efficiency, and increased total sleep time [18]. In pooling the 15 studies examined, Brzezinski calculated that the sleep latency decreased by 3.9 min (95% CI 2.5, 5.4), sleep efficiency by 3.1% (95% CI 0.7, 5.5), and total sleep time by 13.7 min (95% CI 3.1, 24.3) [19]. These studies used polysomnography and actigraphy to assess sleep parameters. The majority (14) used either a crossover design or a Latin squares design. There was a mixture of participants between studies as some enrolled only healthy volunteers while others included those suffering from insomnia. Dosages ranged from 0.1 to 5 mg of melatonin, and not all studies included a placebo control. Finally, the length of treatment varied from 1 to 4 weeks of treatment. While these are modest changes clinically, subjects reported perceived improvement in sleep. Buscemi and colleagues reported in their systematic review that the changes in sleep duration and sleep onset latency were not statistically significant [19]. Differences between these two reviews could be due to inclusion of different studies and participants, data extraction methods, and methods by which the data were analyzed. Brzezinski and colleagues only searched one database (Medline 1980–2003) whereas Buscemi and colleagues searched 13 electronic databases from 1999 to early 2004 and hand searched abstracts from the Associated Professional Sleep Society from 1999 to 2003. Both reviews did state that the side effects/adverse effects from melatonin were rare. The melatonin preparation and dosage varied among all the studies included in the systematic reviews.

In children with chronic insomnia, melatonin demonstrated improved sleep. Smits and colleagues enrolled 62 children from 6 to 12 years of age who had suffered from idiopathic insomnia for at least 1 year. Subjects were enrolled, completed sleep diaries along with functional health status questionnaires for 1 week, and then were randomized to receive either placebo or 5 mg of melatonin at 7 pm for 4 weeks. Sleep onset was significantly advanced (e.g., fell asleep earlier) by 57 min, sleep latency by 17 min, and increase in the time that the child awoke by 9 min when compared to placebo [20]. Side effects of melatonin are rare, but there is a concern about inducing precocious puberty in children given melatonin, and then the melatonin is withdrawn [21].

Melatonin can also be used for the treatment of Delayed Sleep Phase Syndrome (DSPS) [22]. DSPS is a condition where an individual can have sleep onset insomnia and also extreme difficulty arising when they attempt to conform with socially acceptable activities (e.g., going to work or school) [22]. If melatonin is given at the time the person wishes to fall asleep over a number of days, then eventually the body will be able to initiate sleep at that time. This process though takes a number of days to weeks. Also in some patients, the sleep time can revert back to the later sleep time once the melatonin is stopped [22].

Valerian

Valerian is derived from plants of the species *Valeriana* [15]. Several randomized control trials have used valerian (in different preparations) as a treatment for insomnia. For example, in 2000, Doth and colleagues examined 16 healthy subjects with insomnia and then randomized them to receive either 600 mg of valerian at nighttime or placebo for 14 days and used a visual analogue scale to assess improvement in insomnia. Ten percent of the valerian group reported improvement in sleep while 15% of the placebo group reported improved sleep [23]. In 2004, Diaper and colleagues examine two different doses of valerian (300 vs. 600 mg) and control on one night of sleep in 16 subjects in a crossover design. The study team used a visual analogue scale to assess improvement in sleep, and there were no statistical differences between the three conditions [24]. Finally, in 2005, Jacobs and colleagues examined the effect of valerian on 270 adults and randomized them to receive either 600 mg of valerian at night or placebo for 28 days and asked if the subjects thought that they slept better. Eighty-nine percent of those who had received valerian stated that they perceived better sleep, but 86% of those who received placebo also reported better sleep [25]. In some studies, valerian has been found to decrease sleep latency by self-report from subjects' sleep diaries. However, objective data measuring different sleep parameters (such as sleep latency using actigraph) is lacking [15]. Overall, what little data that is available on valerian, this biologically based product does not demonstrate any efficacy in treatment of insomnia [26]. Two systematic reviews demonstrate that valerian does not improve insomnia but does not have any identified adverse side effects [27, 28]. There was no discussion of the potential of placebo effect in taking either herbs or actually placebo. The concept that there is a placebo effect in taking herbal supplements needs to be researched.

Manipulative and Body-Based Practices

Acupuncture is a therapeutic procedure in which specific body areas called meridian points are pierced with fine needles. Acupuncture treats illnesses by recreating the balance between Yin and Yang forces along with restoration of normal Qi [29]. Acupressure is the application of firm pressure of fingers placed on the meridian points. Auricular therapy is the use of acupuncture needles, seeds, or magnetic peels to stimulate acupoints located on the auricles [28].

Acupuncture and its subcategories are the most studied of the manipulative and body-based practices in the treatment of insomnia. Multiple studies have examined acupuncture use in patients with insomnia. Most studies reviewed in this chapter have a heterogeneous sample of subjects. Many of these studies also do not control for other medical conditions, other sleep disorders (such as obstructive sleep apnea), treatment for other sleep disorders, or have objective measures of sleep. Thus, it is difficult to evaluate the "pure" response of the participants to acupuncture. Further, issues with the quality of these papers include inconsistent definitions of insomnia and the lack of standardized outcomes for the measurement of sleep.

Suen and colleagues published in 2002 and then in 2003 a study examining the use of magnetic pearls to specific meridian points in elderly subjects with insomnia. Two control groups used different types of seeds taped to the same areas as the magnetic pearls. A total of 120 subjects were enrolled all greater than or equal to 60 years of age with insomnia complaints of at least 6 months (some up to 20 years) with no severe medical or psychiatric conditions. Objective data using wrist actigraphy was used along with a sleep questionnaire and sleep diaries. Initial results during the 3-week treatment phase demonstrated significant improvement in sleep efficiency as recorded on actigraphy and increase in overall nocturnal sleep. Also there was a significant decrease in sleep latency and wake after sleep onset [30]. In 2003, these researchers reported on a long-term follow-up study of these same subjects. Fifteen subjects who had been in the original intervention group were followed at 1, 3, and 6 months after intervention. No subject continued with the intervention after the initial 3 weeks. Total nocturnal sleep time and sleep efficiency were still significantly increased at the 6-month point, and sleep latency and total wake time after sleep onset were all significantly decreased at the 6-month point, thus demonstrating a sustained effect for the intervention [31].

In 2009, a Cochrane systematic review, authored by Cheuk, Yeung, Chung, and Wong, was published examining acupuncture and related techniques as an intervention for insomnia [29]. Twenty-six studies (all in English) were identified, but only seven met criteria for inclusion into review. All of the reviewed studies had high risk of bias, heterogeneous samples, and used different controls or comparisons such as medication, sham acupuncture/pressure, lack of control over diagnosis of insomnia (patient report vs. medical diagnosis), and length of treatment. The authors felt that overall, the results of the meta-analysis were favorable for the use of acupuncture and its related techniques for treatment of insomnia. However, the authors note that the quality of the data is lacking and that further highly rigorous studies are needed to answer the questions of the use of acupuncture for insomnia. There was only one study that reported a single withdrawal to the actual treatment (slight pain upon needle insertion) [29].

A meta-analysis, authored by Cao and colleagues, was also published in 2009 [32]. The authors had access to Chinese data that the authors of the 2009 Cochrane review did not. Of the 46 included trials, 43 were published in Chinese and most were not available to English-speaking countries. The authors reported that while all the studies demonstrated that acupuncture was effective in "treating" insomnia (specifically sleep quality and duration) compared to sham, no treatment, or medication, most of the studies were flawed as has been described in the above paragraphs and that the benefit of acupuncture could be overvalued [32] . The authors did note though that side effects or risks of acupuncture are very minimal although they did not list the side effects of risks of acupuncture in the review.

Since the publication of the two systematic reviews, two studies were published in 2010 using acupressure in subjects who reside in long-term care facilities. Reza et al. reported that there was significant improvement in sleep quality, duration, and efficiency as measured by the PSQI. Also there was significant decrease in sleep latency when compared to either the sham acupressure or a control group [33]. Also sleep logs that were maintained by the staff (blinded to subject's group) demonstrated a significant decrease in the number of nighttime awakening by the subjects. The subjects ($N=90$) studied were elderly residents in an Iranian nursing home who were reported to have moderate to marked sleep disturbances [33].

Sun et al. reported using acupressure in subjects who were residents of long-term care facilities. Twenty-five subjects were in each group (intervention vs. control). The intervention of 5-s pressure followed by a 1-s rest for 5 min was conducted every night for 5 continuous weeks. The control group only received a very light touch with no pressure with the same timing scheme. Outcome measures were the Athens insomnia scale-Taiwan (AIS-T) form which measures different characteristics of insomnia. There was a significant decrease in the score on the AIS-T which continued for 2 weeks after the intervention was ended [34]. Both of these studies begin to address some of the methodological concerns with previous studies, such as sample size calculations and objective data measurements that have been problematic [29, 32].

Restless Leg Syndrome

The issues surrounding methodology to support the use of acupuncture in treatment of insomnia such as inability to blind the practitioner and subject, questionable use of control conditions, and lack of control of comorbid conditions are also true with the treatment of restless leg syndrome. Restless leg syndrome is the strong uncontrollable desire to move legs after sitting still due to the feeling of uncomfortable sensations. Causes can range from comorbid medical conditions to low iron stores to unknown causes. Reported incidence ranges from 2 to 15% of the US population [35]. A Cochrane Review in 2008 only included two studies out of 14 in the analysis of the effect of acupuncture as a treatment for restless leg syndrome. Both studies were heavily flawed and contained high bias, poor or no randomization, and poor selection of outcome measures. The authors concluded that the effectiveness of acupuncture for the treatment of RLS is not supported by rigorous and comprehensive evidence. Further research is needed before routine use of acupuncture can be recommended in the treatment of RLS [36].

Obstructive Sleep Apnea

Only one study to date has examined the use of acupuncture in the treatment of obstructive sleep apnea (OSA). OSA is the repetitive complete or partial closing of the airway during sleep, leading to disrupted sleep patterns and other cardiovascular and metabolic risk. It is estimated that from 3 to 28% of the western population suffer from OSA [37]. This one study evaluated 36 adults with moderate OSA (apnea hypopnea index (AHI) 15–30 events per hour) and randomized them to one of three groups: acupuncture, sham acupuncture, or control. The intervention acupuncture was provided for ten sessions; the sham acupuncture was applied at the same intervals but located about 1 cm from the actual point and not in acupoints or meridians. Those in the intervention group had a significant decrease in AHI compared to the other two groups (AHI 19.9+4.1 pre vs. 10.1+5.6 post; $p<0.05$). The difference was in the apnea index and not the hypopnea index. There was no difference in body mass index (BMI) or neck circumference in the three groups. Also there was no difference in AHI between the three groups. The authors attribute the improvement in AHI changes in the serotonergic pathway which has been shown in other studies to be influenced by acupuncture [38]. There was no assessment of whether or not the "sham" group could actually feel the needle inserted and if there was any actual manipulation of the sham needles. Finally, these results have not been reproduced in other studies by independent investigators; thus, acupuncture is not a known effective treatment of OSA.

Energy Medicine

Little data is available for the use of energy medicine in relation to sleep complaints. One study examined using Tai Chi Chin with older adults who had poor sleep quality [39]. Tai Chi Chin is a series of movements focused on the development of intrinsic energy called Chi [40]. In this study, 112 healthy older (59–86 years of age) were randomly assigned to either Tai Chi Chin (intervention) or health education (active control) for a total of 25 weeks. Sleep issues were assessed using the PSQI. For those subjects with high scores on the PSQI, there was a significant decrease in the overall score between the intervention group and the active control group ($p<0.05$). For those with low PSQI scores, there were no significant differences. When examining the sleep quality portion of the PSQI, there was significant improvement in sleep quality, duration, and efficiency and decrease in sleep latency and sleep disturbances between the intervention and the active control group ($p < 0.05$) [39]. There were no reported safety issues within the study. The technique of Tai Chi Chin evaluated in this study shows promise as an integrative therapy for treatment of insomnia in older adults. Additional research is needed.

Implications of the Evidence and Science for Practice

The evidence for most of the integrative therapies used for sleep disturbances is lacking. Other than melatonin which has been extensively studied, no other therapy can be recommended with confidence. That is not to say with further rigorous study, some of the integrative therapies addressed in this chapter will be shown in the future to be effective treatments for different sleep disorders especially in the area of insomnia. While most of the integrative therapies discussed in this chapter have little to no side effects (except herbal preparation), reported efficacy is also poor. For clinicians, this is important as patients may come in to an office visit and request the use of integrative therapies for treatment of a sleep disorder expecting either complete resolution of the problem or at least a decrease in symptoms. However, the clinician cannot feel confident that the integrative therapies will be effective. The clinician must council the patient on this fact. Also qualified practitioners of the integrative therapy (such as acupuncture/pressure) may not be available in the community. The clinician has the responsibility to have an up-to-date list of qualified practitioners in the community for any specific therapy if he or she is going to recommend the patient use integrative therapies. With herbal preparations, there is the added risk of herb-drug interactions which cannot be overlooked. Use of herbal preparations needs to be assessed at each office visit and before prescribing a pharmaceutical. Also if the clinician and patient mutually agree on the use of an herbal preparation, then the patient must be counseled on potential herbal-drug interaction. An excellent website for keeping up to date on these interactions is http://www.nlm.nih.gov/medlineplus/druginformation.html.

Directions for Future Research

Future research in the use of integrative therapies for sleep issues needs to be rigorous and well controlled. The most prominent and significant limitation of the current research is the lack of rigor. In many of the reviewed studies, either the sample size is not large enough to detect an effect, the control within the research is lacking, or the overall study design is not appropriate. Concerns about safety and efficacy of certain treatments especially involving herbal remedies need to be addressed before wide-scale acceptance within the healthcare community can be obtained. Research conducted in this area needs to be well controlled (e.g., patient population, sleep diagnosis), defined parameters, objective measures of outcome variables, and in the case of herbal preparations, control of quality and purity of a specific product. This includes the application of established criteria (e.g., DSM-IV or ICSD criteria) and objective measures of sleep and other variables so that studies can be replicated and validated for results.

Summary and Conclusions

The evidence for use of integrative therapies in sleep disorders is lacking except in the case of melatonin for insomnia. Melatonin has been used and reviewed across age groups, types of insomnias, and other sleep disorders and is felt to be safe and effective by the sleep community [18, 20, 22, 23]. Further research to demonstrate the effectiveness of other integrative therapies is needed. The most success with integrative therapies will probably be in the treatment of insomnia, and therefore, well-designed and controlled studies are needed. For the clinician, keeping up to date on research in the use of integrative therapies is important as the field is expanding rapidly.

References

1. http://www.psychiatryonline.com/content.aspx?aID=311891&searchStr=insomnia#311891. Accessed 16 Jan 2011.
2. http://www.psychiatryonline.com/content.aspx?aID=442167&searchStr=insomnia%2c+transient#442167. Accessed 16 Jan 2011.
3. http://consensus.nih.gov/2005/insomniastatement.pdf. Accessed 13 Jan 2011.
4. http://www.sleepfoundation.org/sites/default/files/2005_summary_of_findings.pdf. Accessed 16 Jan 2011.
5. http://nccam.nih.gov/health/sleep/ataglance.html. Accessed 12 Jan 2011.
6. http://nccam.nih.gov/health/sleep/ataglance.html. Accessed 16 Jan 2011.
7. http://www.ncbi.nlm.nih.gov/sites/entrez?orig_db=PubMed&db=pubmed&cmd=Search&term=166%5Bvolume%5D%20AND%2016%5Bissue%5D%20AND%201775%5Bpage%5D%20AND%202006%5Bpdat%5D. Accessed 16 Jan 2011.
8. Winbush N, Gross CR, Kreitzer MJ. The effects of mindfulness based stress reduction on sleep disturbances: a systematic review. J Sci Healing. 2007;3:585–91.
9. Heidenreich T, Tuin I, Pflug B, Michchal M, Michalak J. Mindfulness-based cognitive therapy for persistent insomnia: a pilot study. Psychother Psychosom. 2006;75:188–9.
10. Vera FM, Manzaneque JM, Maldonado EF, Carrannque GA, Rodriguez FM, Blanca MJ, Morell M. Subjective sleep quality and hormonal modulation in long-term yoga practitioners. Biol Psychol. 2009;81:164–8.
11. Khalsa SB. Treatment of chronic insomnia with yoga: a preliminary study with sleep-wake diaries. Appl Psycholphysiol Biofeedback. 2004;29:269–78.
12. Harmat L, Takacs J, Bodizs R. Music improves sleep quality in students. J Adv Nurs. 2008;62(3):327–35.
13. Ziv N, Rotem T, Arnon Z, Haimov I. The effect of music relaxation versus progressive muscular relaxation on insomnia in older people and their relationship to personality traits. J Music Ther. 2008;3:360–80.
14. Lazic SE, Ogilvie RD. Lack of efficacy of music to improve sleep: a polysomnographic and quantitative EEG analysis. Int J Psychophysiol. 2007;63:232–9.

15. Meoli AL, Rosen C, Kristo D, Kohman M, Gooneratne G, Aguillard RN, Fayle R, et al. Oral nonprescription treatment for insomnia: an evaluation of products with limited evidence. J Clin Sleep Med. 2005;1(2):173–87.
16. Altun A, Ugur-Altunn B. Melatonin: therapeutic and clinical utilization. Int J Clin Pract. 2007;61(5):835–45.
17. http://www.ahrq.gov/clinic/epcsums/melatsum.html. Accessed 16 Jan 2011
18. Brezezinski A, Vangel MG, Wurtman RJ, Norrie G, Zhdanova I, Ben-Shuchan A, Ford I. Effects of exogenous melatonin on sleep: a meta-analysis. Sleep Med Rev. 2005;9(1):41–50.
19. http://www.ncbi.nlm.nih.gov/pmc/articles/PMC1490287/?tool=pubmed. Accessed 16 Jan 2011
20. Smits MG, VanStel H, Van Der Heijden K, Meijer AM, Coenen A, Kerkhof GA. Melatonin improves health status and sleep in children with idiopathic chronic sleep-onset insomnia: a randomized placebo-controlled trial. J Am Acad Child Adolesc Psychiatry. 2003;42(11):1286–93.
21. http://www.ncbi.nlm.nih.gov/pubmed/8106956. Accessed 27 March 2011 at 12:00
22. Sack RL, Auckley D, Auger R, Carskadon M, Wright K, Vitiello M, Zhdanova I. Circadian rhythm sleep disorders: part II advanced sleep phase disorder, delayed sleep phase disorder, free-running disorder and irregular sleep-wake rhythm. Sleep. 2007;30(11):1484–501.
23. Donnnath F, Quispe S, Diefennbach K, Maurer A, Fietze I, Roots I. Critical evaluation of the effect of valerian extract on sleep structure and quality. Pharmacopsychiatry. 2000;33:47–53.
24. Diaper A, Hindmarch I. A double blind, placebo-controlled investigation of the effects of two doses of valerian preparation on the sleep, cognitive and psychomotor function of sleep-disturbed older adults. Phytother Res. 2004;18:831–6.
25. Jacob BP, Brent S, Tice JA, Blackwell T, Cummings SR. An internet based randomized, placebo-controlled trial of kava and valerian for anxiety and insomnia. Medicine. 2005;84:197–207.
26. Taibi DM, Vitiello M, Barsness S, Elmer GW, Anderson GD, Landis CA. A randomized clinical trial of valerian fails to improve self-reported, polysomnographic and actigraph sleep in older women with insomnia. Sleep Med. 2009;10:319–28.
27. Bent S, Padula A, Moore D, Patterson M, Mehling W. Valerian for sleep: a systematic review and meta-analysis. Am J Med. 2006;119:1005–12.
28. Taibi DM, Landis CA, Petry H, Vitiello MV. A systematic review of valerian as a sleep aid: safe but not effective. Sleep Med Rev. 2007;11(3):209–30.
29. Cheuk DKL, Yeung J, Chung KF, Wong V. Acupuncture for insomnia. Cochrane Database Syst Rev. 2009;2:1–46.
30. Suen LK, Wong TK, Leung AW. Effectiveness of auricular therapy on sleep promotion in the elderly. Am J Chin Med. 2002;30(4):429–49.
31. Suen LK, Wong TK, Leung AW, Ip WC. The long-term effects of auricular therapy using magnetic pearls on elderly with insomnia. Complement Ther Med. 2003;11(2):85–92.
32. Cao H, Pan X, Li H, Liu J. Acupuncture for treatment of insomnia: a systematic review of randomized controlled trials. J Altern Complement Med. 2009;15(11):1171–86.
33. Reza H, Kian N, Pouresmail Z, Masood K, Bagher M, Cheraghi M. The effect of acupressure on quality of sleep in Iranian elderly nursing home residents. Complement Ther Clin Pract. 2010;16:81–5.
34. Sun J, Sung M, Huang M, Cheng G, Lin C. Effectiveness of acupressure for residents of long-term care facilities with insomnia: a randomized controlled trial. Int J Nurs Stud. 2010;47:798–805.
35. http://www.nhlbi.nih.gov/health/prof/sleep/res_plan/section5/section5d.html. Accessed 27 Mar 2011
36. Cui y, Wang y, Liu Z. Acupuncture for restless leg syndrome. Cochrane Database Syst Rev. 2008;4:1–18.
37. http://ajrccm.atsjournals.org/cgi/content/full/165/9/1217. Accessed 27 Mar 2011.
38. Freire A, Sugai G, Chrispin F, Togeiro S, Yamamura Y, Mello L. Tufik. Treatment of moderate obstructive sleep apnea syndrome: a randomized, placebo-controlled trial. Sleep Med. 2007;8:43–50.
39. Irwin M, Olmstead R, Motivala S. Improving sleep quality in older adults with moderate sleep complaints: a randomized controlled trial of Tai Chi Chih. Sleep. 2008;31(7):1001–8.
40. http://www.taichichih.org/overview.php. Accessed 10 Jan 2011.

Part IV
Integrative Therapies to Promote Lung Health

Chapter 13
Integrative Therapies for Tobacco Cessation

Kate M. Hathaway and Yvette Erasmus

Abstract The use of integrative therapies for the treatment of nicotine addiction and tobacco dependence is limited, and what studies exist are fraught with methodological difficulties such as small sample sizes, no controls, and no long-term data. What research does exist suggests that some mind–body practices, yoga, and physical exercise may be of some benefit in treating tobacco dependence, especially when used in combination with nicotine replacement therapy (NRT). Other integrative therapies may be of help in reducing symptoms of withdrawal (such as anxiety, muscle tension, and mood shifts) but are not established as efficacious treatments for tobacco dependence per se. To date, treatment of choice remains strong and consistent counseling and use of NRT.

Keywords Smoking cessation • Integrative therapies • Tobacco dependence • Withdrawal symptoms • Combined treatment approaches

According to recent surveys on drug use and health, approximately 70.9 million individuals in the United States use tobacco; 60.1 million of these (24.2% of the US population) are smokers, and despite earlier gender differences, prevalence rates are now very similar for men and women [1]. Tobacco use rates decreased significantly between 1960 and 2000, but they have remained relatively stable over the past

K.M. Hathaway, PhD, LP (✉)
Center for Spirituality and Healing, University of Minnesota,
Minneapolis, MN 55455, USA

Department of Clinical Psychology, American School of Professional Psychology,
Twin Cities,1515 Central Parkway, Eagan, MN 55121, USA
e-mail: hatha001@umn.edu

Y. Erasmus, MEd
Department of Clinical Psychology, American School of Professional Psychology,
Twin Cities, 1515 Central Parkway, Eagan, MN 55121, USA

L. Chlan and M.I. Hertz (eds.), *Integrative Therapies in Lung Health and Sleep*,
Respiratory Medicine 4, DOI 10.1007/978-1-61779-579-4_13,

5–10 years, despite increasing evidence and public education about the negative health effects of tobacco use. Tobacco use remains the single leading preventable cause of death in the United States, and annual direct and indirect societal costs attributed to smoking approximate near $193 billion per year. The purpose of this chapter is to briefly introduce to the reader the physiological mechanisms and health complications involved in nicotine addiction, discuss the limited research on integrative therapies for treatment of nicotine dependence and tobacco cessation, and briefly introduce the evidence-based, "state-of-the-art" treatments available for tobacco cessation.

Nicotine Addiction

Although tobacco is used in various forms, the focus of this chapter will be on integrative therapies used to achieve smoking cessation. The nicotine ingested by smoke inhalation reaches peak levels in the bloodstream very rapidly. Smokers report pleasurable sensations that include mood elevation, relaxation, increased focus and attention, and—among regular users—reduction in withdrawal symptoms. These acute effects, however, dissipate quickly, and the smoker is then driven to ingest more nicotine. When an individual is attempting to quit, nicotine receptors in the brain continue to be present and do not approach the levels of nonsmokers for more than a month after quitting [2], making smoking cessation complex and dynamic. Smoking also leads to an increase in blood pressure, respiration, and heart rate. Smokers of tobacco expose themselves to significant health risks, particularly lung and cardiovascular diseases, including chronic obstructive pulmonary disease [3].

The relationship between sleep and tobacco use is complicated; sleep disturbance is often seen as a withdrawal symptom as quitters reduce and eliminate nicotine. Several neuropeptides are thought to mediate the sleep-nicotine relationship. The orexin/hypocretin system, for example, is one of the systems that has been proposed as a modulator for breathing, influences chemosensitivity in the brain, and may affect sleep-wakefulness cycles in humans [4]. Orexin, leptin, and other neuropeptides have also been implicated as potential links between tobacco inhalation, craving, and the psychophysiological "reward" associated with smoking; blocking these neuropeptide receptors in rats appeared to both eliminate the stimulating properties of nicotine and decrease motivation to use nicotine [5]. Neuropeptide activity is also tied to the dopaminergic transmission in mesolimbic systems associated with reward pathways and may offer a partial explanation for emotional challenges with nicotine withdrawal and for the high comorbidity of nicotine dependence with mood and anxiety [6].

Nicotine Addiction, Emotionality, and the Smoking Experience

The exact nature of the nicotine dependence-emotionality relationship is unclear; however, the comorbidity of tobacco use and emotionality is significant.

Nondepressed smokers report changes in mood from smoking, and research reviews report high comorbidity between tobacco smoking and emotional disturbances, which is particularly robust with schizophrenia, depression, and anxiety. An estimated 44% of all purchased cigarettes in the United States are bought by individuals with psychiatric disorders, rates of smoking are 2–4 times greater in individuals suffering from depression and anxiety, and some studies have suggested that 90% of individuals with schizophrenia are smokers. For these individuals in particular, smoking may serve, to some extent, as both a direct anxiolytic and palliative intervention for these conditions, contributing to difficulty quitting. For some smokers who suffer from depression, smoking may essentially act as an antidepressant agent, due to its direct or indirect effect on dopamine and serotonin activity [7].

Smoking tobacco is also a multisensory experience, involving the senses of taste, smell, touch, and vision. As with other types of chemical use, the rituals of buying, unpackaging, touching, lighting up, sharing, and socializing with cigarettes are all associated with the pleasurable effects of nicotine use, including intense and immediate physiological (increased heart rate, respiratory changes, neurological impact) and psychological (mood alteration, decreased anxiety) effects. The act of smoking, even apart from the physiological effects of nicotine, appears to alleviate negative feelings, irritability, and anxiety in many smokers [8]. This effect may be due to the sensory experience of smoke inhalation, not nicotine, as cigarettes with only trace (or no) amounts of nicotine produce similar responses [8]. Many environments and activities are associated with smoking, and conditioned responses may be signaled by these situations (e.g., a stressful argument with someone triggers the desire for mood elevation, achieved by cigarette smoking), thus allowing the cigarette use to serve as future discriminative stimuli [9]. These cued associations make tobacco cessation even more difficult to achieve. In addition, the disincentives for smoking are generally delayed and subtle, providing little comparison to the incentives resulting from the rapid rewarding effects of nicotine via smoke inhalation.

Despite the physiological, behavioral, and emotional challenges involved in quitting, approximately 50% of smokers will eventually quit, and the vast majority of smokers desire to quit [10]. Among smokers who attempt to quit independently, however, estimates are that the vast majority (up to 85% in some studies) will relapse [11]. The complicated relationships between nicotine dependence, sensory stimulation, sleep disturbances, widely conditioned behavioral and societal cues, and emotion regulation challenges may offer an explanation for why tobacco dependence is particularly resistant to treatments that attempt to address only one aspect of the smoking experience. General success rates from tobacco cessation treatment programs are modest at best, and single intervention programs are considerably less successful than those designed to address the multidimensional experiences of smoking. Despite this, much of the research in tobacco cessation has focused on single interventions. Individually, these treatments have had some success in helping smokers quit. Of particular note are nicotine replacement therapies (NRTs), pharmacological interventions, behavioral counseling, and psychoeducational interventions. Combined treatment approaches (making use of these treatments in concert) are proving to be even more successful in the quitting attempts.

These interdisciplinary treatment approaches attempt to address the physiological cravings and withdrawal symptoms and the psychological and behavioral mechanisms underlying the addiction process, as well as the various symptoms and obstacles cited as reasons for relapse (including cravings, weight gain, and increased symptoms of anxiety and depression). NRTs and use of varenicline (a partial $\alpha 4\beta 2$ nicotinic receptor agonist) and bupropion (an antidepressant), which are recommended as first line pharmacological interventions for smoking cessation, appear to be most effective when used in combination with behavioral, social, and psychoeducational support.

Integrative Therapies for Tobacco Cessation

Integrative therapy treatments are discussed in the following sections. With few exceptions (e.g., if a patient experiences negative effects from combining different pharmacological interventions or using herbs with drugs), clinicians should be encouraged to consider using these treatments in a combined treatment (simultaneously administered) manner, tailoring the specific interventions to the individual needs of the smoker; available evidence suggests that multiple interventions can be more effective than single treatments [12].

As an introductory statement, the reader should be aware that very little research has been conducted on the use of integrative medicine treatments for tobacco cessation. What research does exist is often flawed methodologically, with small numbers of subjects and limited or no control groups. Despite this, many patients use these treatments when they attempt to quit smoking. In a recent survey of 1,175 patients seen at an outpatient tobacco treatment clinic in the Midwest, 27% of patients reported previous use of complementary and alternative medicine (CAM) or integrative therapies for tobacco cessation, most commonly reporting the actual use of hypnosis, relaxation, acupuncture, and meditation. In addition, they reported perceiving yoga, relaxation, meditation, and massage therapy as the most efficacious treatments, and 67% of patients seen expressed an interested in future use of CAM for tobacco cessation [13]. Although the research is lacking, integrative, complementary approaches are perceived by smokers as potentially helpful adjunctive approaches in nicotine cessation, especially in addressing withdrawal symptoms, comorbid or related anxiety or depression, and relapse prevention. In general, there is currently little support for the claim that integrative or CAM approaches are effective in achieving tobacco cessation. When a scientific perspective is taken and meta-analyses of the available studies is conducted, the research on integrative therapies in general does not support their use for direct treatment of tobacco use and nicotine dependence, as the principle outcome of treatment in this regard is total abstinence from smoking. These interventions do not seem to consistently or reliably achieve this goal. While integrative therapies may aid in reducing withdrawal symptoms, assist in reducing the number of cigarettes smoked, or address concurrent struggles with mood, there is no compelling evidence to suggest that any one of these therapies is an effective treatment for complete cessation. The very limited research that does exist is reviewed below.

Mind–Body Practices

Perhaps the only integrative mind–body therapy for which there has been some support for its use with tobacco cessation is hypnosis. Use of hypnosis for smoking cessation has shown some positive results, particularly when used in combination with other therapies. An independent review of 11 studies comparing hypnotherapy to 18 different control interventions concluded that, due to the lack of methodologically sound research with hypnosis, there is not enough evidence to support hypnosis as a sole treatment for smoking cessation [14]. When used as an adjunctive therapy, however, it appears that hypnosis may offer advantages over single treatment or some other integrative treatment strategies. Results from a small controlled study of 67 patients showed that hypnosis with NRT was more effective than NRT alone in achieving tobacco cessation [15]. Carmody et al. found that hypnosis, in combination with use of a nicotine patch, may be more helpful for patients attempting to quit than use of behavioral counseling and nicotine patch, especially for those suffering from comorbid depression [16]. However, the 2008 Clinical Practice Guidelines for Treating Tobacco Use and Dependence [12] concluded that there were insufficient studies with hypnosis, that hypnosis procedures varied widely among the various studies, and that the methodological limitations of these studies limited the ability to embrace hypnosis as a viable treatment for tobacco use. According to the authors of the guidelines, the strength of evidence (multiple, well-designed, randomized clinical trials) for hypnosis was not present [12]. While intriguing, support for the use of hypnosis as a solo treatment is not compelling at this time.

Similarly, the number and breadth of studies on the use of acupuncture is low, and the results of these studies are equivocal. Some early research suggested that acupuncture is an effective intervention for smoking, but more recent, rigorously designed studies have not supported the use of acupuncture for tobacco cessation. Both the Clinical Practice Guidelines and the Cochrane Review concluded that the available evidence was insufficient to recommend acupuncture. White and Moody's 2006 meta-analysis of acupuncture for tobacco cessation suggested that location of acupuncture points did not appear to matter in the effectiveness outcomes, bringing into question the possibility that the positive outcomes achieved with acupuncture are more consistent with patient expectations than with the direct procedure of acupuncture [17]. A recent review of 33 randomized controlled trials did not show a long-term benefit from acupuncture as a treatment for smoking cessation [18].

Energy Medicine

There is no available research literature that suggests the use of energy-based therapies to be effective with nicotine withdrawal or tobacco cessation.

Biologically Based Practices

There is no conclusive empirical data that suggest that biologically based practices such as herbs and supplements are effective treatments for tobacco cessation. As discussed below, several herbal combinations and some herbs show promise in reducing the severity of withdrawal symptoms and/or concomitant anxiety; however, their efficacy for tobacco cessation per se is not supported in the literature.

Manipulative and Body-Based Practices

Massage, chiropractic, and osteopathic therapies all offer treatments that are also designed to assist with symptoms of muscle tension, irritability, anxiety, and restlessness and can be considered on an individual basis for those smokers interested in integration of these therapies into their quitting program. Empirical support for the use of these therapies for tobacco cessation directly is not found. The use of these practices for treatment of withdrawal symptoms is encouraging, however.

Integrative Therapies to Aid Relaxation and Reduce Anxiety

As an introduction to this section on the use of integrative therapies to aid relaxation and reduce anxiety, it should be noted that while some tobacco cessation therapies report effectiveness in reducing the *use* of tobacco, there does not appear to be a consistently strong relationship between short- or long-term *reduction* in tobacco use and tobacco *cessation* (except in the case of NRTs) [19, 20]. This is likely to also be the case with integrative treatments.

Integrative approaches, however, may be helpful in aiding relaxation and decreased use of nicotine. Many smokers experience considerable anxiety prior to and during reduction efforts, and many have comorbid anxiety conditions. A recent student of 1,504 smokers found that anxiety diagnoses were not only common among treatment-seeking smokers but were also related to elevated withdrawal symptoms, lack of response to pharmacotherapy, and increased motivation to smoke [21]. The treatments reviewed below may assist in the reduction of negative symptoms such as anxiety or depression (and, in some case, in number of cigarettes smoked) experienced by patients attempting to quit smoking; there is no clear evidence, however, that this in turn results in total cessation from tobacco use.

Mind–Body Practices

Relaxation and Hypnosis

There is a good body of evidence that mind–body practices such as relaxation therapies are helpful for treatment of symptoms of anxiety in populations that suffer from a variety of anxiety disorders and anxiety symptoms. These practices involve instruction in physical (progressively relaxing body parts), cognitive (decrease catastrophic or negative thoughts), and emotional (elicit peaceful feelings) activities. Their use in treating anxious symptoms in the smoking population is also partially supported in the literature [21–25]. Mindfulness, meditation, guided imagery, and relaxation techniques have all been proposed as useful integrative therapies for tobacco cessation. While theoretically different, mind–body and relaxation therapies all involve attention to physical sensations and may use visualization and imagery, regulation of breathing, and systematic muscle contraction/relaxation as a means of achieving deep relaxation. The research is not strong enough to date, however, to include these treatments as evidence-based *stand-alone* therapies for tobacco cessation; as solo treatments, their effectiveness has not been consistently shown to be significantly greater than no treatment. However, they may prove to be particularly helpful in reducing the tobacco withdrawal symptoms and nicotine cravings, especially when combined with education and NRTs. At this time, they can be considered second-line, nonpharmacological interventions for treatment of anxiety symptoms related to nicotine withdrawal and may work best in concert with other treatments. As with other nonnicotine therapies, it is difficult to ascertain whether these therapies have a direct impact on neurophysiological activity associated with nicotine withdrawal and/or are helpful indirectly by promoting relaxation and symptom reduction.

Ussher et al. reported that use of a brief (10-min body scan) guided relaxation exercise with smokers significantly reduced the desire to smoke and aided with symptoms of irritability and tension. Recent research involving the integration of relaxation techniques with isometric exercises provided some evidence for the effectiveness of this combination of therapies for tobacco cessation [24]. This study reported only on short-term effectiveness, and no data currently exist to support this combination of therapies as efficacious in aiding long-term abstinence.

Physical Exercise

Some studies have attempted to determine whether regular exercise can help people sustain a quit attempt by moderating withdrawal symptoms and cravings and helping to control weight gain. A Cochrane review of 13 studies on the use of physical exercise as an aid to smoking cessation reported that, due to methodological concerns and the limited number of available studies, findings from these studies were inconclusive and needed further investigation [26]. Some research has suggested that physical exercise may have an additive effect on treatment success when used in combination with NRTs. Results from an early randomized controlled study of 281 healthy female smokers suggested that the exercise component of an intervention program more than doubled the likelihood of long-term tobacco cessation, and participants had gained less weight than the control group [27]. In another randomized controlled trial with 86 women, researchers found that vigorous exercise was associated with acute improvements in withdrawal symptoms, cravings, and negative affect [28]. The long-term cessation rate, however, was not reported. Recently, a pilot study examining the effect of moderate-intensity exercise on smoking cessation found a moderate effect size for exercise and suggested that, given adequate participant compliance, moderate-intensity exercise may enhance short-term smoking cessation [29].

A limitation of this research is the lack of available evidence regarding the long-term benefit of exercise on smoking cessation. Kinnunen et al., however, found that both exercise and health and wellness education conditions (social support) double the cessation rates (over standard care) in female smokers [30]. Above and beyond the potential benefits of exercise on tobacco cessation, these researchers wisely discussed the advantages of introducing physical exercise into smokers' lifestyles as a potential harm-reduction strategy, improving overall morbidity and mortality related to sedentary lifestyle and smoking. Exercise has also been found to be effective in alleviation of some of the symptoms of both anxiety and depression, which may indirectly aid in reduction of withdrawal symptoms and assist in cessation [31]. Given the generally accepted negative relationship between smoking and physical activity [32], exercise should be considered both as a component of integrative tobacco cessation programs and tobacco use prevention models.

Yoga

Yoga (in a general sense) can be considered as an alternative to traditional aerobic and anaerobic exercise and is comprised of breathing, particular postures, and focused attention. These elements may enhance stress reduction and improve well-being and mood, which are in turn associated with successful smoking cessation [33]. Studies have suggested that regular yoga practice reduces perceived stress, reduces negative effect, and can improve weight control [34–37]. In a study examining the impact of Hatha Yoga (a combination of slower stretching and balancing poses with breathing and meditation) on smokers' desire to stop smoking, 30% of the participants reported a positive shift and increased desire to stop smoking after engaging in breath awareness and stretching exercises focusing on pulmonary health [38]. Tobacco cessation rates, however, were not significant. Due to a combination of yoga's aerobic involvement (physical exercise), meditative components (relaxation), and breath work, yoga may prove to be efficacious as an integrative therapy for tobacco research, but the research is limited at this time. Ongoing studies are being conducted to look at long-term benefits (including decreased withdrawal symptoms and sustained cessation) of yoga for tobacco cessation [22].

Acupuncture

Although the efficacy of acupuncture as a smoking cessation treatment is inconclusive and the quality of studies varies widely, some studies suggest that, rather than a direct impact on nicotine receptors, acupuncture may have benefit in reducing side effects of withdrawal such as irritation, cravings, and headaches. Furthermore, some studies suggest that acupuncture may increase the levels of endorphins, enkephalin, epinephrine, norepinephrine, serotonin, and dopamine in the central nervous system and may help encourage smoking cessation by decreasing the desire to smoke and by mediating various symptoms experienced as a result of cessation [39].

Although limited in scope and number, some studies suggest that true acupuncture may be more effective than placebo, at least in the short term, in helping people quit smoking by reducing cravings [18]. In a small pilot study using a research design to compare acupuncture with nonspecific treatments for stress reduction, Huang et al. found a small but significant trend toward improved stress symptoms after acupuncture treatment [40]. Other researchers have suggested that acupuncture may alleviate some of the autonomic responses to visual cues related to smoking [41]. When used in combination with other treatment approaches, acupuncture may prove to be of additive benefit. In a study combining acupuncture with patient education, Bier et al. conducted a randomized, quasi-factorial study examining the efficacy of auricular acupuncture and education on smoking cessation and found significant reductions in smoking and posttreatment cigarette use; acupuncture and education showed a 40% cessation rate that was significantly greater than the control group and was maintained at 18 months posttreatment [42].

Biologically Based Practices

Herbs and Nutritional Supplements

Both herbs and nutritional supplements have been used for centuries as remedies for some of the physiological and psychological symptoms such as anxiety and irritability. Lemon balm, lavender, chamomile, orange oil (*Camellia sinensis* oil), and peppermint have all been used with reported success to assist with relaxation, gastrointestinal distress, headaches, and agitation. Melatonin, kava kava, and valerian have been used as relaxation aids (reducing symptoms associated with smoking cessation such as anxiety, restlessness, irritability, and cigarette craving). The anxiolytic-like effect of these substances has been supported in some literature [43], and, for any given individual, the conditioned or direct relaxation experiences associated with these substances and smells may be helpful in reducing anxiety and aiding relaxation during the quitting process. A systematic review of the use of some of these natural remedies for treatment of anxiety and depression is not the purview of this chapter, but some evidence exists for the use of herbs, particularly passionflower and kava, in solo or combination. Lysine and supplements also appear to be promising in the treatment of anxiety, and St. John's wort, inositol, and omega-3 fatty acids have received some initial support as likely efficacious adjunctive therapies for symptoms of depression [44]. Safety concerns limit the recommended use of kava at this time, however, and clinicians are cautioned to consider drug-herb interactions when recommending herbal supplements to patients [45].

Hakim et al. suggested that use of antioxidants might aid in reducing some of the negative oxidative damage related to tobacco smoking [46]. Lee and Lee used an herbal tea made with plants high in antioxidant and nicotine degradation activity to aid in conversion of nicotine to cotinine; they reported reduced cravings and three times the smoking cessation rate compared to placebo [47].

Aromatherapy

Use of aromatherapy for tobacco cessation may prove helpful as well, as it potentially addresses the sensory experience of smell (countering the odor of tobacco), has neuropharmacological properties associated with emotions, and may be used to trigger odor-cured memories and responses associated with relaxation. The olfactory system is closely linked to the emotion and memory centers in the limbic system, and memories associated with smell have been found to be more emotionally evocative than those associated with other types of memories; this can be potentially used to link specific odors to relaxation and nonsmoking behavior. Some early research has suggested that inhalation of black pepper essential oil may reduce cravings and physical symptoms associated with cigarette smoking cessation [48], and more research is needed to investigate these claims. Many essential oils (particularly lavender, lemon balm, and neroli) have pharmacological actions consistent with changes in central nervous system activity (specifically triggering the release of neurotransmitters) and have proved beneficial in aiding relaxation. Recent research has begun to investigate the neuropharmacological properties of essential oils and the potential for their use in treatment of anxiety symptoms [49].

Energy Medicine

Reiki and healing touch have been suggested as useful interventions for anxiety but are not, to date, well substantiated in the literature [49].

Manipulative and Body-Based Practices

Massage and chiropractic treatments have not been substantiated as treatments for irritability and anxiety, although they may be helpful for physical symptoms such as headaches and muscle tension that may be associated with nicotine withdrawal.

Summary: Integrative Treatments for Tobacco Cessation

It should be noted that some guidelines suggest that integrative therapies or treatment methods may be helpful primarily for individuals only for whom more conventional interventions have failed. Given the more recent research suggesting that interdisciplinary, simultaneously applied interventions of other types (e.g., NRT plus counseling [12, 50, 51]) appear to be more successful than single treatment approaches (nicotine replacement alone), integrative therapies may be found to be good treatments for tobacco cessation when used in combination with other therapies. Studies investigating the use of these combined approaches are lacking yet are sorely needed. Integrative CAM treatments used by smokers in concert with other therapies, particularly given no contraindications for their use, should not be discouraged despite the lack of current evidence for their unilateral effectiveness on tobacco cessation.

The scope of this chapter does not allow for review of the complete literature supporting the use of various integrative therapies for all of the physical and emotional symptoms that might accompany withdrawal from nicotine. Given patient interest in these therapies, however, and the clinical observation that individual differences also predict outcome and satisfaction with treatment, it appears that patient preference for integrative therapies can usually be considered in tobacco cessation treatment efforts.

State-of-the-Art Treatments for Tobacco Cessation

A brief review of the nonintegrative, "state-of-the-art" therapies and treatments for nicotine dependence and tobacco cessation follows. Their inclusion in this chapter is designed to assist the reader in consideration of the use of integrative therapies with these more typical nicotine dependence/tobacco cessation treatments. These "state-of-the-art" treatments have generally been subjected to rigorous study and have been found to be efficacious for use in this population. It should be noted, however, that if integrative therapies are considered for use with individuals using nicotine replacement or pharmacological treatments, careful consideration needs to be given to possible negative interactions between these treatments, particularly with biologically based therapies.

Treatments That Directly Affect Nicotine Dependence

Although tobacco, not nicotine, is responsible for the majority of negative health effects related to smoking, nicotine is the addictive substance that sustains tobacco use. Evidence-based research suggests that the most successful interventions for nicotine dependence are NRTs; other pharmacotherapy interventions may directly affect dependence or may impact physiological and psychological symptoms of withdrawal. Effective pharmacological treatments can significantly increase the rates of both quitting and long-term abstinence [12]. A variety of medications are available to support people in attempting to quit smoking and can be offered to all tobacco users, except for pregnant women or for those for whom it is medically contraindicated. There is, however, currently insufficient evidence of medication effectiveness with smokeless tobacco users, light smokers, and adolescents [12].

Nicotine Replacement Therapy

NRTs aim to decrease withdrawal symptoms associated with smoking cessation by providing nicotine from slower, more controlled sources than cigarettes. These include patches, chewing gum, tablets (not sold in the United States), lozenges, inhalers, and spray. Wide evidence suggests that NRTs help smoking cessation and that various forms of NRT may be similarly effective [12, 50] (see Table 13.1). Concurrent use of several types of NRTs may improve treatment even more; success rates are higher, for example, when the nicotine patch is used to establish a background level of nicotine, and nasal spray, inhalers, or gum are subsequently used to respond to cravings [52, 53].

Nonnicotine Replacement Pharmacotherapies

Varenicline is a nicotine receptor partial agonist that provides some nicotine-like effects but also blocks the effects of nicotine. Unlike NRTs, which require the patient to cease smoking, varenicline causes a decline in the sense of satisfaction a person experiences while smoking [12]. Research suggests that varenicline may be more effective than bupropion in achieving tobacco cessation [52]. A recent study of 412 cases found that short-term smoking cessation rates were higher with varenicline than NRTs; no differences in cessation rates were found between patients with or without mental illness [54].

Studies show that use of 0.1–0.45 mg/day of clonidine, a central alpha adrenergic agonist that has been used primarily as an antihypertensive, can also lead to an increase in smoking cessation [55]. Clonidine is only recommended as a second-line therapy for people who have not found NRTs, bupropion, or varenicline helpful [55].

A variety of antidepressants appear to have beneficial effects for smoking cessation. Research suggests that bupropion and nortriptyline aid long-term smoking cessation, while selective serotonin reuptake inhibitors (SSRIs) such as fluoxetine, sertraline, and paroxetine are not effective [56]. These findings suggest that although serotonin modulation may be involved in maintenance of smoking, it may not be as important as tobacco cessation and that the dopaminergic or noradrenergic effects of bupropion and nortriptyline may account for their positive effects [56].

Table 13.1 Summary of pharmacotherapies for use with tobacco cessation

Medication	Support for use Y/N	Recommended dose	Side effects	Average cost
Nicotine gum[a]	Y	2 and 4 mg	Rapid chewing may lead to gastrointestinal side effects and headaches	$48 (for 2 mg boxes of 100–170 pieces)
		9–12 pieces daily, every 1–2 h Maximum 20–30 pieces daily Rate of nicotine release depends on speed of chewing	Also hiccups, burping, nausea, mouth soreness	$63 (4 mg boxes of 100–110 pieces)
Nicotine inhaler	Y	6–16 cartridges daily for up to 6 months 1 dose = 1 puff A cartridge delivers 4 mg of nicotine dispersed over about 80 puffs	Mild side effects include mouth and throat irritations, coughing, and rhinitis, which decrease with continued use	Box of 168 10 mg cartridges is about $196
Nicotine lozenges[a]	Y	2 and 4 mg Weeks 1–6 every 1–2 h Weeks 7–9 every 2–4 h Weeks 10–12 every 4–8 h	Hiccups, heartburn, cough	$34–39 per box of 72 lozenges
Nasal spray	Y	A dose of spray consists of a 0.5 mg squirt to each nostril (1 mg total) at 1–2 doses per hour, maximum dosage of 5 doses per hour or 40/day	Highest dependence potential. Irritation of the nose and throat, watery eyes, runny nose, coughing, and sneezing Severity usually decreases to mild after a few days of use	$49 per bottle
Nicotine patch	Y	Step-down dosage Weeks 1–4: 21 mg/24 h	Local skin irritation/reaction	7 mg box ($37), 14 mg box ($47), or 21 mg box ($48)
		Weeks 5–6: 14 mg/24 h Weeks 7–8: 7 mg/24 h	Insomnia, vivid dreams	

(continued)

Table 13.1 (continued)

Medication	Support for use Y/N	Recommended dose	Side effects	Average cost
Varenicline	Y	Days 1–3: 0.5 mg once daily Days 4–7: 0.5 mg twice daily Day 8–12 weeks: 1 mg twice daily	Nausea (30–40%), insomnia, vivid dreaming, changes in behavior, increased hostility, mood changes, depression, suicidal ideation, anxiety, and restlessness. Greater side effects for smokers with severe kidney disease	1 mg, box of 56 (30 day supply) $131
Bupropion SR	Y	Begin treatment a week before actually quitting smoking Days 1–5: 150 mg once daily for 3–5 days Then for 7–12 weeks: 150 mg twice daily	Insomnia, dry mouth	A box of 60 (150 mg) tablets $97 per month (generic) or $197–210 (brand name). Treatment may be extended up to 12 months
Clonidine	Not FDA-approved for smoking cessation	Initiate up to 3 days before quit date. 0.10 mg b.i.d. PO or 0.10 mg/day transdermal. Increase by 0.10 mg/day per week if needed. Duration 3–10 weeks	Significant dry mouth, sedation, postural hypotension, and dizziness Abruptly stopping clonidine can cause rebound withdrawal and hypertension	Oral 0.10 mg box of 60, $13 Transdermal 4 pack TTS $106
Nortriptyline	Not FDA-approved for smoking cessation	25 mg/day increasing gradually to target does of 75–100 mg daily. Duration from 12 weeks to 6 months	Sedation, blurred vision, light-headedness, shaky hands, constipation, urinary retention, and cardiac problems Patients need to be very closely monitored	25 mg, box of 60: $24

SSRIs	N	Studies suggest SSRIs do not significantly increase smoking cessation
Anxiolytics/ benzodiazepines/ beta-blockers	N	Inconclusive evidence and lack of sufficient data. No conclusions have been drawn regarding the effectiveness of these drugs in encouraging smoking cessation
Opioid antagonists/ naltrexone	N	Inconclusive evidence and not enough studies
Silver acetate	N	Several studies have shown no beneficial effects on smoking cessation
Mecamylamine	N	Inconsistent results. No conclusions have been drawn

Data for this table were based upon the 2008 Clinical Practice Guideline: Treating Tobacco Use and Dependence, US Public Health Service, June 2008

[a]Prescription not needed

Use of bupropion has been shown to double the odds of long-term quitting and works equally well with depressed and nondepressed smokers [56]. Research also suggests that bupropion may be as effective as NRT, but it is currently unclear whether or not combining bupropion with NRT increases quit rates, compared to using NRT or bupropion alone [56]. A recent review of research suggests that use of integrative pharmacotherapy (i.e., the nicotine patch with the gum or spray, the nicotine patch with the inhaler, or the nicotine patch with bupropion) is more effective than the medications alone in achieving cessation [12].

A meta-analysis of nine trials using nortriptyline, a tricyclic antidepressant, suggests a significant long-term benefit for tobacco cessation [56]. It is not clear whether or not nortriptyline is more or less effective than bupropion or whether using it in conjunction with NRT improves cessation rates. Although nortriptyline appears to be helpful in aiding smoking cessation efforts, until more research addresses the side effects and safety of this drug, it is currently recommended only as a second-line treatment for smoking cessation [57].

SSRIs and other drugs are promising for smoking cessation, but the research, to date, does not support their use at this time. Similarly, lobeline, anxiolytics, and silver acetate are not well established as useful aids in tobacco cessation [12, 56]. While they may be of help in treatment of comorbid conditions of depression or anxiety for individuals who suffer from these conditions and may be of some palliative help for withdrawal symptoms in nondepressed smokers, their use as direct agents of change for tobacco cessation is not supported at this time.

Psychological and Behavioral Interventions

A great deal of research has been conducted on the potential benefits of counseling and psychotherapy for treatment of nicotine dependence, particularly those therapies that address the physical, cognitive, emotional, and social concomitants of smoking. There are many psychological (conditioned) processes involved in the initiation, maintenance, and cessation of tobacco use, and smokers have developed strong associations between smoking, emotion regulation, pleasure, and social cues. Habit reversal techniques, cognitive therapies and group therapies have all been suggested as helpful adjunctive therapies in cessation efforts. These approaches aid people trying to quit by helping them recognize internal and external trigger situations (such as drinking caffeine or alcohol or being around other tobacco users) and develop cognitive and behavioral coping skills (such as learning cognitive strategies that will reduce negative thinking about quitting and avoiding triggering situations) to help themselves during the quitting process.

Of these, direct behavioral interventions have been shown to be most effective in supporting smoking cessation; these interventions may include gradual cessation programs, motivational interviewing techniques, contingency contracting, extratreatment social support, exercise, aversive smoking, and computerized treatments. Four specific kinds of counseling and behavioral therapy have yielded statistically significant increases in abstinence rates when compared to untreated control conditions: practical counseling including problem-solving and skills training, inclusion of social support as part of treatment, provision of help in securing social support outside of treatment, and utilization of aversive smoking procedures [12].

Combined approaches are particularly helpful for smokers. A meta-analysis by Baillie et al. [58] found a twofold increase in successful quitting when behavioral treatments were added to medical advice for quitting. They also noted a significantly greater treatment effect when more treatment formats were used than when only one intervention was tried, with increasing effectiveness as more treatments (multiple visits) were added. Face-to-face clinical interventions delivered for four or more sessions were particularly helpful in increasing abstinence rates [12].

It should be noted that while these interventions have proved to be helpful in initial tobacco cessation efforts, relapse prevention skills training has not yet been proven efficacious for long-term outcomes, and further research is needed to study effective relapse prevention strategies. However, behavioral approaches that include education regarding quitting, cognitive and behavioral strategies to deal with triggers to smoke, relaxation techniques for symptoms of anxiety, and development of social support for quitting have proved to be particularly beneficial, especially for those quitters who also suffer from depression [59].

Interventions That Educate

Due to the clear health benefits associated with smoking cessation, the importance of encouraging and helping people to quit successfully cannot be overstated [60]. Whether one's orientation is to integrative or traditional treatments for tobacco cessation, the educational component of treatment appears critically important for tobacco cessation. Studies have shown that even limited tobacco dependence interventions can be effective for many smokers. In meta-analyses of over 20 trials, even receiving brief advice from a primary care physician to quit smoking during routine office visits has been shown to increase the number of smokers who quit [61]. Interventions of even 5–10 min (which typically include simple opportunistic advice to stop, an assessment of the person's commitment to quit, an offer of pharmacotherapy and/or behavioral support, provision of self-help materials, and referral to more intensive support) are likely to significantly increase smokers' willingness and motivation to quit [12, 62].

Self-help materials are also effective in assisting tobacco cessation. A review of 68 trials found that providing standard self-help materials was more likely to increase quit rates than no interventions and that tailored or targeted self-help materials were more effective than standardized self-help materials [63]. Early research on tailored materials for quitting smoking suggest strong support for combined treatment approaches involving use of these materials in combination with pharmacological interventions such as NRT [64].

Studies examining telephone quit-line access and counseling show that these interventions also increase quitting success rates, are effective with diverse populations, and are able to reach many different people. In a randomized controlled trial in the Midwest, researchers found that telephone counseling and support increased the use of behavioral and pharmacologic assistance and subsequently led to higher smoking cessation rates than health-care provider information alone [51]. A systematic review of literature from 1990 to 2008 analyzed 11 randomized controlled trials examining the efficacy of online, interactive interventions for smoking cessation. Results indicated that these interventions may be effective in aiding smoking cessation but that more research is needed to compare static websites that offer advice and education to interactive web-based interventions that can offer more tailored and individualized approaches to quitting [65].

Although counseling and medication are both effective when they are used by themselves for smoking cessation, the combination of counseling and medication is more effective than stand-alone treatments. Recent reviews have found that when counseling and medication are combined, a 1-year abstinence rate of about 25% can be expected [66]. It is also possible that educationally based counseling or medication, combined with integrative treatments, holds promise for smokers.

Clinical Recommendations

The available literature on effective tobacco cessation suggests that tobacco use and nicotine dependence are difficult to treat, and relapse rates are high. Integrative, complementary treatments have not, to date, offered any particular advantages to the "state-of-the-art" treatments. A summary of these treatments and the support for their use as primary treatments, combined treatments, or adjunctive treatments for withdrawal symptoms is provided in Table 13.2.

The available research ("state of the art") is clear that all health-care providers should strongly advise patients to stop smoking and refer, as appropriate, to specialist services for aid in quitting. Instructions to quit should be repeated often, and information should be provided regularly about the risks of smoking and benefits of quitting. Smokers (particularly those smoking ten or more cigarettes daily) should be encouraged to use NRT as a smoking cessation aid. In addition, to aid in the likelihood of successful quitting, patients should be offered *interdisciplinary, simultaneously delivered, and integrated* interventions that include, at the very least, individual, group, or telephone counseling. Intensive interventions are more effective than brief interventions and should be offered wherever possible. Smoking cessation interventions should include problem-solving and skills training to help deal with conditioned behaviors associated with quitting and withdrawal symptoms. Integrative approaches should be provided as part of treatment. Relaxation interventions and physical exercise should be considered for all smokers unless there are medical contraindications; evidence-based use of herbals for treatment of anxiety secondary to nicotine withdrawal can also be considered but must be monitored for

Table 13.2 Summary of empirical support for use of integrative therapies with tobacco cessation

Intervention	Support for use as solo treatment	Support for use as combined treatment	Support for use as adjunctive treatment for symptoms of withdrawal
Acupuncture	C	C	B
Aromatherapy	D	C	C
Biologically based practices such as herbs and supplements	D	C	C
Brief intensive clinical interventions advising to quit	B	A	N/A
Counseling and behavior therapy	A	A[a] (very strong when combined with medication)	N/A
Energy medicine	D	D	C
Hypnosis	C	C	B
Manipulative, body-based practices including massage, chiropractics, and osteopathic therapies	D	D	C
Mind–body and relaxation therapies (guided imagery, meditation, mindfulness)	D	C	B
Motivational interviewing	C	B	N/A
NRTs, bupropion, and varenicline	A	A[a] (very strong when combined with counseling)	A
Physical exercise	C	B	B
Yoga	C	B	B

A: strong support, evidence based upon randomized controlled studies; B: good support; C: limited support, inconsistent findings needing further research; D: no support or no available research yet; N/A: not applicable or not focus of intervention

[a]Providing medication in addition to counseling significantly enhances treatment outcomes. "Medication and/or counseling are effective and should be provided as stand-alone interventions when it is not feasible to do both or the patient is not interested in both. By combining medication and counseling, however, the clinician can significantly improve abstinence rates" [12]

potential interactions if used with NRTs. Organizationally, clinic systems should expand attempts to identify and monitor tobacco use among patients.

Additionally, the US Task Force on Community Preventive Services (TFCPS) recommends the following community strategies to increase tobacco use cessation:

- Increase the unit price for tobacco products (strongly recommended).
- Use mass media campaigns combined with other interventions such as education, assistance with withdrawal symptoms, and counseling.
- Provide health-care provider reminders to identify tobacco users and advise on cessation. Techniques include chart stickers, vital sign stamps, medical record flow sheets, and checklists. Provider reminders combined with provider education are strongly recommended.
- Reduce patient out-of-pocket cost for effective cessation therapies.
- Offer multicomponent patient telephone support (strongly recommended).

As a minimum, telephone support should be combined with patient education materials.

Research Needs

There is considerable research needed in the area of integrative therapies and their contributions to achieve tobacco cessation. Methodological rigor (multiple, well-designed, RCTs with larger populations) in these studies is critical. Research and treatment paradigms that focus on concurrently offered, interdisciplinary, and transdisciplinary interventions are greatly needed, such as those previously proposed by the Transdisciplinary Tobacco Research Centers initiative [67]. These include more studies investigating how the combined contributions of behavioral interventions, pharmacotherapies, and CAM treatments for smokers can enhance treatment effectiveness. Of some promise for integrative therapy appears to be the integrative use of exercise, yoga, and hypnosis with NRTs; many more studies are needed to investigate their combined effectiveness for tobacco cessation. Investigation of optimal sequencing of treatments and treatment combinations, with attention to stage of change-specific interventions, will be valuable. Identification of organizational features of health-care systems that support the delivery of appropriate interventions, improving access to care for all smokers, development of efficacious treatment for smokers with comorbid (e.g., psychiatric) conditions, and improving proactive means by which to prompt quitting in more smokers is also sorely needed.

Because relapse rates are so high with nicotine users, much more research is needed to investigate strategies for long-term cessation. Relapsers have been found to be more likely than sustained quitters to experience emotional distress and high levels of tobacco use/nicotine dependence; they drink more alcohol and report more general health difficulties [68]. Efficacious interventions for individuals with these characteristics will be very important. Studies that target lower socioeconomic status (SES) populations, women, and individuals from a variety of racial and cultural backgrounds and that test interventions for adolescent smokers are also of great importance. Smoking rates are higher among individuals who are of American Indian/Alaskan native descent and whites, among individuals living in the southern United States, and among individuals who are blue-collar workers or have a lower annual household income [69]. Significantly, more research is needed to test and develop interventions that will be particularly effective for these high-risk populations. Genetic markers of nicotine dependence may differ for individuals from different racial groups as well, and interventions may need to be tailored to selectively attend to the strength and salience of their effect on related nicotine receptors [70]. Gender and age differences are also important considerations in tobacco cessation treatment and research. There is some debate regarding the efficacy of NRT for women [71], and women appear to face different stressors in quitting than do men. Additionally, female smokers are more likely than male smokers to have comorbid depression, compromising successful treatment outcome [72]. Smoking prevalence is also higher among those who started smoking as teenagers. To date, there is little research concerning efficacious treatment of smoking in youth, despite evidence that onset of smoking during adolescence is likely to contribute to more difficulties quitting later in life; however, it is hopeful that, in contrast to other age groups, cigarette use among teenagers appears to have declined over the past 10 years [73].

In sum, individuals from various cultures, races, SES, age, and gender groups are likely to respond differently to treatments designed to aid and achieve tobacco cessation. The research reviewed in this chapter strongly supports the use of integrated assessment, treatment, and long-term follow-up approaches that involve interdisciplinary and individually tailored interventions. These approaches are likely to significantly improve success rates of tobacco cessation efforts.

Conclusion

Integrative therapies (CAM) for tobacco cessation among tobacco users is a field with growing interest but little research or evidence regarding effectiveness. However, relapse rates for people trying to quit tobacco are high and anxiety, irritability and depression, strong and prolonged withdrawal symptoms, and weight gain are threats to long-term tobacco cessation [12]. Some limited research has suggested that various integrative, complementary interventions can be helpful with these symptoms. How or if these adjunctive therapies work directly on the nicotine cravings, neurophysiological effects of nicotine, and/or cognitive-sensory experience of smoking has yet to be determined. In the interim, the demonstrated interventions that promote the highest success rates for tobacco cessation are NRTs, behavioral interventions, and strong, consistent counseling.

References

1. Department of Health and Human Services. The health consequences of smoking: a report of the surgeon general. Atlanta: Department of Health and Human Services CfDCaP, National Center for Chronic Disease Prevention and Health Promotion, Office on Smoking and Health; 2004.
2. Cosgrove KP, Batis J, Bois F. Beta2-nicotinic acetylcholine receptor availability during acute and prolonged abstinence from tobacco smoking. Arch Gen Psychiatry. 2009;66:666–76.
3. Yolton K, Xu Y, Khoury J, Succop P, Beede DW, Owens J. Associations between secondhand smoke exposure and sleep patterns in children. Pediatrics. 2010;125(2):e261–8.
4. Gestreau C, Bévengut M, Dutschmann M. The dual role of the orexin/hypocretin system in modulating wakefulness and respiratory drive. Curr Opin Pulm Med. 2008;14(6):512–8.
5. Hollander JA, Qun L, Cameron MD, Kamenecka TM, Kenny PJ. Insular hypocretin transmission regulates nicotine reward. Proc Natl Acad Sci USA. 2008;105(49):19480–5.
6. Koopmann A, Dinter C, Richter A, et al. Orexin and leptin are associated with nicotine craving: a link between smoking, appetite and reward. Psychoneuroendocrinology. 2010;35(4):570–7.
7. Mineura YS, Picciottoa MR. Nicotine receptors and depression: revisiting and revising the cholinergic hypothesis. Trends Pharmacol Sci. 2010;31(12):580–6.
8. Perkins KA, Ciccocioppo M, Conklin CA, Milanak ME, Grottenthaler A, Sayette MA. Mood influences on acute smoking responses are independent of nicotine intake and dose expectancy. J Abnorm Psychol. 2008;117(1):79–93.
9. Fisher EB, Brownson RC, Health AC, Luke DA, Sumner WA. Cigarette smoking. In: Boll TJ, Raczynski JM, Leviton LC, editors. Handbook of clinical health psychology. Washington: American Psychological Association; 2004. p. 75–120.
10. Oncken C, Gonzales D, Nides M, et al. Efficacy and safety of the novel selective nicotinic acetylcholine receptor partial agonist, varenicline, for smoking cessation. Arch Intern Med. 2006;166(15):1571–7.
11. Brown RA, Lejuez CW, Kahler CW, Strong DR, Zvolensky MJ. Distress tolerance and early smoking lapse. Clin Psychol Rev. 2005;25:713–33.
12. Fiore MC, Jaen CR, Baker TB, et al. Treating tobacco use and dependence: 2008 update. Rockville: Public Health Service; 2008.
13. Sood A, Ebbert JO, Sood R, Stevens SR. Complementary treatments for tobacco cessation: a survey. Nicotine Tob Res. 2006;8(6):767–71.
14. Barnes J, Dong C, McRobbie H, Walker N, Mehta M, Stead LF. Hypnotherapy for smoking cessation. Cochrane Database Syst Rev. 2010;6(10):CD001008.
15. Hasan F, Pischke K, Saiyed S, Macys N, McCleary N. Hypnotherapy as an aid to smoking cessation of hospitalised patients: preliminary results. Chest. 2007;132(4):527a.
16. Carmody TP, Duncan C, Simon JA, et al. Hypnosis for smoking cessation: a randomized trial. Nicotine Tob Res. 2008;10(5):811–8.
17. White A, Moody R. The effects of auricular acupuncture on smoking cessation may not depend on the point chosen—an exploratory meta-analysis. Acupunct Med. 2006;24:149–56.
18. White AR, Rampes H, Liu JP, Stead LF, Campbell J. Acupuncture and related interventions for smoking cessation. Cochrane Database Syst Rev. 2011;1:CD000009.
19. Broms U, Korhonen T, Kaprio J. Smoking reduction predicts cessation: longitudinal evidence from the Finnish adult twin cohort. Nicotine Tob Res. 2008;10(3):423–7.
20. Hughes JR, Cummings KM, Hyland A. Ability of smokers to reduce their smoking and its association with future smoking cessation. Addiction. 1999;94(1):109–14.
21. Taylor CB, Chang VY. Issues in the dissemination of cognitive-behavior therapy. Nord J Psychiatry. 2008;62(47):37–44.
22. Bock BC, Morrow KM, Becker BM, et al. Yoga as a complementary treatment for smoking cessation: rationale, study design and participant characteristics of the Quitting-in-balance study. BMC Complement Altern Med. 2010;10(1):14.

23. Wynd CA. Guided imagery for smoking cessation and long-term abstinence. J Nurs Scholarsh. 2005;37(3):245–50.
24. Ussher M, Cropley M, Playle S, Mohidin R, West R. Effect of isometric exercise and body scanning on cigarette cravings and withdrawal symptoms. Addiction. 2009;104:1251–7.
25. Vidrine JI, Businelle MS, Cinciripini P, et al. Associations of mindfulness with nicotine dependence, withdrawal, and agency. Subst Abus. 2009;30(4):318–27.
26. Ussher MH. Exercise interventions for smoking cessation. Cochrane Database Sys Rev. 2008;(4):CD002295.
27. Marcus BH, Albrecht AE, King TK, Parisi AF, Pinto BM, Roberts M. The efficacy of exercise as an aid for smoking cessation in women: a randomised controlled trial. Arch Intern Med. 1999;159:1229–34.
28. Bock BC, Marcus BH, King TK, Borrelli B, Roberts MR. Exercise effects on withdrawal and mood among women attempting smoking cessation. Addict Behav. 1999;24(3):399.
29. Williams DM, Whiteley JA, Dunsiger S, et al. Moderate intensity exercise as an adjunct to standard smoking cessation treatment for women: a pilot study. Psychol Addict Behav. 2010;24(2):349–54.
30. Kinnunen T, Leeman RF, Korhonen T, et al. Exercise as an adjunct to nicotine gum in treating tobacco dependence among women. Nicotine Tob Res. 2008;10(4):689–703.
31. Carek PJ, Laibstain SE, Carek SM. Exercise for the treatment of depression and anxiety. Int J Psychiatry Med. 2011;41(1):15–28.
32. Kaczynski AT, Manske SR, Mannell RC, Grewal K. Smoking as a physical activity: a systematic review. Am J Health Behav. 2008;32(1):93–110.
33. McCarthy DE, Fiore MC, Baker TB, Piasecki TM. Have we lost our way? The need for dynamic formulations of smoking relapse proneness. Addiction. 2002;97(9):1093–108.
34. Emery CF, Blumenthal JA. Perceived change among participants in an exercise program for older adults. Gerontologist. 1990;30(4):516–21.
35. Bera T, Rajapurkar M. Body composition, cardiovascular endurance and anaerobic power of yogic practitioner. Indian J Physiol Pharmacol. 1993;37:225–8.
36. Malathi A, Damodaran A, Shah N, Patil N, Maratha S. Effect of yoga practices on subjective well-being. Indian J Physiol Pharmacol. 2000;44(2):202–6.
37. Mahajan AS, Reddy KS, Sachdeva U. Lipid profile of coronary risk subjects following yogic lifestyle intervention. Indian Heart J. 1999;51(1):37–40.
38. McIver S, O'Halloran P, McGartland M. The impact of hatha yoga on smoking behavior. Altern Ther Health Med. 2004;10(2):22–4.
39. Cabioglu MT, Ergene N, Tan U. Smoking cessation after acupuncture treatment. Int J Neurosci. 2007;117(5):571–8.
40. Huang W, Howie J, Taylor A, Robinson N. An investigation into the effectiveness of traditional Chinese acupuncture (TCA) for chronic stress in adults: a randomised controlled pilot study. Complement Ther Clin Pract. 2011;17:16–21.
41. Chae Y, Park H-J, Kang OS, et al. Acupuncture attenuates autonomic responses to smoking-related visual cues. Complement Ther Med. 2011;19 Suppl 1:S1–7.
42. Bier ID, Wilson J, Studt P, Shakleton M. Auricular acupuncture, education, and smoking cessation: a randomized, sham-controlled trial. Am J Public Health. 2002;92(10):1642–7.
43. Larzelere MM, Campbell JS, Robertson M. Complementary and alternative medicine usage for behavioral health indications. Prim Care. 2010;37(2):213–36.
44. Lakhan SE, Vieira KF. Nutritional and herbal supplements for anxiety and anxiety-related disorders: a systematic review. Nutr J. 2010;9(42). http://www.nutritionj.com/content/pdf/1475-2891-9-42.pdf. Accessed 3 Jan 2010.
45. Brazier NC, Levine MA. Drug-herb interaction among commonly used conventional medicines: a compendium for health care professionals. Am J Ther. 2003;10(3):163–9.
46. Hakim IA, Harris RB, Brown S, et al. Effect of increased tea consumption on oxidative DNA damage among smokers: a randomized controlled study. J Nutr. 2003;133(10):3303S–9.
47. Lee H, Lee J. Effects of medicinal herb tea on the smoking cessation and reducing smoking withdrawal symptoms. Am J Chin Med. 2005;33(1):127–38.

48. Rose JE, Behn FM. Inhalation of vapor from black pepper extract reduces smoking withdrawal symptoms. Drug Alcohol Depend. 1994;34(3):225–9.
49. Perry N, Perry E. Aromatherapy in the management of psychiatric disorders: clinical and neuropharmacological perspectives. CNS Drugs. 2006;20(4):257–80.
50. Stead LF, Perera R, Bullen C, Mant D, Lancaster T. Nicotine replacement therapy for smoking cessation. Cochrane Database Syst Rev. 2008;20:CD000146.
51. An LC, Zhu S-H, Nelson DB, et al. Benefits of telephone care over primary care for smoking cessation: a randomized trial. Arch Intern Med. 2003;166(5):536.
52. Fagerström K, Hughes J. Integrating varenicline into treatment for tobacco dependence. Neuropsychiatr Dis Treat. 2008;4:353–63.
53. Henningfield JE, Fant RV, Buchhalter AR, Stitzer ML. Pharmacotherapy for nicotine dependence. CA Cancer J Clin. 2005;55:281–99.
54. Stapleton JA, Watson L, Spirling LI, et al. Varenicline in the routine treatment of tobacco dependence: a pre-post comparison with nicotine replacement therapy and an evaluation in those with mental illness. Addiction. 2008;103:146–54.
55. Gouraly SG, Stead LF, Benowitz N. Clonidine for smoking cessation. Cochrane Database Syst Rev. 2004;(3):CD000058.
56. Hughes J, Stead L, Lancaster T. Antidepressants for smoking cessation. Cochrane Database Syst Rev. 2007;(1):CD000031.
57. Hughes J, Stead L, Lancaster T. Nortriptyline for smoking cessation: a review. Nicotine Tob Res. 2005;7:491–9.
58. Baillie A, Mattick R, Hall W, Webster P. Meta-analytic review of the efficacy of smoking cessation interventions. Drug Alcohol Rev. 1994;13:157–70.
59. Hall S, Munoz R, Reus V. Cognitive-behavioral intervention increases abstinence rates for depressive-history smokers. J Consult Clin Psychol. 1994;62:141–6.
60. Burke MV, Ebbert JO, Hays JT. Treatment of tobacco dependence. Mayo Clin Proc. 2008;83(4):479–84.
61. Lancaster T, Stead LF. Physician advice for smoking cessation. Cochrane Database Syst Rev. 2004;7.
62. Brief interventions and referral for smoking cessation in primary care and other settings. In: Excellence NIfHaC, ed. Public Health Intervention Guidance; 2006.
63. Lancaster T, Stead LF. Individual behavioural counselling for smoking cessation. Cochrane Database Syst Rev. 2005;2:CD001292.
64. Strecher VJ. Computer-tailored smoking cessation materials: a review and discussion. Patient Educ Couns. 1999;36:107–17.
65. Shahab L, McEwen A. Online support for smoking cessation: a systematic review of the literature. Addiction. 2009;104(11):1792–804.
66. Tonneson P. Smoking cessation: how compelling is the evidence? A review. Health Policy. 2009;91 Suppl 1:S15–25.
67. Transdisciplinary tobacco use research centers initiative. http://dccps.nci.nih.gov/tcrb/tturc/. Accessed 7 Feb 2011.
68. Augustson EM, Wanke KL, Rogers S, et al. Predictors of sustained smoking cessation: a prospective analysis of chronic smokers from the alpha-tocopherol beta-carotene cancer prevention study. Am J Public Health. 2007;98:549–55.
69. Lawrence D, Fagan P, Backinger CL, Gibson JT, Hartman A. Cigarette smoking patterns among young adults aged 18–24 years in the United States. Nicotine Tob Res. 2007;9(6):687–97.
70. Muller DJ, Likhodi O, Heinz A. Neural markers of genetic vulnerability to drug addiction. Curr Top Behav Neurosci. 2010;3:277–99.
71. Cepeda-Benita A, Reynoso JT, Erath S. Meta-analysis of the efficacy of nicotine replacement therapy for smoking cessation: differences between men and women. J Consult Clin Psychol. 2004;72:712–22.
72. Gritz ER, Thompson B, Emmons K, Ockene JK, McLerran DF, Nielsen IR. Gender differences among smokers and quitters in the Working Well Trial. Prev Med. 1998;27:553–61.
73. National Institute on Drug Abuse. InfoFacts: nationwide trends. In: Services NIoHUDoHaH, ed.; 2010.

Chapter 14
Integrative Therapies to Support Palliative and End-of-Life Care in Lung Disease

Sandra W. Gordon-Kolb

Abstract Patients with advanced lung disease are living longer. They constitute a significant proportion of the US population suffering with serious chronic illness whose quality of life (QOL) is suboptimal due to inadequately assessed or addressed high symptom burden from their disease. Early integration of palliative care's interdisciplinary approach can improve the illness experience of these patients and their families. It can improve their satisfaction with care and facilitate transition of care to less aggressive interventions when appropriate. Timely hospice care referral can minimize patient and family suffering at end of life. Improved clinician identification of symptom burden and communication of prognosis are skills needed to permit earlier palliative and hospice care. Evidence-based integrative or complementary therapies can be utilized to effectively supplement allopathic palliative treatment of multidimensional symptoms expressed by seriously ill patients and families. Further research is needed to strengthen the evidence base for integrative therapy in chronic lung disease and to determine the most optimal point and delivery method for integration of palliative approaches into treatment plans for these patients.

Keywords Caregiver stress • Chronic lung disease • Complementary therapies • Illness coping • Integrative therapies • Palliative care • Prognosis • Suffering • Symptom burden

Overview

Serious and chronic pulmonary disease affects a significant proportion of the US population and is the fourth leading cause of death in this country. Considered alone, chronic obstructive pulmonary disease (COPD) accounts for more than one million

S.W. Gordon-Kolb, MD, MMM (✉)
Department of Palliative Medicine, Fairview Health Services, Minneapolis, MN, USA
e-mail: sgordon4@fairview.org

L. Chlan and M.I. Hertz (eds.), *Integrative Therapies in Lung Health and Sleep*, Respiratory Medicine 4, DOI 10.1007/978-1-61779-579-4_14,

emergency department visits yearly, often resulting in frequent hospital admissions as the disease becomes advanced. Patients' breathlessness, fatigue, other physical symptoms, and emotional distress—as well as their caregivers' distress—are under-recognized or often inadequately assessed and managed. As lung disease advances with limited available opportunities for effective disease treatment, patients and families are frequently unprepared to consider end-of-life care until prompted by frequent readmissions or crisis care. This population is also known to underutilize the hospice benefit available to them for improved end-of-life care. Incorporating palliative care, which includes integrative therapies, to improve patients' distressing symptom burden and enable patients and their families to cope and live better with chronic pulmonary disease is the focus of this chapter.

As a result of advances in medical care, patients with serious lung disease are living longer but not necessarily with improved quality of life (QOL). Previously, diseases that would have been terminal early in their courses now have treatments that allow patients to live with a chronic illness process. This longer life usually involves a slowly progressive illness course for many years but, as in the case of transplantation for a variety of lung processes, may include periods of prolonged disease remission. Patients and their families have exchanged imminently "life-threatening" for "life-altering" diagnoses and illness courses, each with their attendant multidimensional symptom burden. The content, context, and impact of this symptom burden on patients and families are now being recognized as critical components of the illness care process. This process requires improved understanding of the illness experience of both patients and caregivers through additional qualitative and quantitative research and the development of additional evidence-based therapies for a more comprehensive and integrated processes of illness care.

Integrative medical care seeks to optimize health and healing from a multidimensional focus. It utilizes multidisciplinary therapeutic approaches, combining conventional medical–surgical therapies with evidence-based "complementary" therapies to achieve a holistic perspective of care, with the potential of maximizing the benefits of while reducing the adverse effects of mainstream care [1].

Since its inception, palliative care has been fundamentally integrative in its approach to care. The discipline utilizes conventional and alternative therapies, often in innovative ways, to achieve desired outcomes of care. More than 15 years ago, US palliative care evolved as a care discipline out of the hospice movement to address serious discrepancies in end-of-life care identified by the 1995 SUPPORT study regarding the suffering of dying cancer patients [2]. In 2006, Hospice and Palliative Medicine was recognized as an official medical subspecialty by the American Board of Medical Specialties. The discipline is dynamic and rapidly evolving in its standardized principles and approaches to care. As currently conceived, Hospice and Palliative Medicine consists of an interdisciplinary approach to patient- and family-centered care that is focused on assessing and relieving the suffering from illness consequences. It seeks to optimize function and QOL, as possible, within the illness context. Its approach requires illness experience assessment and management from an individualized, multidimensional symptom perspective, including physical, psychosocial, and spiritual components. This care process adjusts supportive and palliative elements of the care approach as appropriate to illness progression and patient and family goals of care. By focusing on the *illness experience,* palliative care addresses the *life-altering* aspects of illness care, seeking to restore meaning, control, and a sense of well-being to patients and their families.

As thus conceived, palliative care is applicable throughout any serious illness continuum from the time of diagnosis through the period of end-of-life care. The evidence base and experience of palliative care integration into comprehensive cancer care suggests that incorporating this model of care into the comprehensive care plan of any serious illness process should offer similar significant benefits. Research related to the palliative aspects of symptom burden in other diseases, but relevant to lung disease, support the beneficial use of incorporating palliative and integrative therapies in chronic lung disease management. Appropriate areas of palliative focus include lung cancer, COPD, pulmonary fibrosis, cystic fibrosis, and lung transplant care.

General Palliative Assessment and Management

The targeted global outcomes for patient symptom assessment and management in palliative care are QOL, coping capacity, functional capacity, and sense of well-being. Recent studies have shown patients with chronic illness commonly present with complex, multivariate symptom profiles that cluster according to causal relationships with specific disease manifestations, treatment effects, or interactions with each other. Persistent, unmanaged, clustered symptoms have been noted to define high levels of patient distress and create symptom management difficulties in cancer patients [3]. Patients' perceived inability to manage their symptoms has been associated with reduced QOL outcomes in cancer survivors. Based on this observation, consistent symptom relief without improvement in patients' perceived self-efficacy for continued symptom management likely will not optimize QOL impact [4]. Simple, rapid tools are available to facilitate primary treating teams to identify distressed, chronically ill patients and trigger referral of those with more complex palliative needs to a palliative consult team. Currently, the *distress thermometer* is the most commonly used tool [5]. A newly developed and validated *General Symptom Distress Scale* shows promise in identifying not only distressed patients but also their symptom ranking and ability to manage their symptoms. Improved physician–patient communications about chronic symptoms and improved patients' ratings of QOL and emotional functioning have been the observed impacts of provider attention to illness symptoms among cancer patients [4].

Complex symptom assessment and management optimally requires a palliative-trained, interdisciplinary team, minimally including a physician and/or advanced practice nurse, psychosocial provider (licensed clinical social worker and/or psychologist), and chaplain. The team applies validated, quantitative measures and qualitative descriptions of core physical and emotional symptoms common to chronic illnesses to assess and document symptoms serially over time. Descriptions of a patient's sense of spirituality, its importance, and the assessment of potential existential distress are included. To identify family-related issues, caregiver or child distress—including grief, loss, and coping dysfunction—are explored for focused support. Patient and family understanding of the patient's disease, current status, proposed treatment options, and prognosis are reviewed. Goals of care are defined. The latter may include advanced care planning information if appropriate and desired. A palliative and supportive plan of care is developed through a shared decisional dialogue for subsequent interdisciplinary team implementation. All processes of care are recommended or comanaged in collaboration with the patient's primary treating provider.

Definition and Supportive Data for Integrative Therapies Used for Palliative and Supportive Care

Integrative therapies including complementary and alternative medicine (CAM) techniques are used by a large proportion of the US population for a variety of reasons: to control symptoms, to enhance QOL and sense of well-being, and to promote healing and self-efficacy. Complementary techniques are considered evidence-based and used adjunctively with conventional medical therapies in palliative and other treatment approaches. In contrast, alternative therapies are not evidence-based and widely used by the public without clear benefit and often harm, if substituted as a therapeutic process for conventional treatments. Inquiring about use, correcting misinformation, and channeling or initiating safe and effective therapies for palliative treatment is a necessary component of palliative assessment [1, 6].

The National Institutes of Health (NIH) National Center for Complementary and Alternative Medicine (NCCAM) is charged with the directive to investigate CAM therapies for safety and effectiveness in given clinical situations. The organization categorizes CAM therapies into whole medical systems and four practice-based domains. The complex theories and practices of nonallopathic whole systems evolved separately from conventional medicine. Examples include homeopathic medicine, Ayurvedic medicine, and traditional Chinese medicine. Practice-based domains include (1) biologic-based approaches, (2) body-manipulative systems, (3) energy-based treatments, and (4) mind–body therapies [1]. Biologic-based botanicals, comprising aromatherapy, are variably used in palliative care. Techniques in the latter three domains are most commonly used. Techniques that are relevant to patients with lung diseases are explored in detail in the following text.

Biologic-Based Approaches

Aromatherapy

Botanical combinations in essential oil form are mixed in carrier lotions or oils for use in massage, inhalation, and bath therapies. For inhalation use, oils may be dripped onto absorptive materials such as cotton balls, tissue, or gauze placed near the nose, dabbed onto body pulse points, or sprayed/vaporized into a patient care area. Various botanicals are promoted as acting centrally and locally on soft tissues to induce analgesia, relaxation, immunostimulation, and antiemesis. These therapies are generally safe, easy to use by patients, not viewed as medical interventions by patients, and enhance a sense of control and self-efficacy in treatment. However, the evidence base for their effectiveness is limited [1, 6, 7].

Body-Manipulative Therapies

Massage

Multiple types of massage techniques exist. Therapists apply pressure to muscles and connective tissues with the intent to reduce tension and pain, increase circulation, improve range of motion, and promote relaxation for a general increase in well-being. The American College of Chest Physicians recommends massage as a complementary technique in lung cancer patients. Manual lymph drainage in combination with compressive bandaging is considered standard practice in lymphedema care, a common problem in advanced lung cancer and lung disease. Massage has also been shown to be effective for nonmalignant back pain. A recent randomized controlled trial (RCT) in cancer patients has shown that massage therapy results in an immediate improvement in mood and pain but has not verified sustained effects. Early evidence from preclinical studies suggests that massage affects physiologic processes that are relevant to pain modulation.

Trained therapists with clinical experience are able to adjust their techniques to avoid harm to diseased or treatment-affected areas. Allodynia from neuropathic pain and significant thrombocytopenia are relative contraindications to the use of massage [1, 6].

Energy-Based Techniques

Reiki, Healing Touch, Therapeutic Touch

Bioenergy manipulation therapies do not involve physical touch but an energy connection with a trained therapist. These techniques attempt to restore harmony and balance in a patient's energy system to promote self-healing. Though studies are limited, current data supports positive effects on pain, stress reduction, relaxation, sleep, chemotherapy-induced nausea, and a sense of "safeness." These effects appear to allow reductions in analgesic usage. No significant placebo effect related to pain treatment was identified. Effectiveness of the symptom improvement appears to vary directly proportional to the experience of the therapist [1, 6, 8].

Tai Chi, Qigong, and Related Techniques

Physical movement, breath control, and meditation are practiced in slow, balanced, choreographed movements during these therapies. The literature suggests general health benefits of cardiopulmonary fitness, balance and fall prevention improvement, increased QOL, and higher sense of self-efficacy; all of which are areas of symptom distress in chronic lung disease patients. A specific study in breast cancer patients demonstrated improved aerobic capacity, strength, and flexibility and increased their reported rates of QOL and self-esteem [1, 6].

Yoga

Yoga is a practice that incorporates physical movement, breath control, and various forms of meditation to improve spirituality and well-being. Different practices vary in their degree of physical difficulty. Evidence supports global improvements along with reductions in specific symptoms of nausea, anxiety, depression, and stress perception. Protective effects on NK cell levels and DNA damage postsurgery, chemotherapy, and radiation treatment in cancer patients have been reported [1, 6].

Acupuncture and Acupressure

This CAM approach utilizes strategically placed thin needles and heat or pressure application to one or several of the 12 principle meridians of the body to regulate the flow of *qi* (vital energy), as conceptualized in traditional Chinese medicine. Acupuncture may be combined with electrostimulation to enhance effects. The proposed mechanism of action of acupuncture or acupressure effect is centrally mediated through the release of neurotransmitters. Changes on functional magnetic resonance imaging (MRI) have been documented during acupuncture treatment that may correspond to such effects. A recent report in *The Journal of Pain* documented correspondence of the anatomic distribution of the 3,000+-year-old meridians to currently defined myofascial trigger points and referred pain patterns used for contemporary acupuncture treatment, suggesting a physiologic basis for this therapeutic approach [9]. Reasonable levels of evidence support the use of both approaches as adjunctive therapies for multiple types of pain and nausea/vomiting, including postoperative and chemotherapy-induced symptoms. Acupuncture appears more definitive than acupressure effects for the latter symptom process. Preliminary evidence exists for positive effects in cancer-related fatigue and for dyspnea in lung disease. When applied by trained, experienced practitioners, acupuncture is considered safe, although pneumothoraces may occur when needles are placed in the chest. Safety is enhanced by the regulation of acupuncture needles as medical devices in the United States [1, 6, 10].

Mind–Body Therapies

Hypnosis

This clinical technique involves a therapist-induced, altered level of awareness similar to daydreaming. During this state, the patient is more receptive to suggestions. It requires a safe environment, trust in the therapist, and an induction period of relaxation. A patient is then guided to focus on targeted objects or thoughts with the therapeutic intent of reducing symptoms or reactions related to the point of focus. Then the patient is returned to a normal waking state by the therapist. Sessions may be audiotaped for continued self-use by the patient. Evidence supports improvement in pain, nausea/vomiting, fatigue, anxiety, and sleep difficulties. In end-of-life care, hypnosis can be used to ameliorate the fear of death through a process of death preparation [1, 6].

Guided Imagery

Guided imagery induces a therapeutic meditative state that involves directing thoughts towards images that can create a state of relaxation, sense of well-being, and safety. After initial training, this is a self-use technique, which fosters a sense of patient self-efficacy. The method has proven to be adjunctive in controlling symptoms such as pain and in inducing positive attitudes during illness [1, 6].

Progressive Muscle Relaxation

This related technique utilizes focused concentration by the patient to produce progressive relaxing or tensing/relaxing of the entire body from head to toe. The process is slowly paced and deliberate. It is easy to learn and can be used independently by patients, contributing to a sense of control over treatment. Continued practice is required to maintain the sustained effects of this technique [1, 6].

Meditation

This approach is a form of mindfulness that focuses a person's mental attention on increasing awareness of all experiences or sensations that flow through the mind moment to moment. It is similar to a stream-of-consciousness effect. Data is limited but supports the use of the technique for improved mood, sleep, and QOL with stress reduction. It may have sustained effects. Immune function parameters also have been documented to increase in cancer patients. After initial training, meditation becomes a patient-controlled method of symptom management, contributing to an increased sense of self-efficacy [1, 6]. Clinicians' use of meditation has been shown to increase their sense of empathy [11].

Prayer

Prayer involves direct, meditative communication with a spiritual energy or higher being. It may occur individually, be facilitated by a spiritual mentor, or be practiced in a group setting. Prayer includes silent or verbalized expressions of gratitude or requests for help in managing a difficult life situation. The process may not necessarily involve formal religious content. Reports indicate that 50–90% of US and Canadian patients with cancer view spirituality as important to them in their illness. Prayer may be part of their spiritual practices. The *Brief Measure of Religious Coping Scale* and the *Religious Coping Activities Scale* have distinguished positive and negative coping and problem-solving strategies in illness related to spiritual beliefs. A clinical chaplain is trained to help patients discern which strategies patients practice and can help them utilize these strategies most effectively in their illness process. Physical healing has not been supported by the limited evidence available for prayer's clinical impact, but significant improvements in anxiety, psychological distress, and QOL have been demonstrated. Prayer and other spiritual coping strategies may provide patient guidance for advanced care planning and treatment preferences [1, 6, 12].

Music Therapy, Other Expressive Arts Therapies

In music therapy, a trained therapist involves a patient in listening to music, playing instruments, discussing music, or writing lyrics or musical scores with the intention of addressing an identified emotional issue or physical symptom. Often, it allows communication of feelings not able to be expressed in other media by patients. Existing evidence suggests that reduction of anxiety, pain, stress, fatigue, nausea, and insomnia results from this form of intervention [1, 6]. The Cochrane Collaboration reviewed studies that applied music listening interventions in mechanically ventilated patients but did not utilize a trained music therapist in the process. The eight studies reviewed showed reductions in heart and respiratory rates and anxiety. Whether application by a trained therapist could elicit more profound effects requires further study [13].

Other forms of expressive therapies employ various media such as poetry, art, and writing. All therapies are most effective when administered by a therapist trained in the supportive medium deployed. Nonverbal expressive therapies may be most effective for patients who have difficulty expressing their emotions or are more socially isolated. Such therapies offer an alternative method for patients to communicate their thoughts, emotions, fears, and beliefs about their illness experience and prognosis and have demonstrated improved coping and modulation of dysphoria.

The interdisciplinary palliative team's or the primary physician's narrative engagement with the patient and family can be restorative in itself. The narrative process provides "witnessing" of the suffering endured and the life or illness story expressed. This active listening process facilitates the patient or family's ability to find meaning in their illness process and improve illness coping [14]. This communication skill of "narrative competency" is integral to all palliative clinical interventions.

Palliative Approach to Common Symptoms in Lung Disease

Dyspnea

Dyspnea (breathlessness) is commonly defined as the subjective experience of an unpleasant or uncomfortable awareness of the need to breathe. As such it has both sensory and intensity components similar to the pain experience. It should be assessed and approached similar to pain. Psychosocial factors strongly shape an individual patient's experience of the symptom. The descriptor found most common to dyspnea across disease categories is "I cannot get enough air." Reportedly, patients and caregivers alike experience dyspnea as frightening and very distressing. It may present as chronic and/or incidental in occurrence and be difficult to control despite aggressive underlying disease management [15, 16]. Persistence suggests an advanced lung process that may have become minimally responsive to active disease treatment. Its debilitating effects have significant impact on functional capacity, QOL, and sense of well-being. Dyspnea is present in 94% of chronic lung disease patients in their last year of life [17].

Frequent symptoms clustered with dyspnea include anxiety, depression, fatigue, insomnia, and anorexia. Due to the frightening and distressing nature of dyspnea, anxiety may be both anticipatory and resultant in effect [16]. Objective respiratory parameters do not correlate with the subjective sense of dyspnea and should not be used to determine if a patient is or is not experiencing dyspnea. A tachypneic patient may not experience dyspnea subjectively. Dyspnea may also occur in the absence of hypoxemia. In such cases, oxygen supplementation may not optimally relieve the sense of dyspnea.

The pathophysiologic mechanisms of dyspnea are poorly understood and defined, as are the effects of the palliative methods used to manage the symptom. Opioids and benzodiazepines are the primary pharmaceutical classes shown to be effective in the palliation of dyspnea, regardless of disease etiology. Most recent palliative studies favor the use of opioids over benzodiazepines as first-line pharmacologic palliation [18]. Integrative techniques have been shown to be effective in dyspnea management. These techniques may be employed as a single method in less severe dyspnea but generally require combination with pharmacologic methods when dyspnea is more severe. Hypnosis, progressive muscle relaxation, guided imagery, meditation, and possibly healing touch and prayer are effective integrative techniques with an evidence basis for dyspnea relief.

Other complementary techniques with evidence-based effectiveness for dyspnea in COPD patients, both at rest and with exertion, include a handheld fan directed at the face and the nasal flow of cooled room air. These techniques have been documented to significantly lower minute ventilation and improve peak exercise performance and end-exercise dyspnea ratings. They induce a relative hypoventilatory pattern suggesting reduction in neural respiratory drive as the operative mechanism. This process is surmised to be mediated by the trigeminal nerve and/or nasal sensory receptors. Improved diaphragmatic electromechanical coupling has been proposed as an additive mechanism. Reduced diaphragmatic electromyographic activity/tidal volume ratios have been seen in healthy volunteers using facial fans during episodes of hypercapnia-induced dyspnea. These parameters have not been studied in diseased patients [19].

Fatigue and Insomnia

Fatigue is the most common symptom in advanced illness and is commonly underreported by patients. It is a multidimensional symptom that has physical, cognitive, and affective components [20]. Frequent descriptors of fatigue include a sense of generalized weakness, a lack of energy, tiredness, and a lack of sense of feeling "rested," despite patient-perceived adequate sleep. Difficulties getting to sleep, staying asleep, or frequent nocturnal awakenings all characterize insomnia. Both sleep disturbance and fatigue are commonly linked symptoms in chronic lung disease. They are multifaceted in both cause and effect, with disease process, treatment, and psychological aspects affecting their presentation. Unrecognized pain or depression is frequently associated and may be etiologic factors. A detailed patient narrative of their symptom experience coupled with clinical details of disease status and current treatment regimen is necessary to adequately assess the two symptoms and design optimal patient-specific, palliative interventions. The treatment plan should be guided by patient goals of care. Its primary focus should be modulation of reversible causes, within disease limitations and consistent with patient preferences. This plan should include adequate treatment of pain and depression, if symptoms are determined to be interfering with sleep or impacting fatigue [21].

Nonpharmacologic, integrative techniques with evidence bases for fatigue and insomnia management include (1) mind–body therapies of hypnosis, meditation, and guided imagery; (2) cognitive behavioral counseling including sleep hygiene approaches; and (3) patient/caregiver education about symptom knowledge and management. Active, low-level exercise and combined exercise/mind–body therapies of yoga and Tai Chi have evidence-based effectiveness in improving energy, mood, and sleep. Less evidence-based, but safe with some demonstrated benefits, are prayer and healing touch, acupuncture and acupressure, music therapy, and aromatherapy administered by an experienced practitioner [1, 6].

Anxiety, Altered Mood, Grief, and Loss

Grief and loss are normal responses to progressively debilitating disease, which commonly reduces independent functioning, changes social relationships, creates prognosis uncertainty, and alters physical or emotional self-images. Provider inquiry about these effects plus acknowledgement of these reactions as normal is often enough to promote adequate patient and family acceptance and facilitate coping strategies.

Patients and families with identified dysfunctional coping strategies will benefit from supportive grief counseling, during which more complex coping strategies can be ascertained and taught. Left unrecognized or unaddressed, these normal reactions may evolve into clinical depression or other manifestations of complicated grief. Addressing loss of meaning through cognitive or spirituality-based techniques or through life legacy work may reframe and restore hope and improve QOL. The ability of persons to find meaning in their suffering facilitates their capacity to cope with it [22]. Given their particular focus on feelings and meaning, art or poetry therapy and expressive writing are complementary techniques that may be effective adjunctive approaches [23].

Depressed mood and reduced QOL have been associated with shortened survival in metastatic lung cancer patients; whereas, addressing these issues has improved survival [24]. Clinical depression may be induced by uncontrolled physical symptoms and may improve with adequate physical symptom management alone. For those patients requiring behavioral intervention, cognitive–behavioral and supportive counseling may be required and may be effective without the need for drug therapy. Conventional antidepressant agents should be added in accordance with psychiatric clinical practice guidelines. Individual drug response is unpredictable. Choice of drug should be based on prior usage experience; concomitant symptoms such as pain, anxiety, fatigue, or sedation; and potential adverse interactions with existing treatment regimens or disease processes.

Similarly, clinically significant anxiety may be triggered by uncontrolled symptoms, especially pain and dyspnea. Adequately controlling these symptoms may sufficiently relieve anxiety without other treatment. When pharmacologic measures are required, benzodiazepines may be used safely in small doses in many cases of lung disease. Proactive use should be considered in anticipatory anxiety when clear triggers can be identified. Longer acting agents may be more helpful in sustained anxiety. Antidepressant agents with anxiolytic effects may be an alternative or synergistic drug choice when sedation is a significant concern. Traditional mind–body techniques have proven effectiveness in calming anxiety with potentially additive effects from prayer. Energy-based healing touch has less evidence to support its use but may be beneficial as well. When physically possible, mild active exercise and Tai Chi have demonstrated anxiolytic effects [6].

Cough and Secretions

Cough is common in many chronic lung disease patients. Studies have documented cough as the most prevalent symptom noted by adult cystic fibrosis (CF) patients, occurring with a >80–90% incidence. Its prevalence correlates with CF disease severity and exacerbations. Patients express cough as physically and emotionally distressing and often interfering with sleep. This latter effect contributes to other associated symptoms of fatigue and irritability. Cough may drive patients to socially isolate themselves due to perceived social stigma. This may be compounded when excessive secretion production is also present [25]. Cough may also be a significant symptom in lung cancer patients, with less prominence in other chronic lung processes. When active disease management including steroids inadequately controls cough distress, then palliation with combined benzonatate, a nonnarcotic antitussive, and low-dose opioids have proven effective. Some CF patients have reported effective symptom relief with the ingestion of water or hot liquids or with the use of distractive activities [26]. Mind–body techniques or spiritual interventions may reduce the symptom distress without overt cough reduction.

Palliative secretion management in lung disease may improve cough, dyspnea, and distress but must be balanced against the negative effects of increased sputum or oral secretion viscosity. Antisecretory agents act via anticholinergic effects. Sedation can be minimized by the use of agents that do not cross the blood–brain barrier including glycopyrrolate and hyoscamine. In bronchoalveolar cancer patients with severe bronchorrhea, case reports of improvement with inhaled indomethacin or octreotide at 300–500 μg/day via continuous aerosol administration have been published [27].

Pain

Pain in chronic lung disease is common but variably recognized and controlled. Both disease and treatment sources can cause pain: examples include musculoskeletal pain from vest treatment, intrinsic lung pain from disease or infection, skin and mucosal damage from radiation therapy, and neuropathy from disease or chemotherapy. Lung cancer patients benefit from the experience of clinicians' recognition and management of cancer-related pain in general [28]. Pain in nonmalignant lung disease is commonly underrecognized and inadequately treated. Fear of opioid-induced respiratory depression in the presence of lung compromise compounds this problem. Even with respiratory compromise, opioids can be safely used if initiated with low doses and titrated slowly under adequate monitoring. Under- or untreated pain creates significant physical and emotional distress which impacts other associated symptoms and reduces functional capacity and QOL [28].

Integrative, multimodality pain management approaches targeted to suspected sources and types of pain (somatic, visceral, neuropathic) minimize adverse therapeutic effects. Drug and complementary therapies being used for other symptoms or active treatment may improve pain with titration of doses or other enhancements. Examples include (1) duloxetine and tricyclic antidepressant effects on chronic and neuropathic pain and (2) steroid effects on inflammatory somatic, compressive visceral, or neuropathic pain types. All previously noted mind–body therapies improve pain symptoms. Acupuncture, acupressure, and transcutaneous nerve stimulation have proven effective in some types of somatic and neuropathic pain [6, 10].

Topical pharmaceutical agents have proven effective in relieving some types of pain. Minimal systemic absorption significantly diminishes drug class, adverse reactions. Common topical agents include lidocaine patches for neuropathic and visceral pain, mentholated or nonsteroidal anti-inflammatory gels or patches for somatic pain, gabapentin gel for peripheral neuropathy, and topical opioids for open wound pain or oral/esophageal mucositis [29, 30]. Some of these are available as commercial prescriptions; others must be compounded for use in appropriate delivery vehicles relevant for the specific site of pain.

Palliative Aspects of Selected Lung Diseases

Chronic Obstructive Lung Disease

Three recent studies in both Britain and the United States have documented that advanced COPD patients have a symptom burden and QOL comparable to or worse than that of advanced non-small-cell lung cancer (NSCLC) patients, who more routinely receive palliative care. Habraken et al. noted the most prominent care issues to be (1) management of dyspnea, (2)reduced functional status with perceived increased dependency, (3) lack of information about the disease and its prognosis, (4) depression, and (5) illness coping. They evaluated a more stable group of COPD patients than have previous studies; those with first-second expiratory volume (FEV1) parameters of less than 30% of predicted and greater than or equal to 60 years of age. They then compared this cohort to a similarly aged group of stages IIIb or IV NSCLC patients. Twenty-three percent of the COPD cohort died within 1 year of the study, and 50% required hospitalization for pulmonary exacerbations. Bausewein et al. studied stage III–IV COPD patients all with reported dyspnea during daily activities and compared them to matched stage III–IV NSCLC patients. The COPD patients had a median of 14 symptoms and global symptom distress equal to the cancer patients but a median survival five times longer. This study demonstrated a high morbidity and mortality in this COPD population and a clear need to address symptom burden earlier in their protracted illness trajectories. To meet this need, the authors advised integrating a palliative approach into the general care process of these patients well before the need for end-of-life care. Blinderman et al. demonstrated similar findings and conclusions in a prospective observational study of an advanced COPD population [31–33].

In both a 2008 and 2010 study of British COPD patients with daily dyspnea, Gysels and Higginson corroborated the need for palliative care in a similar population. These studies noted that current care processes in Britain were focused on the management of acute COPD exacerbations. In the care of this population, the recognition, assessment, and management of associated symptom burden, QOL, and expected decline were more often overlooked. In these studies, patients expressed feeling ill-prepared for both their disabling decline and the terminality of their disease. Most indicated a desire for earlier prognostic discussions with their physicians, better education about what symptoms they might experience, how symptoms might affect their QOL, and how such symptoms could be managed [15, 34]. In a 2011 BJM editorial, Thorns reiterated this integrative theme, noting that, "an accurate holistic assessment of need can guide the delivery of care more effectively than projected longevity, so that those with the greatest need receive the specialist palliative care that they require" [35].

In the United States, current COPD care is more often similarly disease- and crisis-focused. There remains insufficient attention to symptom burden, QOL, or communication about prognosis to promote early palliative care integration in this patient group. Palliative intervention is often postponed until at or very near the end of life. The American Thoracic Society's policy statement on palliative care in respiratory diseases strongly supports integrating palliative care into all stages of lung-related illness [36].

Attention to studies such as these is needed to increase primary and subspecialty COPD clinicians' awareness of patients' large and distressing symptom burden and the critical effect on their QOL. Such studies provide tools for clinicians to identify and address these issues at a more optimal phase of illness using palliative and integrative techniques.

Cystic Fibrosis

With treatment advances, CF is now a chronic pediatric and young adult illness process with the median predicted survival for CF patients now 39 years. Survivors, even those with mild pulmonary disease, have been documented as having a significant symptom burden affecting QOL. The three most prominent symptoms identified have included pain, cough, and dyspnea. Secondary symptom consequences have been noted as disturbed sleep and fatigue. On average, most patients have reported greater than two locations of pain with headache and abdominal pain most frequently described. Dyspnea has been noted to be present despite normal or mildly impaired pulmonary function and limited daily activities. Patients have been found to minimize their report of dyspnea, unless prompted by effort-described symptom inquiry. Study authors have theorized that minimization has occurred as an adaptive disease response in patients who have coped with chronic background dyspnea for years by reducing their activity levels and expectations [25, 26].

A 2008 Harvard study using data from the prospective, longitudinal *Project on Adult Care in Cystic Fibrosis* confirmed a similar symptom burden and defined psychological consequences more specifically. Patients studied had a predicted survival of less than or equal to 5 years. Sinus pain and discharge were identified as additional prominent symptoms with these likely accounting for headache reported as a frequent location of pain noted in other studies. In these patients, distress levels appeared more related to fatigue and psychological symptom burden and did not correlate with the degree of other physical symptoms. Over 50% of sampled patients most frequently described such distress using symptoms of "worrying, feeling irritable, and feeling sad" [25].

Dying CF patients frequently receive aggressive treatments at the end of life. This appears due to inadequate exploration of preferences prior to the active dying period when it is more difficult to elicit such preferences. Dellon assessed bereaved caregivers of deceased CF patients and reported that 81% endorsed discussing treatment preferences with patients during a stable period of disease when it was more likely that their wishes could be better understood by families and unwanted treatments could be minimized [37].

As with COPD patients, the CF population has an extended illness survival with a progressively disabling symptom burden and negative QOL impact. Earlier and more definitive symptom assessment and management using palliative and integrative techniques should positively impact the quality of care and lives of this patient group. Earlier advanced care planning also seems accepted and desired by patients and families based on the studies above.

Lung Transplantation

Lung transplantation is an increasing frequent option to extend life in a variety of chronic lung diseases. Approximately 1,300 patients receive lung transplants in the United States annually. A survival rate of 52% at year 5 is lower than other solid organ transplant survival rates. Despite this lower survival rate, studies have consistently shown surviving lung transplant patients have marked improvement over QOL and symptoms than other solid organ transplant patients. This seems related to a greater symptom burden prior to transplant than other organ diseases [38, 39]. The chronic immunosuppression required for transplantation creates multiple comorbid conditions that may reduce survival due to life-threatening complications. Chronic rejection, manifested as bronchiolitis obliterans syndrome (BOS), occurs in up to 64% of lung transplant patients by 5 years after transplant [39]. It results in frequent hospitalizations and intensive care unit stays. Both immunosuppression-related complications and BOS reduce QOL during the shortened survival period. Patients have reported the experience of high levels of psychological distress and an average physical symptom burden of 17 symptoms. Due to the complex care needs and unpredictable trajectory of these patients, their caregivers report similarly high levels of distress, as well as logistic and financial concerns. Studies have confirmed their desire for improved communication and psychological support during the illness experience [40].

BOS poses a particularly difficult period of care for both providers and patients/families in which the integration of palliative approaches could offer significant benefit. Although BOS often predicts a terminal decline, this decline is prolonged, with a median survival of 12.6 months after onset. Frequent hospitalizations and periods of aggressive acute care occur during this period. Song et al. surveyed major US lung transplant centers and reported a lack of involvement with palliative care services until all treatment options had been exhausted. They reported both provider and patient/family factors as barriers to palliative support in this population. Caregivers were noted to express disappointment that their care "investment" in preventing rejection in the recipient had failed. Due to the unpredictability of the rejection course, caregivers maintained hope that continued aggressive treatment would offer extended stabilization and postpone the inevitable. The option of retransplantation seemed to particularly reinforce this hope and treatment demand. Authors noted physician reluctance to discuss a poor prognosis as likely reinforcing such potentially false hope and the continued focus on an aggressive treatment model. Unawareness was evident that palliative care integration in this period of care might alleviate this distress. Proposed process changes included earlier symptom management and support concurrently with stabilizing treatments with later facilitation of more appropriate care as the patient declined. The authors concluded that transplant programs needed to be more informed about palliative care integration options to better address patients/family care needs as transplant recipients decline [40].

All lung transplant patients and caregivers have palliative needs but especially those with the complications noted above. Adjusting from a chronically ill to a wellness role requires substantial psychosocial change for both patient and caregiver. Pretransplant anxiety levels have been shown to persist for at least 6 months after transplant, even in patients who do well [38]. Integrative techniques could be significantly beneficial in reducing both physical and psychosocial symptom burden and this role adjustment process. Currently, there is limited integration of palliative approaches or services into post–lung transplant care despite this apparent need. The optimal design of such integration requires further definition. Song et al. in their study on meaning in lung transplant chronic rejection suggest some rational time points for palliative integration [40].

Lung Cancer

Despite advances in treatment, lung cancers have limited survival trajectories with an increasingly severe symptom burden as the disease progresses. Lung cancer patients report higher levels of distress than other cancer populations. Suffering appears not only related to physical symptoms but also to psychological, social, and existential distress. Uncontrolled symptom burden increases psychological angst and reduces the sense of hope. Anxiety and depression have been correlated with reduced QOL and coping capacity in this population [41]. Palliative approaches for optimal symptom control include the pharmacologic and integrative techniques reviewed above. Integrative strategies to improve coping skills may further impact QOL. Cognitive–behavioral techniques to improve illness coping are an integral part of palliative treatment; consistent patient use of these techniques after training optimizes coping skills. As disease severity increases, patients use these skills less consistently, and caregiver involvement in symptom management is more likely to insure its success. Porter et al. have shown that training lung cancer patients and caregivers together rather than separately may increase this consistency of use and sustain their impact. They demonstrated improved symptom-related communication between patient and caregiver, increased ability of caregivers to prompt and reinforce patients' use of learned skills, and enhancement of caregivers' sense of self-efficacy. Supportive intervention and education seem most appropriate for stage I lung cancer patients and caregivers. A focus on coping skills training appears more beneficial for latter stage cancer cases [28, 42–44].

Possessing higher levels of spirituality may reduce the impact of lung cancer symptom burden distress. This was suggested by a preliminary study that correlated greater levels of spirituality with less global distress and less specific distress about breathing symptoms, body image changes, worry, and fear. Assessing and maneuvering spiritual strengths in patients, when they exist, may positively impact cancer patient QOL outcomes [45].

As previously noted, early integration of palliative care into chronic lung disease management has been demonstrated to improve QOL. A recent study of stage III–IV NSCLC patients has now also established that early ambulatory palliative integration improves survival. Even when combined with more appropriate but less aggressive care, patients with early palliative care had extended survival beyond usual oncology care patients by as long as 3 months. This included significantly improved QOL and mood compared with the usual care cohort [24]. A recent study on prognostic perceptions and goals of therapy of metastatic NSCLC patients revealed inaccurate patient prognosis understanding. The study demonstrated that early palliative care in these patients significantly improved their prognosis understanding and positively impacted decisions near the end of life [46].

End-of-Life Care in Pulmonary Disease

Palliation of symptoms and improvement in QOL and sense of well-being become the primary foci of care in advanced lung disease patients as they approach the end of life. This includes the increased importance of the application of the integrative and complementary therapies discussed previously. The benefits of a palliative approach become more important than its risks as patients struggle to be comfortable and most often desire QOL over quantity of life at this point in their illness. As always in palliative care, treatment at the end of life is governed by the wishes and goals of care of the patient or their surrogates, if patients are incapacitated for decisions of care. Primary treating providers can facilitate the transition to end-of-life care by having earlier conversations with patients and their family in preparation for this period of illness. The earlier in the disease continuum that palliative care is integrated as a concomitant process of care, the more likely that preparation for this period of care will occur [1, 24, 37, 40]. The completion of healthcare directives and the newer physician order for life-sustaining treatment (POLST) should be encouraged as part of this preparation to help insure that patients' care wishes are more likely to be followed in a fragmented healthcare system [47]. Contrary to some physicians' fears, most patients wish to have their prognosis honestly discussed. Studies have shown hope is not destroyed through these conversations but reframed in ways that allow meaning to be maintained and anticipatory grief and loss expressed and supported to sustain this meaning. Life legacy work with an interdisciplinary team, using any of the integrative expressive art therapies, can enhance the meaning of this care process [48]. Recent studies have shown that families who are involved in a supported end-of-life care process are more satisfied with the care their loved one received and are less likely to have a difficult or complicated grief process.

Hospice care is the formalized delivery process of end-of-life care in the United States. Parameters for this care benefit were established by Medicare in 1982, and commercial insurances generally follow Medicare benefit criteria. Eligibility criteria require a prognosis of <6 months if the disease follows its natural expected course of decline. This criterion was based on cancer, which has a predictable trajectory of decline. Nonmalignant chronic diseases have a less predictable trajectory, often punctuated with frequent exacerbations with some degree of recovery and a slower decline. These altered trajectories create uncertainty for providers and patients and families as to when end-of-life care is appropriate and hospice referral should be considered. This ambiguity translates into underutilization of hospice care for nonmalignant disease or delayed referral until the last few days or weeks of life when the full benefits of hospice care are unable to be realized. It also increases the probability that inappropriately aggressive care is continued late into the illness trajectory with death occurring in ICUs or hospitals when most patients wish to die at home.

Hospice care is most commonly delivered at home, if a safe and adequate caregiving situation can be arranged. With widely dispersed contemporary families and the lack of hospice benefit coverage for paid caregivers, home hospice care may be difficult to manage. Facility care in a skilled nursing facility or a residential hospice facility is an alternative care option, but rooming charges are not covered under the hospice benefit and often make this option unaffordable. Facilities are also not where most patients wish to die. State Medicaid benefits usually will cover this cost at skilled facilities but not private residential hospice facilities. Few charitable residential hospices exist in the United States. National palliative and hospice organizations are recommending Congress to revamp the archaic funding and eligibility criteria of the existing hospice benefit to meet the care needs of contemporary chronic illness trajectories [49].

Future Areas for Palliative Care Research in Lung Disease

Challenges continue to exist in palliative and integrative therapies research in general. RCTs are the gold standard for evidence-based research. However, the application of this type of research approach is problematic in the palliative population which has limited longevity and difficulty participating in such trials due to illness-based debility. The complexity of the outcomes sought is also problematic. Desirable outcomes should encompass measures of wholeness and healing from palliative and integrative interventions. Currently, there is a lack of qualitative research about illness experiences and lack of validated tools to measure such outcomes in order to proceed to a quantitative process. Also, there are economic barriers to translating the clinical use of integrative techniques into a palliative approach. Specifically, measures of cost-effectiveness to demonstrate economic worth and support of integrative interventions depend upon proven clinical effectiveness and safety for which there is limited evidence to date.

Though both NIH CAM and palliative research efforts have made considerable strides in these areas, much remains to be done.

General themes identified for the applications of interventions and outcomes measures include the following:

- Determining the optimal therapeutic relationship, including narrative competency and relational empathy
- Assessment of the clinical impact of treatment methods to enhance self-concept, self-efficacy, and self-regulation
- Assessment and management of existential distress including hope, spirituality, and dignity
- Assessment and management of patient-centered symptoms and concerns
- Impact of palliative and integrative processes on survival and QOL [50]

Specific needs related to lung diseases may include:

- Identifying unique symptom clusters characteristic for each disease process and which integrative interventions most positively impact their management.
- Measuring the illness experience of specific lung disease impact on caregivers as well as patients, and determine how best to support caregivers during the illness process.
- Determining whether increased caregiver illness-related education and support impacts patient illness experience outcomes.
- Discerning the most optimal points in specific disease processes when prognostic discussions and advanced care planning will be most acceptable to patients and families and have a positive impact on subsequent care decisions as the patient declines. Particular impact on end-of-life care including place, cost, and satisfaction with such care will be important to continue to define.

Conclusions

Evidence is rapidly evolving that demonstrates the clinical and experiential value of applying palliative supportive and integrative interventions as concurrent collaborative processes of care in multiple types of chronic lung disease and after lung transplantation. Earlier integration of these interventions and the need for more aggressive and earlier symptom burden identification and management are emerging as critical to QOL, treatment tolerance, and perhaps survival in lung disease. Provider narrative competency and empathic assessment of illness experience are crucial components in most successfully impacting a positive patient and family illness experience, regardless of disease entity. Identifying and addressing caregiver suffering and support is increasing being shown to have an important impact on the patient illness experience and treatment process. In order to develop optimal care protocols, further research is needed regarding which palliative and integrative interventions have clinical benefit and translational practicality for patient and caregiver experience during specific lung disease courses.

References

1. NIH National Center for Complementary and Alternative Medicine.
2. The SUPPORT Principle Investigators. The study to understand prognoses for outcomes and risks of treatment. J Am Med Assoc. 1995;274:159–98.
3. Molassiotis A, Wengström Y, Kearney N. Symptom cluster patterns during the first year after diagnosis with cancer. J Pain Symptom Manage. 2010;39(5):847–85.
4. Badger TA, Segrin C, Meek P. Development and validation of an instrument for rapidly assessing symptoms: the general distress scale. J Pain Symptom Manage. 2011;41(3):535–48.
5. Lynch J, Goodhart F, Saunders Y, O'Connor SJ. Screening for psychological distress in patients with lung cancer: results of a clinical audit evaluating the use of the patient distress thermometer. Support Care Cancer. 2011;19(2):193–202.
6. Deng GE, Frenkel M, Cohen L, Cassileth BR, Abrams DI, Capodice JL, Courneya KS, Dryden T, Hanser S, Kumar N, Labriola D, Wardell DW, Sagar S. Evidenced-based clinical practice guidelines for integrative oncology: complementary therapies and botanicals. J Soc Integr Oncol. 2009;7(3):85–119.
7. Price S, Price L, editors. Palliative and supportive care, Chap. 15. Aromatherapy for health professionals. 3rd edn. London: Churchill Livingstone/Elsevier; 2007. p. 313–30.
8. So PS, Jiang Y, Qin Y. Touch therapies for pain relief in adults. Cochran Database Syst Rev. 2008;(4):CD 006535.
9. Dorsher PT. Myofascial referred pain data provides physiologic evidence of acupuncture meridians. J Pain. 2009;10(7):723–31.
10. Ernst E, Lee MS. Acupuncture for palliative and supportive cancer care: a systematic review of systematic reviews. J Pain Symptom Manage. 2010;40(1):e3–5.
11. Ludwig DS, Kabat-Zinn J. Mindfulness in medicine. JAMA. 2008;300(11):1350–2.
12. Van Laarhoven HWM, Schilderman J, Vissers KC, Verhagen C, Prins J. Images of god in relation to coping strategies of palliative cancer patients. J Pain Symptom Manage. 2010;40(4):495–501.
13. Bradt J, Dileo c, Grocke D. Music interventions for mechanically ventilated patients. Cochrane Database Syst Rev. 2010;(12):CD006902.
14. Romanoff BD, Thompson BE. Meaning construction in palliative care: the use of narrative, ritual, and the expressive arts. Am J Hosp Palliat Care. 2006;23(4):309–16.
15. Gysels M, Higginson IJ. The experience of breathlessness: the social course of chronic obstructive pulmonary disease. J Pain Symptom Manage. 2010;39(3):555–61.
16. Wilcock A, Crosby V, Hughes A, Fielding K, Corcoran R, Tattersfield AE. Descriptors of breathlessness in patients with cancer and other cardiorespiratory diseases. J Pain Symptom Manage. 2002;23(3):182–9.
17. Pan CX, Morrison S, Ness J, Fugh-Berman D, Leipzig RM. Complementary and alternative medicine in the management of pain, dyspnea, and nausea and vomiting near the end of life: a systematic review. J Pain Symptom Manage. 2000;20(5):374–87.
18. Simon ST, Higginson IJ, Booth S, Harding R, Bausewein C. Benzodiazepines for the relief of breathlessness in advanced malignant and non-malignant diseases in adults. Cochrane Database Syst Rev. 2010;20(1):CD007354.

19. Galbraith S, Fagan P, Dip G, Perkins P, Lunch A, Booth S. Does the use of a handheld fan improve chronic dyspnea? A randomized, controlled, crossover trial. J Pain Symptom Manage. 2010;39(5):831–8.
20. LeGrand SB. Fatigue. Palliative medicine. 1st edn. Chap. 161. Philadelphia: Saunders; 2009. p. 886–90.
21. Del Fabbro E, Dalal S, Bruera E. Symptom control in palliative care—part II: cachexia/anorexia/fatigue. J Palliat Med. 2006;9(12):409–22.
22. Fegg MJ, Brandstätter M, Kramer M, Kögler M, Haarmann-Doetkotte S. Meaning in life in palliative care patients. J Pain Symptom Manage. 2010;40(4):502–9.
23. Clary PL. Poetry and healing at the end of life. J Pain Symptom Manage. 2010;40(8):796–88.
24. Temel JS, Greer JA, Muzikansky A, Gallagher ER, Admane S, Jackson VA, Dahlin CM, Blinderman CD, Jacobsen J, Pirl WF, Billings JA, Lynch TJ. Early palliative care for patients with metastatic non-small-cell lung cancer. N Engl J Med. 2010;363:733–42.
25. Sawicki GS, Sellers DE, Robinson WM. Self-reported physical and psychological symptom burden in adults with cystic fibrosis. J Pain Symptom Manage. 2008;35(4):372–80.
26. Stenekes SJ, Hughes A, Grégoire M-C, Frager G, Robinson WM, McGrath PJ. Frequency and self-management of pain, dyspnea, and cough I cystic fibrosis. J Pain Symptom Manage. 2009;38(6):837–84.
27. Hudson E, Lester JF, Attanoos RL, Seamus JL, Byrne A. Successful treatment of bronchorrhea with octreotide in a patient with adenocarcinoma of the lung. Letter to the editor. J Pain Symptom Manage. 2006;32(3):200–2.
28. Henoch U, Bergman B, Gustafsson M, Gaston-Johansson F, Danielson E. The impact of symptoms, coping capacity, and social support on quality of life experience over time in patients with lung cancer. J Pain Symptom Manage. 2007;34(4):370–9.
29. Gairard-Dory AC, Schaller C, Mennecier B, Molard A, Gourieux B, Beretz L, Quoix E. Chemotherapy-induced esophagitis pain relieved by topical morphine: three cases. J Pain Symptom Manage. 2005;30(2):107–9.
30. LeBon B, Zeppetella G, Higginson I. Effectiveness of topical administration of opioids in palliative care: a systematic review. J Pain Symptom Manage. 2009;37(5):913–7.
31. Habraken JM, ter Riet G, Gore JM, Greenstone MA, Weersink JM, Bindels PJE, Willems DL. Health-related quality of life in end-stage COPD and lung cancer patients. J Pain Symptom Manage. 2009;37(6):973–81.
32. Bausewein C, Booth S, Gysels M, Kühnbach R, Haberland B, Higginson I. Understanding breathlessness: cross-sectional comparison of symptom burden and palliative care needs in chronic obstructive pulmonary disease and cancer. J Palliat Med. 2010;13(9):1109–18.
33. Binderman CD, Homel P, Billings AJ, Tennstedt S, Portnoy RK. Symptom distress and quality of life in patients with advanced chronic obstructive lung disease. J Pain Symptom Manage. 2009;38(1):115–23.
34. Gysels M, Higginson IJ. Access to services for patients with chronic obstructive pulmonary disease: the invisibility of breathlessness. J Pain Symptom Manage. 2008;36(5):451–60.
35. Thorns A. Palliative care in people with chronic obstructive pulmonary disease. Br Med J. 2011;342:d106.
36. American Thoracic Society End of life Care Task Force. An Official American Thoracic Society clinical policy statement: palliative care for patients with respiratory diseases and critical illnesses. Am J Respir Crit Care Med. 2008;177:912–27.
37. Dellon EP, Shores MD, Nelson KI, Wolfe J, Noah TL, Hanson LC. Family caregiver perspectives on symptoms and treatments for patients dying from complications of cystic fibrosis. J Pain Symptom Manage. 2010;40(6):829–37.
38. Santana MJ, Santana MJ, Feeny D, Jackson K, Weinkauf J, Lien D. Improvement in health-related quality of life after lung transplantation. Can Respir J. 2009;16(5):153–8.
39. Orens JB, Garrity Jr ER. General overview of lung transplantation and review of organ allocation. Proc Am Thorac Soc. 2009;6:13–9.
40. Song MK, DeVito Dabbs AJ, Studer SM, Arnold RM, Pilewski JM. Exploring the meaning of chronic rejection after lung transplantation and its impact on clinical management and caregiving. J Pain Symptom Manage. 2010;40(2):246–55.

41. Kroenke K, Theobold D, Wu J, Loza JK, Carpenter TS. The association of depression and pain with health rated quality of life, disability, and healthcare use in cancer patients. J Pain Symptom Manage. 2010;40(3):327–41.
42. Porter LS, Keefe FJ, Garst J, Baucom DH, McBride CM, McKee DC, Sutton L, Carson K, Knowles V, Rumble M, Scipio C. Caregiver-assisted coping skills training for lung cancer: results of a randomized clinical trial. J Pain Symptom Manage. 2011;41(1):1–13.
43. Berendes D, Keefe FJ, Somers TJ, Kothadia SM, Porter LS, Cheavens JS. Hope in the context of lung cancer: relationship of hope to symptoms and psychological distress. J Pain Symptom Manage. 2010;40(2):174–82.
44. Lobchuk MM, Kristjanson L. Perceptions of symptom distress in lung cancer patients: II behavioral assessment by primary family caregivers. J Pain Symptom Manage. 1997;14(3): 147–56.
45. Dedert EA, Ghate S, Floyd A, Banis P, Weissbecker I, Hermann C, Studts J, Salmon P, Sephton S. Spirituality suffers symptom distress in patients with lung cancer. J Psychosom Res. 2003;55:169–70.
46. Temel JS, Greer JA, Admane S, Gallagher ER, Jackson VA, Lynch TJ, Lennes IT, Dahlin CM, Pirl WF. Longitudinal perceptions of prognosis and goals of therapy in patients with metastatic non-small-cell lung cancer: results of a randomized study of early palliative care. J Clin Oncol. 2011;29(17):2319–26.
47. Citko J, Alvin H, Carley M, Tolle S. The National POLST Paradigm Initiative, 2nd Edition #178. J Palliat Med. 2009;14(2):241–2.
48. Boston P, Bruce A, Schreiber R. Existential suffering in the palliative care setting: an integrated literature review. J Pain Symptom Manage. 2011;41(3):604–18.
49. Casarett DJ. Rethinking hospice eligibility criteria. JAMA. 2011;305(10):1031–2.
50. Thompson EA, Quinn T, Paterson C, Cooke H, McQuigan D, Butters G. Outcome measures for holistic, complex interventions within the palliative care setting. Complement Ther Clin Pract. 2008;14:25–32.

Chapter 15
Whole Medical Systems in Lung Health and Sleep: Focus on Traditional Chinese Medicine

Guoqin Li, Fang Wang, Shihan Wang, Yi Tian, Yongjun Bian, Lei Wang, Guangxi Li, Jie Wang, and Amy T. Wang

Abstract Integrative medicine has emerged as an increasingly useful and complementary approach to allopathic medicine. Over the last few decades, Traditional Chinese Medicine (TCM) as a whole medical system has become a well accepted and integral component of integrative medicine. This chapter serves as a tutorial illustrating modalities widely used in China, focusing on TCM philosophy and common practices for lung health and sleep.

Keywords Lung health • Pulmonary • Sleep • Traditional Chinese medicine • Whole medical systems

Overview and Introduction

Disorders of the respiratory tract affect millions of Americans every year. Respiratory infections, such as influenza and pneumonia, are among the leading causes of death worldwide. In addition, the incidence of asthma, chronic obstructive pulmonary disease (COPD), interstitial pulmonary fibrosis (IPF), and sleep disorders are on the rise. The scientific community has continued to gain insight into the pathophysiology and treatment of various respiratory processes, leading to more accurate diagnoses and improved management of many respiratory conditions. However, there are still

G. Li, MD (✉) • F. Wang, MD, PhD • S. Wang, MD, PhD • Y. Tian, MD, MSc • Y. Bian, MD, PhD • L. Wang, MD, PhD • J. Wang, MD, PhD
Guang An Men Hospital, China Academy of Chinese Medical Science,
No. 5 Bei Xian Ge St., Beijing 100053, China

G. Li, MD • A.T. Wang, MD
Mayo Clinic, 200 First St. SW, Rochester, MN 55905, USA
e-mail: li.guangxi@mayo.edu

L. Chlan and M.I. Hertz (eds.), *Integrative Therapies in Lung Health and Sleep*,
Respiratory Medicine 4, DOI 10.1007/978-1-61779-579-4_15,

numerous pulmonary processes that are poorly understood and for which treatments are lacking.

Allopathic medicine has enabled significant improvements in the prevention and treatment of pulmonary and sleep pathology worldwide but there is still significant progress to be made. Combining the practice of Traditional Chinese Medicine (TCM) as a Whole Medical system with allopathic medicine can offer new and valuable perspectives and techniques to improve both lung and sleep health. The purpose of this chapter is to define Whole Medical Systems and to present information specifically on one whole medical system: TCM. The information presented is based on available Chinese literature, our own experiences with TCM, and limited Western-published investigations. Common lung and sleep disorders that could be treated from a TCM perspective are highlighted in this chapter, including lung infections, asthma, COPD, interstitial lung disease (ILD), and selected sleep disorders.

Overview of Whole Medical Systems: Focus on TCM

Whole medical systems are comprehensive schools of thought and medical practices that developed independently from and often trace back further than allopathic medicine. Examples of whole medical systems include Ayurvedic medicine, TCM, and homeopathy. This chapter will focus exclusively on TCM.

The origination of TCM dates back to 2,000 BC. In TCM, the body is viewed as two opposite but united energies of yin and yang. In simple terms, yin symbolizes cold forces while yang symbolizes hot forces. Achieving balance between these two systems is one of the driving forces behind the therapies of TCM. The vital energy or qi is also another guiding principle in TCM. Imbalances between yin and yang are believed to block the smooth and natural flow of qi. Thus, the mainstays of therapies of TCM revolve around restoring harmony between these two life forces.

The main function of the lung is to facilitate gas exchange between the human body and the natural environment. As air from the environment enters the lung, potentially hazardous microorganisms and particles are often inhaled, and may pose a threat to lung health. Though the human body is designed to filter many of these particles, this remains a common entry point for bacteria and viruses, causing respiratory conditions from the common cold to historic pandemics such as the 1918 Spanish flu [1] and the 2009 H1N1 influenza outbreak [2]. The diagnosis and treatment of infectious respiratory illnesses dates back thousands of years. An ancient Chinese medical text *Shang Han Lun,* by Zhang Zhongjing, describes symptoms and diagnosis of respiratory infections and treatments including herbal formulas, acupuncture, and other mind-body practices used 2,000 years ago. Another book, *Wen Bing Tiao Bian,* published in 1798, also delineated respiratory infections including symptoms, diagnosis, and treatment. Many other ancient cultures also date back over 2,000 years, including the Egyptians and Greeks who described treatment of respiratory infections with concoctions of botanical components, including molds and plants.

Historical Perspective of Whole Medical Systems for Respiratory System Infections

While theories in the approach to respiratory infections may differ among TCM, Ayurvedic medicine, Homeopathic medicine, and other whole medicine systems, the historical success and thousands of years of experience inherent to these systems suggest that they may serve as important adjuncts to the Western medical system. The use of natural plants to treat infectious disease can be traced back to many ancient cultures. Acupuncture has been described as an important method in the treatment of respiratory infections in many antiquated Chinese Medicine books. Pricking out blood therapy is one of the oldest acupuncture techniques, which uses needles to pierce particular points on the body to let out blood therapeutically. This method was historically used to drain fever caused by infectious diseases and was described in *Yellow Emperor's Classic of Internal Medicine* [3].

Although treatment of disease is often thought to be the focus of alternative medical systems, the central philosophy in TCM is the *prevention* of disease. It is believed that disease is often caused by imbalance present within the body. Thus, a prime focus for therapies is to prevent disease by maintaining balance within the body and averting imbalance. This is the one of the principles common to Qigong, Tai chi, Yoga, and other mind-body medicine techniques, which promote balance and are believed to aid in disease prevention. Whole medical systems, including TCM, have successfully treated illnesses for thousands of years with an emphasis on maintaining balance within the body.

Asthma

TCM has a long history in treating asthma. In TCM, asthma is often thought of in terms of *xiao* and *chuan*; wheezing and dyspnea, respectively. It is also divided into heat-, cold-, deficiency-, or mucus-type asthma depending on symptoms. These classifications help to shape corresponding treatments. In recent years, TCM has been increasingly recognized and utilized as an adjunctive therapy for asthma. Modalities of TCM including acupuncture, acupoint application with medicines to various acupuncture points on the body, and ingestion of oral Chinese medicines.

While acupuncture has been used to treat asthma in China since ancient times, the practice has evolved over time, yielding some differences in acupoint selections between the ancient and more modern traditions. We reviewed the important peer-reviewed papers published in major Chinese Medicine Journals from 1990 to 2010 for this section. There are two major outcome evaluation systems used in TCM research to rate asthma control: Chinese Medicine Symptom Evaluation for Asthma (CMSEA) (Table 15.1) and the Global Initiative for Asthma (GINA) (Table 15.2) (Full text available at http://www.ginasthma.org). CMSEA is an individual symptom-based evaluation system in which the efficacy rate is evaluated by the score.

Table 15.1 Chinese medicine symptom evaluation for asthma

Level of severity Symptom	Severe (3)	Moderate (2)	Mild (1)	None (0)
Panting	Dyspnea with significant activity limitation	Dyspnea with moderate activity limitation	Dyspnea without activity limitation	No dyspnea
Coughing	Cough very often; no sleep	Cough often but not in the night	Cough occasionally	No cough
Wheezing	Loud noise wheezing	Moderate noise wheezing	Mild noise wheezing	No wheezing
Sputum	Dark purulent yellow sputum	Yellow sputum	Light yellow sputum or white sputum	None

Table 15.2 Global initiative for asthma classification of severity

Classification	Symptoms	Exacerbations	Nocturnal symptoms	Pulmonary function test
Intermittent	Less than once a week	Brief	Not more than twice a month	FEV1 or PEF ≥80% pred; PEF or FEV1 variability <20%
Mild persistent	Symptoms more than once a week but less than once a day	May affect activity and sleep	More than twice a month	FEV1 or PEF ≥80% pred; PEF or FEV1 variability <20–30%
Moderate persistent	Daily	May affect activity and sleep	More than once a week. Daily use of inhaled short-acting β(beta)2-agonist	FEV1 or PEF 60–80% pred; PEF or FEV1 variability >30%
Severe persistent	Daily	Frequent	Frequent nocturnal symptoms; limitation of physical activities	FEV1 or PEF ≤60% pred; PEF or FEV1 variability >30%

The worst score is 12 and the best is 0. At least a four point reduction in symptoms is considered as "effective" in this system, while at least an eight point reduction in symptoms is considered as "significantly effective." The GINA system is a worldwide accepted standard to evaluate the efficacy of asthma control. The Intermittent level is considered as well-controlled asthma; any two-level decrease in the severity is considered as significant, and a one level decrease is deemed effective. No improvement in the severity of symptoms is considered as ineffective.

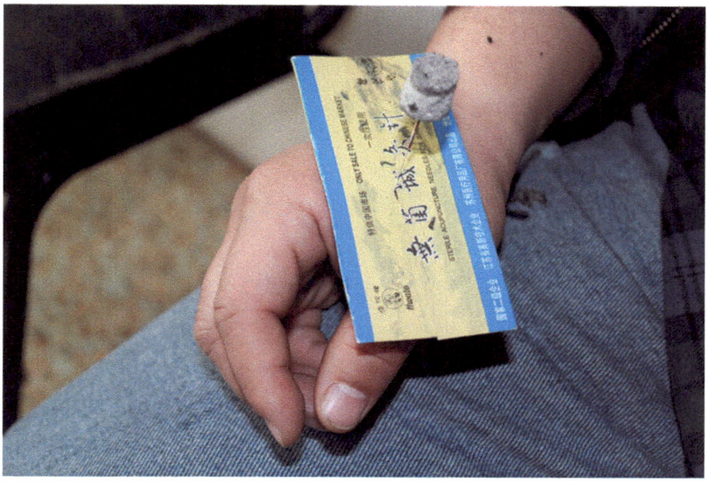

Fig. 15.1 Moxibustion with acupuncture

Acupuncture in Asthma Control

Liu [4] reviewed 353 related writings in 62 ancient books, and found that the commonly used acupoints, or acupuncture points, to treat asthma in ancient TCM traditions are: Tiantu(RN22), Tanzhong(RN17), Zhongwan(RN12), Feishu(BL13), Lieque(LU7), Taiyuan(LU9), Zhusanli(ST36), Fenglong(ST40), Taixi(KI3), etc.; while the commonly used meridians (the pathways in which the acupoints locate) are: Ren meridian, Urinary bladder meridian, Lung meridian, Stomach meridian, Kidney meridian, Large intestine meridian, and Du meridian. Commonly used body parts for acupuncture include the chest, upper abdomen, upper back, interior of arm, exterior leg, head, face, and lower abdomen. These acupoints and meridians are used in many different TCM methods including moxibustion (Fig. 15.1), (a TCM therapy using moxa, or mugwort herb), cauterization, acupuncture, bloodletting, contralateral needling, and hot medicated compress applications.

Qi [5] perused the China modern acupuncture-moxibustion information databank (1970–2002), and collected 495 related papers involving 50,631 clinical cases, and found that the commonly used acupoints to treat asthma in modern times are Feishu(BL13, 38%), Tanzhong(RN17, 28%), Dazhui(DU14, 23%), Tiantu(RN22, 22%), Dingchuan(21%), Shenshu(BL23, 17%), Fengmen(BL12, 15%), Gaohuang (BL43, 14%), and Zhusanli(ST36, 11%), with a variety of treatment methods including acupoint application (19%), acupuncture (9%), hydro-acupuncture (7%), and moxibustion(6%).

Yang [6] treated 174 asthma cases with a combined method named "three acupoints, five needles and one cup" that was mainly applied to Feishu(BL13), Fengmen(BL12), and Dazhui(DU14), and found an efficacy rate of 85% according to CMSEA. Zhang [7] treated 61 asthma cases with Tanzhong, daily for 12 days for

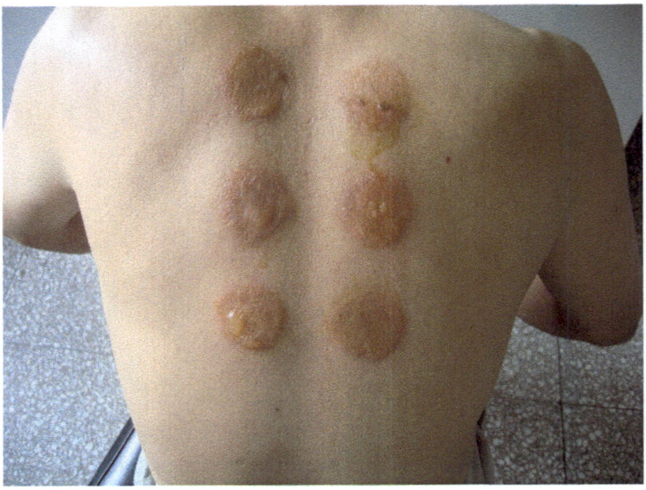

Fig. 15.2 Contact dermatitis resulting from application of Xiao Chuan paste (XCP)

a total of one to five courses of treatment. Hu [8] treated 50 asthma cases in the remission stage with grain-sized moxibustion, utilizing acupoints of Bailao(EX), Dingchuan (Extra Point 17), Feishu(BL13), Gaohuangshu(UB43), Pishu(BL20), Shenshu(BL23), Guanyuan(RN4), and Zhusanli(ST36). Of the 50 moderate to severe persistent asthma patients, 30 patients became mild persistent after the treatment according to the GINA (full text available at 222.ginasthma.org) classification (Table 15.1). Zao [9] treated 36 mild or moderate asthma cases according to GINA asthma classification in the remission stage with mild-warming moxibustion, choosing the acupoints of Dazhui(DU14), Guanyuan(RN4), Zhusanli(ST36), Feishu(BL13), and Lieque(LU7). Moxibustion was applied to the acupoint for 10 min at a time, 3 times a week for 6 weeks. One year follow-up showed that 15 cases were well controlled and became mild persistent after treatment.

Acupoint Application Within TCM: Herbal Paste Application

Xiao Chuan herbal paste application made from mustard seed in the summer with specific back acupoints has been documented as one of the major modalities to prevent asthma exacerbations in the winter. These herbs and natural remedies are thought to have some immune regulation properties as described below.

Li [10] retrospectively studied a group of 531 asthma patients treated with the external herb paste, Xiao Chuan Paste (XCP) to prevent winter asthma exacerbations. These pastes were applied on acupoints of the back (BL13, BL15, and BL17) 4 times over the summer months from July to August. Patient satisfaction rate with panting symptom was 91%, 60% of patients were satisfied after 1 year of treatment, and 75% after 3 years of treatment. The only adverse event related to this treatment was mild allergic contact dermatitis (Fig. 15.2).

Dong [11] treated 223 asthma patients with XCP and followed them for 10 years. 72 of 223 patients were cured, with 86 markedly effective, 35 improved, and 30 ineffective. The total effective rate was 86.5%. Patients categorized as the cold syndrome asthma type had the best result with a total effective rate of 95%, while efficacy rates for the mixed-syndrome asthma type reached 80%, and 73% for the heat-syndrome asthma type. Factors that improved efficacy included longer duration and increased frequency of TCM treatments. The efficacy of this study was evaluated based on CMSEA [12] (Table 15.1). Compared with GINA evaluation system, CMSEA focused more on specific symptoms and the patient satisfaction with their symptom control. The treatment was considered as effective when the stage of disease goes down at least one level, for example, from moderate coughing to mild coughing. Overall efficacy is determined by summarizing the frequency of improvement for the entire sample of patients evaluated in the TCM studies.

Li [13] treated 216 bronchial asthma cases with acupoint application combined with cupping, the therapeutic application of cups onto the skin by suction, which resulted in fewer exacerbations and milder symptoms in 82.4% of patients. Continually applied acupoints achieved a better effect. Fan et al. [14] divided asthma patients into a summer group (application of medicine in summer) of 213 patients and a winter group (application of medicine in winter) of 143 patients. They made an herbal paste with Chinese medicine extracts, and then applied the paste to the summer group patients 3 times during the hottest days of summer. The winter group underwent application of paste 3 times every 10 days in December. Three months later, the total effective rate of the summer group was 89.7%, while the winter group had an effective rate of 76.2% evaluated by Chinese Medicine Symptom Evaluation. Zhang et al. [15] performed a similar study in 986 bronchial asthma cases with acupoint application in the three periods of greatest heat days and the 3, 9-day periods after the winter solstice, choosing the acupoints of Feishu(BL13), Dingchuan(EP17), Gaohuang (UB43), Tiantu (CV22), and Tanzhong(RN17). The results showed that exacerbation frequencies were reduced from 3 times a month to 1 time a month. The laboratory studies before and after treatment, showed higher levels of cluster of differentiation 8 (CD8) ($P<0.01$), lower CD4/CD8 ratios ($P<0.01$), higher CD3 counts ($P<0.05$), and higher IgA levels ($P<0.01$). Thus, acupoint application may be able to affect T-lymphocyte subsets, enhance immunity, decrease the chance of respiratory tract infection, and reduce the recurrence rate of asthma.

TCM Decoctions

Decoction is a method of extraction, by boiling, of dissolved chemicals, or herbal or plant material, which may include stems, roots, bark, and rhizomes. There are three types of decoctions used in the TCM tradition for the treatment of asthma: The most popular decoction in TCM is the preparation of an individualized decoction according to the particular syndrome pattern of a patient; the second most commonly used decoction is a fixed decoction of several herbs made by the Chinese Medicine industry ready-to-use like modern medication; and the least used decoction is made with a single herb.

One of the unique features of treating asthma using TCM is that treatment during the remission stage remains a strong focus, in an attempt to enhance immunity, reduce the number of exacerbations, help in symptom relief, and improve quality of life. Further, TCM has also been utilized to help treat side effects of glucocorticoids, including secondary Cushing's syndrome, by using decoctions with warming yang and invigorating kidney therapy in steroid-dependent asthma, or during a steroid taper to prevent the rebound phenomenon.

Individualized Decoctions Applied to Asthma

Wu et al. [16] divided asthma into four types by using syndrome differentiation, and treated 174 patients with mixed herbs including Bupleurum Mume Fruit and Schisandra chinensis. The efficacy was evaluated based on GINA classification (Table 15.2). Results showed that 32 cases were well controlled, 72 cases were significantly effective, 54 cases were effective, and 16 cases were ineffective according to GINA classification; 90.8% were well controlled at the intermittent stage.

Zhang [17] used Pingchuan Yiqi Granule (PYG) to treat 60 patients over 7 days with bronchial asthma exacerbations of qi deficiency cold syndrome type (BS-QDC). Lung function testing showed a statistically significant change in forced expiratory volume in 1 s (FEV_1) after treatment ($P<0.05$), but no significant difference in peak expiratory flow (PEF, $P>0.05$). No adverse reactions were found over the course of treatment. Thus, PYG used to treat BS-QDC was both effective and safe in this group of patients.

Wu [18] treated 120 asthma cases with strengthened spleen and warming kidney oral paste; the results showed that the pulmonary function FEV1 improved significantly. Long et al. [19] treated 52 cases of asthma in remission with Bufei tablets (including Cordyceps, Ginseng, Gecko) combined with inhaled corticosteroids. After 3 months, the level of CD4 and IgE in the group treated with Bufei tablets was significantly lower than the control group, and CD8 levels were significantly higher than the control group. It is proposed that Bufei tablets can reduce CD4 and raise CD8, reduce IgE levels, control airway inflammation, and decrease airway hyperresponsiveness—thus controlling asthmatic exacerbations.

Cai et al. [20] treated 80 asthma cases in remission stage with spleen insufficiency syndrome, using a syndrome-specific decoction based on Six Gentlemen Decoction that included Ginsen, Poria, Atractylodes, Radix Glycyrrhizae, tangerine, and pinellia. The results showed a significant improvement in pulmonary function (FEV1) and decreased eosinophils; the total effective rate was 81.2%. Zhang et al. [21] treated 85 asthma cases in the moderate stage with Six Gentlemen decoction plus Astragalus and showed that the asthma exacerbations were less frequent at the mild stage according to GINA classification.

TCM Decoction Treatments for Steroid-Dependent Asthma

Cui [22] treated 40 SDA cases with a classic TCM decoction—Wumei Wan. The treatment group ($n=20$) was given Wumei Wan oral decoction, 100 mL orally twice a day, and Pulmicort Turbuhaler 200 μg inhalation twice a day. The 20-case randomized control group was treated with Pulmicort Turbuhaler 400 μg inhalation twice daily. Follow-up was conducted every 2 weeks over a 12-week treatment course. The results showed that in the treatment group two cases were well controlled, six cases were significantly effective, ten cases were effective and two cases were ineffective and the total effective rate was 90%. In the control group, one case was clinically controlled, four cases were significantly effective, nine cases were effective, and six cases were ineffective; total effective rate was 80%. The treatment group effectively reduced the dose of oral glucocorticoid, improved clinical symptoms and pulmonary function (FEV1) of SDA patients without any evident toxic or other side effects when compared to the usual care group.

Gong et al. [23] treated 40 SDA cases with Chaipo Decoction (a combination of Xiaochaihu Decoction and Banxia Houpo Decoction). The overall success rate measured in terms of discontinuing glucocorticoid use was 47.5%, with improvement in both clinical symptoms and pulmonary function. Many side effects from steroid therapy also improved, including acne, moon face, and infections. This study demonstrates that combining Caipu Decoction with glucocorticoid therapy may reduce the volume of corticosteroids and relieve some of the medication side effects. Moreover, in vitro tests have confirmed that Magnolol, the main ingredient of Chaipo Decoction, can reduce concentration of s11β-hydroxysteroid dehydrogenase in the liver homogenate, in order to increase the blood concentration of prednisolone [24].

TCM Food Therapy for Asthma Patients

As asthma is a chronic disease that requires long-term therapy, it is often difficult for patients to take medicines regularly and consistently, particularly when they are feeling well during the remission stage. In TCM, diet therapy may be an alternative and convenient way for some patients to manage their asthma.

In TCM theory, it is believed that "medicine and food come from the same source." Both food and medicine have particular characteristics to induce positive or negative effects on different diseases or different types of patients. For asthma patients in the remission stage, it is advised to consume foods that have a supplementation function, including lily bulb, tremella, honey, gingko, Chinese yam, lotus seed, walnut, Semen sesami nigrum, white turnip, and quail eggs. Food to avoid includes those thought to have a phlegm-producing function, such as egg yolk, fatty meat, and peanuts. Raw or cold foods are forbidden, and sweet food is not recommended [25].

Food therapy is mostly done in summer according to the principle of "treating the winter disease in summer," as many patients in asthma remission stage are generally in summer [26]. Lung deficiency patients can use porridge made from Chinese yam, lily bulb, rice, and crystal sugar [27]. Spleen deficiency patients can use ginger-chicken porridge [28], while kidney deficiency patients are advised to use Cordyceps stewing old duck [29] or dried-persimmon and walnut cake [27].

Summary: The efficacy of whole medical systems such as TCM in the treatment of asthma is well documented in case studies dating back several thousands of years. However, there are few well-controlled studies supporting the efficacy of TCM therapies in asthma. Thus, future well-designed studies of TCM in asthma are needed to provide the high-quality evidence needed for TCM to be widely adopted in Western medical practice.

TCM for Chronic Obstructive Pulmonary Disease

In TCM, COPD is categorized with emphysema, cough, asthma, shortness of breath, and retention of phlegm and fluid in the lung. The main symptoms are chronic cough, expectoration, shortness of breath, gasping, and chest stuffiness. Like asthma, COPD can be divided into two categories, the acute exacerbation stage and the stable stage.

Li [30] divided COPD into three types by clinical manifestations: (1) deficiency syndromes (Syndrome of qi deficiency of lung and spleen, Syndrome of qi deficiency of lung and kidney, Syndrome of qi and yin deficiency of lung and kidney); (2) excess syndrome (exterior cold and interior fluid retention syndrome, syndrome of phlegm-heat obstructing lung, syndrome of turbid phlegm obstructing lung, and syndrome of orifices confused by phlegm), and; (3) Embolism syndrome accompanying symptoms (blood stasis syndrome). Lu [29] viewed the lung as governing qi, which promotes blood circulation; and that deficiency of lung qi leads to the syndrome of blood stasis. Therefore, a syndrome of qi deficiency and blood stasis is the main pathologic mechanism of COPD in TCM. Phlegm-heat and evil qi remain during the stable stage, which can obstruct qi-blood circulation. In the TCM tradition, COPD is treated with internal and external therapies, as described below.

Internal Therapy for COPD

Currently, TCM practitioners focus on eliminating pathogens during the acute COPD exacerbation stage and supporting healthy energy during the stable stage. Excess syndrome plays an important role in the acute stage such as exogenous evil, phlegm, and blood stasis [30]. Practitioners focus on freeing lung qi, eliminating pathogens, repressing upward perversion of qi, warming yang to promote diuresis, blood-activating and stasis-dissolving, and calming wind to cure diseases. The principle of tonifying insufficiency is the main treatment philosophy in the stable COPD phase. During this phase, the spleen and kidney are strengthened by supplementing qi and nourishing yin to cure diseases. Deficiency-excess complications are treated by strengthening body resistance and eliminating evil. Luo [31] considered that TCM practitioners should provide different treatments according to different disease patterns. In the acute stage, syndrome of phlegm-heat obstructing lung should be treated by Ma Xing Shi Gan Decoction, which is effective at clearing the lungs and eliminating phlegm. The syndrome of turbid phlegm obstructing lung is treated with Xiao Qing Long Decoction, which warms the lung to alleviate fluid retention, cough, and asthmatic symptoms. Gua Lou Xie Bai Ban Xia Decoction can be used to treat obstruction of qi in the chest resulting from syndrome of phlegm and blood stasis obstructing lung. Radix Astragalus, Radix Atractylodis Macrocephalae, Fructus Trichosanthis, White Mulberry Root-bark, Lepidium Seed, Peach Seed, Radix Salviae Miltiorrhizae, and Poria cocos, are used to treat the syndrome of phlegm and blood stasis obstructing lung coupled with deficiency of yang in both the spleen and kidney. Other syndromes can accompany and worsen the lung-specific syndromes outlined above. In the syndrome of delirium by phlegm, Antelope's Horn Powder, acorys gramineus is used to resuscitate the brain. If the patient is also affected with the syndrome of sudden collapse of heart yang, Shen Fu Long Mu Decoction is used to rescue the collapse by restoring yang. The syndrome of deficiency of both qi and yin should be treated with lilyturf root, fritillaria cirrhosa, almond, and Common Fleabane to supplement qi and nourish yin. Deficiency of both lung and spleen is treated with Radix Astragalus, Radix Atractylodis Macrocephalae, and poria cocos.

In the stable phase, the syndrome of qi deficiency of spleen and lung is treated with Bu Fei Decoction and Er Chen Decoction. Deficiency of Lung Yin is treated with Bai He Gu Jin Decoction. Fang [32] reported that respiratory muscle fatigue and nutrition disorders are relevant to deficiency of spleen qi and lung qi. Therefore, the spleen should first be reinforced. Li [33] recommended Six Gentlemen Decoction to supply qi and eliminate phlegm, Er Chen Decoction to regulate qi flowing for eliminating phlegm to treat the syndrome of dampness stagnancy due to spleen deficiency, and kidney qi tonifying pill to invigorate the lung and the kidney in the syndrome of qi deficiency of lung and kidney.

External Therapy for COPD

A large amount of information has been recorded in the TCM tradition regarding the use of external herbs to treat COPD [34]. There are more than 400 external therapies which can be divided into two categories: external therapy with herbs; and external therapy without herbs. This section will focus specifically on the treatment of COPD using external TCM therapies.

History of External Therapy of TCM

There are records of external therapy in the oldest Ancient Chinese Medical Literature. The *Synopsis of Golden Chamber* created many external therapies with drugs, such as washing, fumigation, coating with drugs, suppositories, administering drugs through the nose, and cauterization. Ancient TCM practitioners made use of many types of treatments for external use, including ointments, factice, pulvis, pastille, and aqua. The *Compendium of Materia Medica* summarized the experience of external therapy before the Ming Dynasty in 1578, describing details of 40 external therapy methods. Selections of those numerous therapies are reviewed here.

Classification of External Therapy of TCM

Wu [35] summarized the classification of external therapy of TCM in three aspects: Meridian transmission, skin penetration, and mucosal absorption. Li [36] divided external therapy into four categories on the basis of clinical application [33]: (1) human organs and tissues (eye method, sneeze method, plug nose method, plug ear method, aerosol Inhalation); (2) acupuncture points (umbilical therapy, grasping drug method, vesiculation therapy, drug moxibustion); (3) specific body surface (external application, thin-spreading, suppository, fumigation, washing); and (4) others, such as penetration of drug administering ultrasound.

Zhu Qingwen divided external therapy into four categories for clinical application according to their application: whole treatment, skin treatment, meridian, and brain acupoint treatment. Whole treatment focuses on the entire body, as in Dao Yin (Qigong) and music therapy. Skin treatment refers to drugs that are absorbed into part of the body or circulation system through the skin, such as the application of fumigation-washing therapy. Transdermal drug delivery systems (TODS) or transdermal therapeutic systems (TTS) of Western medicinal preparations fall into this treatment category. These preparations are called patches in Western medicine and *tie pian* in China. Meridian and brain acupoint treatment refers to drugs, maneuvers, or instruments that work on meridians and acupoints such as massage, moxibustion, umbilical therapy, and foot massage therapy.

Treating COPD by External Therapies of TCM

Modern medical research has found that acupoints are sensitive to TCM medicines and herbs, with an amplification effect defined as increased effect along the meridians. The meridian system is composed of channels with low resistance. Therefore, applying herbs to specific acupoints could have significant pharmacodynamic effects on certain organs with mono- or biphasic regulation. For effective external therapy in TCM, it is crucial that medicines penetrate the skin barrier. Thus, there are methods employed to promote penetration of the herbs or other skin preparations. The first is through the property of the drug, the encapsulation of the solvent and liposomes (carrier); the second is the application of the physical methods to promote penetration and absorption; and the third is the employment of chemical methods to promote penetration and absorption. The skin should be closely monitored for adverse reactions during the treatment period.

Overview of Acupoint External Therapy for COPD

Acupoint external therapy with herbs was first recorded in Comprehensive Medicine According to old Chinese Medicine book *Zhang Shi Yi Tong* that "this is the method to treat cold wheezing ... there would be good curative effect by applying mustard seed (Semen Sinapis) during the three hottest periods in the summer." The formula is powder of white mustard seed (Semen Sinapis) 1 liang (one of Chinese weight unit), corydalis rhizome (Rhizoma Corydalis) 1 liang, gansui root (Radix Kansui), and Manchurian wild ginger (Radix et Rhizoma Asari) 0.5 liang, respectively. All the herbs are prepared into a fine powder. Then musk (Moschus) 0.5 qian is added and the formula is mixed with ginger juice (Succus Rhizomatis Zingiberis). The prepared medicine is applied to acupoints, including BL 13 (Fei Shu), BL 43 (Gao Huang), and EX-HN15 (Jing Bai Lao). The skin area with application may feel numb and painful [35]. It is said in *Yellow Emperor's Classic of Internal Medicine* that "celestial qi communicates with the lung while earth qi with the pharynx" [3]. First, the yang qi in the human body is corresponding to that in nature during the three periods of greatest heat in the summer. The strengthened yang qi is thought to dispel the phlegm externally and reinforce healthy qi internally. Second, the interstitial spaces are loose and open in this season and it is easy for the medicine to penetrate the skin, reach the specific organ, and travel by way of channels and meridians. According to TCM the relationship between syndromes and curative effect, this therapy is best used for the cold syndromes. Moreover, a better effect can be achieved for COPD patients in the stable phase in the summer to prevent COPD exacerbations in the upcoming colder seasons.

Many experts in Guan An Men Hospital, China Academy of Chinese Medical Science, have been working since 1955 to create the empirical formulas originating from the Qing Dynasty. Their observations suggest that the total effective rate of the therapy in treating COPD is between 60 and 70%. These formulas function to prevent acute exacerbations of COPD. Furthermore, it was found that there was a significant positive correlation between courses of treatment and long-term effects. The treatments not only minimized the respiratory symptoms, but also promoted the immunologic function of the body. The respiratory department of Beijing TCM Hospital has created a new formula, combining traditional and modern herbs composed of Manchurian wild ginger (Radix et Rhizoma Asari), Chinese magnolivine fruit (Fructus Schisandrae Chinensis), white mustard seed (Semen Sinapis), dried ginger rhizome (Rhizoma Zingiberis), pinellia rhizome (Rhizoma Pinelliae), apricot kernel (Semen Armeniacae Amarum), stemona root (Radix Stemonae), ephedra (Herba Ephedrae), angelica root (Radix Angelicae Dahuricae), and borneol (Borneolum Syntheticum). This formula was prepared into a powder and applied to

DU 14 (Da Zhui) on du vessel, BL 13 (Fei Shu) and BL 43 (Gao Huang) on the bladder meridian of foot taiyang and RN 17 (Tan Zhong) on the Ren meridian. According to clinical observations, symptoms, influence on daily activities, frequency of acute exacerbations of COPD, and quality of life were all significantly improved. At Xinjiang Uygur Autonomous Region Hospital of TCM the formula was composed of honey-fried ephedra (Herba Ephedrae), apricot kernel (Semen Armeniacae Amarum), astragalus root (Radix Astragali), and herbs growing in Xinjiang. The herbs were made into a powder and prepared into a paste with azone and glycerin. Three grams of the medicine was applied to BL 13 (Fei Shu), RN 17 (Tan Zhong), BL 20 (Pi Shu), BL 12 (Feng Men), and EX-B1 (Ding Chuan) each morning for 14 days. The results showed that the pulmonary function (FEV1) of COPD patients in the acute stage improved significantly compared to before treatment [37].

Acupuncture and Massage in COPD

Jia [38] randomly divided 66 stable stage COPD patients into three groups: acupuncture, pulmonary rehabilitation including education and exercise, and acupuncture-rehabilitation groups. He found that both acupuncture and rehabilitation could improve the pulmonary function (FEV1) of COPD patients but combining the two therapies created an even better improvement in pulmonary function. Chen [39] randomly divided 30 COPD patients into two groups: 15 received body massage therapy, and 15 were assigned to the control, no-massage group. In addition to routine medical treatment for the two groups, patients in the massage group received five body massage treatments per week for 20 min each over an 8-week period. There was a statistically significant difference ($P<0.05$) in the 6-min walk test (6MWT), and reduced dyspnea [38–40].

Qi Gong in COPD

Respiration is an essential movement of life. The extent and the frequency are relative to respiration efficiency and vital movement. In terms of TCM, Qi Gong is spirit, qi, xing united, mind and body combined, in which the heart is the leader. Qi Gong can improve the ability of the human body to reach a balance of yin and yang, regulating qi and blood, dredge the channel, and foster the genuine qi. Qi Gong has been used to treat neurotic disorders, regulate functions of the human body, and eliminate pathological states. When people enter into a stage of tranquil-ness of their mind, the human body is in low dissipation of energy and in high rehabilitation [41].

Deep and slow breathing can expand the chest volume and amplitude, improving the alveolar gas exchange and tissue respiratory efficiency. These exercises broaden the area between capillary and alveolus, which can help stabilize the internal environment. Bai [42] studied Songjinggong (one Qi Gong exercise) practiced 30 min a day in 13 COPD patients and found that treatment improved the lung function and oxygen saturation after 3 months. It is believed that during these exercises, peak inspiratory pressure is elevated and fresh air enters freely, which improves the partial pressure of oxygen and helps with elimination of carbon dioxide.

Summary: There is a wealth of scientific data in the form of observations and case studies in the Chinese literature, there is still a need for better, high-quality, randomized trials from a Western perspective to provide the evidence for adoption of TCM practices in the management of COPD.

Interstitial Pulmonary Fibrosis

Pulmonary interstitial fibrosis is a broad term to describe a variety of ILDs including idiopathic pulmonary interstitial fibrosis (IPF) and secondary pulmonary interstitial fibrosis (SPF).

In ancient TCM documents, there is no record of pulmonary interstitial fibrosis. According to the characteristics and main clinical manifestations of these lung diseases, they are generally included under the categories of "cough," "breath-holding," and "short of breath." There are, however, a number of perspectives in TCM for treating IPF depending on the pattern of the dyspnea or cough.

The Pathogenesis of Pulmonary Interstitial Fibrosis from a TCM Perspective

It is thought that the invasion of the lung with exopathic factors causes pulmonary interstitial fibrosis. The lung can be easily attacked by exopathic factors such as pollution and heat, which can cause sudden damage to lung fluid and qi. Inhalation of polluted air can directly lead to disharmony of qi movement and blood circulation and eventually to obstruction of lung meridians. Deficiency of lung and kidney make it easier for exopathic factors to invade. Among all the factors, condensation of phlegm, blood stasis, and obstruction of lung meridians are the central contributors to the disease.

Wu and Ren [43] consider the disease as the mixture of syndromes of deficiency and excess; some give priority to deficiency syndrome while others give priority to excess syndrome. The deficiency syndrome refers to deficiency of lung and kidney or qi and yin. The excess syndrome refers to obstruction of phlegm and blood stasis in lung meridians. "Lung bi-complex" and "lung paralysis" are the two stages, and both are considered in TCM as pulmonary interstitial fibrosis. Development from "lung bi-complex" to "lung paralysis" is a process from excess to deficiency and development from "lung paralysis" to "lung bi-complex" is a process from deficiency to excess.

Liu [44] considers deficiency of lung and kidney or lung and spleen to be secondary to nature, improper diet, and overtiredness as the contributors of pulmonary interstitial fibrosis. If the six evils (exopathic factors) attack the organism at this time, the meridians of lung are stagnated because of the unsmooth movement of qi. This results in asthenic fever, deficiency of qi and yin, phlegm-heat and blood stasis blocking the meridians, and the scorched lung.

Wu [45] considers obstruction of lung meridians as the fundamental pathogenesis of the disease. Deficiency of lung and kidney and invasion of evils lead to dystrophy and blocking of phlegm and blood stasis in lung meridians. As a result, movement of qi and blood in the lung become unsmooth.

Kong [46] theorized that IPF belongs to the category of "breath-holding" and "lung bulge." Exopathic factors invade and block lung flow. As time passes, these factors convert fluid to phlegm. The blocked qi movement leads to blood stasis. Then phlegm and blood stasis bond together and damage the kidney vitality. The damaged function of inhalation leads to breath-holding.

Peng [47] and Guan [48] divide pulmonary interstitial fibrosis into three stages. The first stage is pulmonary alveolitis (early stage or acute) in which there is infection and deficiency in vitality. Second, the lung damage stage (a period of change from pulmonary alveolitis to pulmonary interstitial fibrosis) involves bonding together of phlegm and blood stasis. Third, the stage of pulmonary interstitial fibrosis (chronic), which is "upper excess and lower deficiency" meaning the lung, spleen, and kidney are all affected.

Syndrome Differentiation and Treatment of Pulmonary Interstitial Fibrosis from the TCM Perspective

Wu [43] proposed that "Syndrome differentiation and treatment" should be inserted in the process of treatment under the principles of "supplementing lung and kidney, dissipating phlegm and blood stasis, dredging lung meridians." The main points in syndrome differentiation are listed as follows: (1) recognize the different stages of the disease, (2) analyze the inducement, (3) understand the characteristics of exopathic factors, (4) clarify the main aspect of the disease (excess or deficiency), and (5) differentiate between cold and heat of the disease, and its transformation. The stages are the acute exacerbation period, chronic extension period, and critical changeful period.

The common syndromes in the first period involves phlegm, heat obstructing in the lung syndrome, blood stasis blocking in the lung syndrome, wind-coldness invading the lung due to qi deficiency syndrome, and dryness-heat damaging the lung due to yin deficiency syndrome. Treatment is considered according to different stages and "activating blood circulation to dissipate blood stasis, dredging lung meridians" is felt to be the most important part of the treatment of pulmonary interstitial fibrosis. In the acute period, the following measures are commonly used:

(a) releasing exterior, dissipating phlegm and dredging meridians; (b) clearing heat, promoting diuresis and eliminating toxins, and (c) activating blood circulation, dissipating blood stasis and dredging meridians. Small Bluegreen Dragan Decoction (Xiao Qinglong Tang) is usually used to eliminate the exterior factors with pungent-warm herbs, disperse coldness and dredging meridians. Honeysuckle Forsythia Powder (Yin Qiao San) is often used to eliminate the exterior factors with pungent-cool herbs, dissipate phlegm and dredging meridians. Minor Decoction for Relieving Phlegm-Heat in the chest (Xiaoxianxiong Tang) and Chinese Angelica Fritillaria Sophora Flavescens Pills (Danggui Beimu Kushen Pills) are often used to clear heat, promote diuresis, and eliminate toxins.

Qiu [49] divides IPF into six syndromes from the TCM perspective: the wind-heat invading the lung syndrome; phlegm-heat obstructing in the lung syndrome; blood stasis due to qi deficiency of heart and lung syndrome; obstruction of blood circulation due to deficiency of both qi and yin syndrome; excess water and blood stasis due to yang deficiency of heart, spleen, and kidney syndrome; and deficiency of both yin and yang syndrome. Herbs promoting blood circulation and removing blood stasis should be used in the overall treatment process. To treat wind-heat invading the lung syndrome, herbs that work to dispel wind-heat, clear heat, eliminate toxins, promote blood circulation, and remove blood stasis should be used together. To treat phlegm-heat obstructing in the lung syndrome, herbs that work to clear heat, eliminate phlegm, free lung, relieve asthma, promote blood circulation, and remove blood stasis should be used together. To treat blood stasis due to qi deficiency of heart and lung syndrome, herbs that work to supplement heart and lung, eliminate phlegm, and remove blood stasis should be used together. To treat obstruction of blood circulation due to deficiency of both qi and yin syndrome, herbs that work to supplement the vital energy, nourish yin, reduce phlegm, stop cough, promote blood circulation, and remove blood stasis should be used together. To treat excess water and blood stasis due to yang deficiency of heart, spleen, and kidney syndrome, herbs that work to warm yang, promote diuresis and blood circulation, and remove blood stasis should be used together. To treat deficiency of both yin and yang syndrome, herbs that work to restore yang (aconite), rescue yin (long-cultivated field), tonify qi (ginseng), promote blood circulation (safflower), and remove blood stasis (curcuma) should be used together.

Management of Stable and Acute Exacerbation of Pulmonary Interstitial Fibrosis

Cui [50] theorizes that in acute exacerbation periods with infections, eliminating outside factors are usually used together with tonifying qi, yin and dissipating phlegm accordingly. If phlegm-heat obstructs in the lung, Reed Rhizome Decoction (Weijing Tang) and Honeysuckle Forsythia Powder (Yin Qiao San) can be used to clear heat and dissipate phlegm. If phlegm–blood stasis blocks in the lung, Treating Cold Limbs Powder (Sini San), Perilla Seed Decoction for Directing Qi Downward (Suzi Jiangqi Tang), and Three-Seed Decoction for the Aged (Sanzi Yangqin Tang) can be used to regulate vital energy, reduce phlegm, and promote blood circulation. If wind-heat invades the lung due to qi deficiency, Anticough Powder (Zhisou San) and Jade-Screen Powder (Yupingfeng San) can be used to dispel wind, clear heat, descend qi, and relieve asthma. If dryness-heat damages the lung due to yin deficiency, Decoction for Eliminating Dryness and Rescuing the Lung (Qingzao Jiufei Tang), Mulberry Leaf and Apricot Kernel Decoction (Sang Xing Tang), and Decoction of Adenophora Stricta and Radix Ophiopogonis (Shashen Maidong Tang) can be used to clear lung, reduce phlegm, dispel wind, and nourish dryness.

Deficiency of both qi and yin combined with phlegm and deficiency of both qi and yin combined with blood stasis are two common syndromes in the chronic extension period. Deficiency of both qi and yin combined with phlegm can be treated with Jinshui Liujun Jian to tonify lung and kidney, dissipate phlegm, and relieve asthma. Deficiency of both qi and yin combined with blood stasis can be treated with Decoction to Protect Lung (Baofei Tang) to tonify qi, nourish yin, dissipate phlegm, and promote blood circulation. In the later period, there are also two syndromes, excess water due to yang deficiency syndrome and deficiency of both yin and yang syndrome. To treat excess water due to yang deficiency, Diuretic Decoction to Strengthen Yang of Spleen and Kidney (Zhenwu Tang) and Tonifying (supplement) Lung Decoction (Bufei Tang) can be used to tonify yang with warm herbs, produce qi, and promote dampness. To treat deficiency of both yin and yang, Restoring the Right (Kidney) Bolus (Yougui Wan) and Sea Cucumber Clam Powder (Shenge San) can be used to tonify yin and yang, promote blood circulation, and remove blood stasis.

Major TCM Therapeutic Principles Applied to Pulmonary Interstitial Fibrosis

Liu and Liu [44] emphasize the importance of therapeutic methods to treat disease such as supplementing the vital energy and nourishing yin, activating blood circulation to dissipate blood stasis, strengthening body resistance and eliminating evil, softening hard lumps and dispelling nodes, ventilating the lung and resolving phlegm, clearing heat and eliminating toxins, and flexing the lung movement. Supplementing the vital energy and activating blood circulation are common throughout the entire treatment process. In the early stage of pulmonary interstitial fibrosis, there is often deficiency of both lung and spleen, qi deficiency of lung and kidney, and insufficient anti-pathogenic energy especially lack of the lung qi. Yu-Ping feng San is the first herb chosen for reinforcing lung qi and the commonly used herbs of reinforcing qi have Ginseng, CodonoPsis, Radix Astragali, and Large head Atractylodes Rhizome. The treatment method of activating blood circulation to dissipate blood stasis usually consists of herbs for activating blood circulation such as Salvia miltiorrhiza Bunge, Szechuan Lovage Rhizome, Chinese Angelica, Turmeric Root-tuber, Earthworm, Red Peony Root, and often are put into Bitter Orange, sliced perilla stem, and other Chinese herbs to promote blood circulation.

Wu and Zhang [45] proposed the therapeutic method of the collateral disease theory to treat pulmonary interstitial fibrosis. They believe that the best way to treat collateral deficiency is supplementation, which belongs to yin and blood deficiency with the method of "Xin Gan Wen Run," with Angelica, Rehmannia, donkey-hide gelatin, white peony root, Ophiopogon japonicus, North and South Adenophora, cornus, wolfberry fruit, Ligustrum lucidum, and Radix. When the patient with Yang Qi deficiency is treated with the method of the sweet and warm quality supplementing qi, "the herbs of the épicée, the sweet and warm quality is used to supplement the herbs for dredging meridians and collaterals," including the herbs of Codonopsis, Astragalus, Atractylodes, Huang Jing, Chinese yam, Epimedium, Cistanche, Cuscuta, Psoralea, and Morinda. Lu [51] believes that the treatment for pulmonary interstitial fibrosis should be from the root of disease, by healing the lung, spleen, and kidney while working to achieve the purpose of affecting a permanent cure. The purpose of supplementing the lung is to regulate water passage, increase and decrease qi; nourish the kidney at the intersection of yin and yang, to breathe normally. Reinforcing the spleen promotes the production of body fluid and benefits vital energy.

Peng [47] theorized that in the early stage of pulmonary interstitial fibrosis (the alveolar inflammation period) the main treatment is geared toward dispelling evil. The therapeutic methods are tonifying qi and smoothing blood, transforming phlegm and expelling static blood, descending adverse-rising, and alleviating water retention. The prescriptions include Reed Rhizome Decoction, or Minor Decoction for Relieving Phlegm-Heat in the Chest with BuFei Tang. In the later stage of pulmonary interstitial fibrosis, the therapeutic methods are tonifying spleen and kidney, improving inspiration and clearing up phlegm, expelling static blood and dredging collaterals, softening hard lumps and dispelling nodes, and addressing both the symptoms and root causes. The prescriptions include ShenYu Tang, or Corii Asini Decoction for Tonifying the Lung with Major Decoction for Relieving Phlegm-Heat in the Chest.

Jiang [52] considers the occurrence and development of IPF as a lack of righteousness, in particular lung and kidney qi deficiency exists regardless of the symptoms, duration or course of the disease. Therefore, treatment focuses on invigorating the lung and the kidney for treatment of the chronic phase; and reinforcing lung qi is the main treatment method in the early phase. In the middle phase, the therapeutic method is reinforcing lung and kidney. In the later period, the therapeutic methods are reinforcing kidney and lung. Invigorating the lung and the kidney at the same time should focus on regulating functional activities of qi, transforming phlegm and dispelling nodes, activating blood circulation to dissipate blood stasis, dredging collaterals, and dispelling nodes.

External Therapy Applied for Interstitial Lung Disease

There is a long history of treating ILD with acupuncture and moxibustion therapy mainly with feishu point (BL13). Sun [53] stated in Qianjinyifang zhenjiuzhifeibing that the efficacy of feishu point (BL13) was effective for treating cough, feishu point

(BL13) moxibustion to treat shortness, combining feishu point (BL13) moxibustion for 100 times and Taichong point (LR3) for 50 times in order to descend Qi. Li [54] believes that IPF belongs to Luo disease in TCM, feishu point (BL13) and Gaohuang point (BL43) moxibustion, Shaoshang point(LU11), and Shangyang point (LI1) bloodletting, combined with glucocorticoid can achieve effectiveness from the TCM perspective. The means above can improve difficult breathing to a certain extent, and can also delay the progress of pulmonary function (DLCO-Diffusing Capacity of Carbon monoxide) decline. Acupuncture and moxibustion therapy combined with hormone therapy can improve pulmonary function. Li Rong used glucocorticoid combined with bloodletting and moxibustion therapy to treat 22 patients with pulmonary interstitial fibrosis, using three-edged needles puncture Shaoshang point (LU11) and Shangyang point (LI1), kernel-like moxibustion feishu point (BL13) and Gaohuang point (BL43) on both sides. Results showed improved lung function and improved the clinical effects of oral systematic steroids for pulmonary interstitial fibrosis.

Liu [55] treated IPF with a TCM combination of therapy and herbs: Adenophora stricta 30 g, raw Rehmannia 15 g, Radix Ophiopogonis 15 g, Schisandra chinensis 6 g, Astragalus 12 g, donkey-hide gelatin 10 g, radix paeoniae alba 15 g, radix asteris 15 g, white mulberry root-bark 15 g, caulis lonicerae 20 g, Prunus armeniaca 10 g, rhizoma bletillae 10 g, etc. In addition, herbs were mixed for application to the skin, a technique utilizing electric charges as a vehicle for medicinal delivery. A control group received Bailing capsule, ten capsules 3 times daily. The study follow-up lasted for 6 months and showed that TCM supplemented vital energy and nourishing yin, invigorating blood circulation, and dredging meridians can remit cough and asthma symptoms, improve blood gases and pulmonary function tests, and improve the quality of life measured by the SF-36.

Summary: Currently, we only have lower levels of evidence to demonstrate the efficacy of TCM for the treatment of IPF. The lack of reliable diagnostic definitions of IPF lowers the evidence for TCM treatment. Most TCM treatments are not well evaluated since the diagnostic techniques are limited to TCM hospitals in China. Moreover, there are numerous TCM perspectives on the origin and treatment regimens for IPF. Clinical trials are needed to provide the evidence to demonstrate or refute the efficacy and safety supporting the use of the TCM approaches reviewed in this section for treating IPF patients.

Basic Research on Chinese Herbs to Treat Interstitial Pulmonary Fibrosis in TCM

Song [56] performed animal studies using mice and found that TCM prescriptions can reduce alveolar inflammation and pulmonary fibrosis to some degree with several decoctions such as Ophiopogon Decoctong, Trichosanthes, and Allium Decoction; The Kidney-Qi Bolus; Compound Salvia Tablet; Pulse-Activating

Decoction; and WuShe San. Binqing Tang, Wu [57] treated IPF in rodents with FeiXian Jian, and found efficacy of FeiXian Jian mainly in the control of symptoms and stability of the disease on imaging. Prescription of FeiXian Jian includes: Codonopsis 30 g, Astragalus 20 g, Ladybell Root 30 g, Coastal Glehnia Root 30 g, Radixophiopogonis 15 g, Unprocessed Rhizoma Pinelliae 15 g, Baical Skullcap Root 10 g, Common Burreed Rhizome 15 g, Curcuma 15 g, Scorpion 3 g, and Centipede 3 g; all were combined and administered for 1 month.

Lu [58] conducted rat experiments to demonstrate that Fuzhenghuayufang can improve the pathological changes on the lung of rats with pulmonary fibrosis. This formula is a new compound, which is believed to resist pulmonary fibrosis. It reflects the theory of treating different diseases with the same therapy to resist other diseases, including pulmonary interstitial fibrosis.

Li [59] studied moxibustion in rats with IPF and compared them with the prednisone group to evaluate the efficacy of moxibustion. The moxibustion group had lower expression of transformation growth factor-β(beta)1mRN. This indicates that moxibustion may be effective in the treatment of pulmonary interstitial fibrosis in this limited study.

Thus, there are a number of promising animal studies for treating IPF that require additional investigations prior to investigation in humans.

Sleep Disorders from the TCM Perspective

Overview

In view of the multiple factors contributing to sleep disorders, there are multiple approaches to therapy for promoting sleep health. While conventional treatments such as sleep hygiene education, stimulus control therapy, sleep restriction therapy, and pharmacologic treatments may be effective, this section will focus only on approaches to sleep disorders that emanate from a TCM perspective.

Tai Chi

Tai Chi is a low to moderate-intensity Chinese exercise that includes a meditational component. A study of the effects of Tai Chi (consisting of three 60-min sessions per week for 24 weeks) in 118 older adults in comparison to low-impact exercise noted that Tai Chi improved self-reported sleep duration by 48 min [60]. General health-related quality of life and daytime sleepiness levels also improved. No injuries were reported in either group. Of note, 33% of subjects withdrew from the study (no significant difference between the Tai Chi and exercise groups).

These findings are very interesting and if replicated by additional research using objective measures, could add to the treatment options for insomnia with an integrative approach.

Ginseng

Ginseng root has been used for over 2,000 years for its health-promoting properties in China [61]. Results of several studies indicate the effect of ginseng may be, at least in part, related to maintaining normal sleep and wakefulness. Of the several species of ginseng, Panax ginseng (Korean or Asian ginseng), Panax quinquefolius (American ginseng), and Panax vietnamensis (Vietnamese ginseng) are reported to have sleep-modulating effects. Constituents of most ginseng species include ginsenosides, polysaccharides, peptides, olyacetylenic alcohols, and fatty acids [62]. There are few reports of severe side effects secondary to ginseng. The most common reported side effects are nervousness and excitation, but these diminish with continued use or dosage reduction [63]. On the basis of its long-term usage and the relative infrequency of reported significant side effects, it is safe to conclude that ginseng is usually not associated with serious adverse reactions. [64] The recommended daily dosage is 1–2 g of the crude root, or 200–600 mg of extracts. As the possibility of hormone-like or hormone-inducing effects cannot be ruled out, some authors suggest limiting treatment to 3 months. [65]

Acupressure

Another form of manipulative therapy in TCM is acupressure, which is a noninvasive technique that involves stimulation of meridian or acupoints on the body using finger pressing movements. It can be administered by trained nursing staff, or by trained family members of a patient. Acupressure has been studied in a randomized design in institutionalized older adults [66].This study noted statistically significant improvements in both the Pittsburgh Sleep Quality Index (primary outcome measure) and number of nocturnal awakenings in the acupressure group relative to the two placebo arms (sham acupressure and conversation). Another study has replicated these findings [67].

Another form of acupressure is auricular therapy, which involves applying pressure to acupoints either via the fingertips, medicinal seeds, or with magnets [68, 69]. Suen et al. conducted a 3 week randomized, single-blind placebo-controlled study using wrist-activity monitoring to provide an objective assessment of sleep parameters between magnetic auricular acupressure and two matched controls [70]. They observed statistically significant improvements in sleep latency and sleep efficiency, with an overall increase of approximately 35 min in the total sleep time in the auricular therapy group. Adverse effects were not discussed in their manuscript;

however, auricular therapy is generally considered safe. A 6 month follow-up of this cohort was also conducted and found that insomnia symptoms remained ameliorated in the treatment group relative to the control groups [68]. The results of these studies are very intriguing. However, this work needs to be replicated in additional studies among more diverse cohorts before it can be routinely recommended for the management of insomnia.

Acupuncture also acts on meridian points to influence health [70]. Few studies have used polysomnography to evaluate the effects of acupuncture in insomnia [71–74]. While one pilot study demonstrated evidence of improved sleep, it was not placebo-controlled [71]. Zhang et al. conducted a study [73] in which 92 college students suffering from insomnia were randomly divided into a treatment group and a control group. Acupuncture plus cupping was used in the treatment group and conventional differentiation of symptoms and signs was used in the control group. The investigators found a significant difference in sleep efficiency between the two groups ($P<0.05$). For the cases with moderate insomnia, the sleep efficiency was obviously better in the treatment group than that in the control group ($P<0.05$), and for the cases with slight and moderate insomnia, the number need to treat (NNT) was remarkably less in the intervention group ($P<0.01$). Gong et al. conducted a study [74] that randomized 120 patients with insomnia into a wooden needle group and a Western medicine group. In the wooden needle group, the patients were treated with wooden needles to press the plantar reflexing areas, such as cerebellar, thyroid, and cerebral areas. In the Western medicine group, Alprazolam was taken orally. The investigators found that the total therapeutic effect (sleep latency less than half an hour) was 100% in the wooden needle group, while it was 90.7% in the Western medicine group. However, no significant difference was observed between the two groups ($P>0.05$).

In TCM, Chinese medicine herbs are rarely used alone but rather in combination formulas. One open case series of more than 100 patients with either insomnia or neurasthenia reported an improvement in 80–90% of cases with treatment of Liquorice, wheat, and jujuba soup. [75] These studies, however, were limited by the lack of randomization and a control group. A large-scale double-blind case-controlled study of 303 patients with insomnia has also been reported. One hundred and fifty-one patients received a combination "sleep-aid pill" (containing suanzaoren, baishao, Radix bupleuri, Albizziae, etc.), while 152 patients received an "Anshen pill" (ingredients not revealed). More patients receiving the "sleep-aid pill" demonstrated improvement (92.7%) than did patients in the "Anshen pill" group (85.5%) [76]. Although this study used a better research design than earlier studies, the lack of a placebo control group, objective assessment, and the unknown ingredients of the "Anshen pill" limit the interpretation of this study. In a study conducted by Li et al. [77], 33 patients with psychological stress insomnia were assigned to one of four groups: TCM group treated with JXYP, Western medicine (WM) group treated with Estazolam, integrated medicine (IM) group treated with JXYP plus Estazolam, and control group treated with placebo. They found that JXYP, combined with or without Estazolam, can improve the quality of sleep subjectively, and the combination of the two enhanced the efficacy of sleep in patients with psychological stress insomnia.

Qigong

Qigong is a type of mind-body exercise that originated in China. It is a collective label for a number of exercises that involve slow deliberate movements, relaxed breathing, and deep mental focusing [78]. According to TCM, by practicing qigong, one can increase the flow of "qi," the life energy, in the human body to enhance health [79]. Wang et al. conducted the following study [80]: patients with type 2 diabetes accompanied by insomnia ($n=90$) were randomly divided into the Baduanjin Qigong group (routine treatment plus Baduanjin Qigong and Relaxation Qigong) or control, usual care group. They found that Qigong can improve the sleep quality in the patients with type 2 diabetes accompanied by insomnia.

If CAM interventions, particularly those from the TCM perspective, are to be considered as viable stand-alone or adjuvant treatments for sleep disorders, future researchers are urged to use quality methodology, including appropriate sample sizes and adequate controls. RCTs evaluating other untested CAM therapies such as massage, and other whole medical systems such homeopathy or osteopathy are encouraged, as is the exploration of using CAM therapies adjuvantly with conventional therapies resulting in a more integrative approach to sleep disorders. [81]

Review and Future Prospects

Looking back on recent research literature concerning whole medical systems, specifically the use of TCM in pulmonary diseases and sleep disorders, more evidence in support of TCM is coming out from basic science and clinical research (Table 15.3). [60, 66–68, 71–73, 82–84] However, there is still a compelling need for stronger evidence including: robust research designs; reliable data reporting and analysis; and useful and appropriate outcome measurements. It is not until these types of studies are performed in TCM and other whole medical systems that the full potential of integrating these valuable approaches into Western medicine can be fully realized for patients with acute and chronic lung diseases and sleep disorders.

There are a number of TCM practitioners in the United States. A skilled TCM practitioner is knowledgeable about the entire TCM medical system and not only one modality. Thus, a qualified TCM practitioner should provide the best advice from the TCM system standpoint to help patients manage their health, including clinical experience with TCM modalities for managing respiratory diseases and sleep disorders. The reader interested in learning more about TCM should refer to the Further Reading List at the end of this chapter.

Based on the evidence presented in this chapter it is the opinion of the authors that mild or moderate persistent asthma, stable COPD, ILD, chronic cough, and insomnia might receive the most benefit from TCM treatment. Only future, high-quality research will document TCM's benefits.

Table 15.3 Appraisal of all RCTs designed to evaluate the effectiveness and safety of CAM modalities for sleep

References	Participants	Intervention	Objectives	Results	Sample size	Randomization	Blinding	Intention to treat
[82]	Persons of both sexes, over the age of 60 year	Yoga Ayurvedic therapy Wait-list control	To compare the effects of Yoga and Ayurveda on the self-rated sleep in a geriatric population	Yoga group: decrease in the time taken to fall asleep ($P<0.05$); increase in the total number of hours slept ($P<0.05$); and in the feeling of being rested in the morning based on a rating scale ($P<0.05$) after 6 months. The other groups showed no significant change	69	Y	No	Not mentioned
[60]	Persons of both sexes, aged 60–92	Tai Chi 10w-impact exercise	To determine the effectiveness of tai chi on self-rated sleep quality and daytime sleepiness in older adults reporting moderate sleep complaints	Tai chi group: significant improvements in five of the PSQI subscale scores (sleep quality, sleep-onset latency, sleep duration, sleep efficiency, sleep disturbances) ($P<0.01$), PSQI global score ($P=0.001$), and ESS scores ($P=0.002$);sleep-onset latency of about 18 min per night (95% confidence interval (CI)=−28.64 to −7.12) and sleep duration of about 48 min more per night (95% CI = 14.71–82.41); better scores in secondary outcome measures	118	Y	Unclear	Unclear

(continued)

Table 15.3 (continued)

References	Participants	Intervention	Objectives	Results	Sample size	Randomization	Blinding	Intention to treat
[71]	Persons of both sexes from 45 states	Kava with valerian placebo Valerian with kava placebo Double placebo	To determine if kava is effective for reducing anxiety and if valerian is effective for improving sleep quality	The primary outcome measures were changes from baseline in anxiety (STAI-state questionnaire) and insomnia ([ISI]) compared with placebo. Participants receiving placebo had a 14.4 point decrease in anxiety symptoms on the STAI-state score and an 8.3 point decrease in insomnia symptoms on the ISI. Those receiving kava had similar reductions in STAI-state score (2.7 point greater reduction in placebo compared with kava; those receiving valerian and placebo had similar improvements in sleep (0.4 point greater reduction in the placebo than the valerian group	1551	Y	Double-blind	Unclear
[83]	Hospice patients of both sexes with advanced cancer	Combined massage (aromatherapy and massage) Massage No intervention	This study was designed to compare the effects of long-term effect of aromatherapy massage and massage alone on physical and psychological symptoms in patients with advanced cancer	After 4-week courses' intervention, sleep scores improved significantly in both the massage and the combined massage groups. There were also statistically significant reductions in depression scores in the massage group	42	Y	Unclear	Unclear
[84]	Patients of both sexes presenting in general practice suffering from stress	Therapeutic massage Using a relaxation tape in the surgery Relaxation tape to use at home	To compare the effect of six sessions of therapeutic massage with the use of a relaxation tape on stress	Large improvements in sleep index consistent across the three treatment groups, while with no significant benefit of one over the other	79	Y	No	No

[72]	Older men with a cardiovascular illness who were hospitalized in a critical care unit	Back massage Combined muscle relaxation, mental imagery, and a music audiotape Control	To determine the effects of a back massage and relaxation intervention on sleep in critically ill patients	Descriptive statistics showed improved quality of sleep among the back-massage group. Initial analysis showed a significant difference among the three groups in sleep efficiency index. Post hoc testing with the Duncan procedure indicated a significant difference between the back-massage group and the control group; patients in the back-massage group slept more than 1 h long than patients in the control group. However, the variance was significantly different among the three groups, and reanalysis of data with only 17 subjects in each group revealed no difference among groups ($P=0.06$)	69	Y	Unclear	Unclear
[66]	Institutionalized residents of both sexes	Acupressure Sham acupressure Control	To determine the effectiveness of acupressure in improving the quality of sleep of institutionalized residents	There were significant differences in PSQI subscale scores of the quality, latency, duration, efficiency, disturbances of sleep, and global PSQI scores among subjects in the three groups before and after interventions. Furthermore, there was a significant reduction in the frequencies of nocturnal awakening and night wakeful time in the acupressure group compared to the other two groups	84	Y	No	Unclear

(continued)

Table 15.3 (continued)

References	Participants	Intervention	Objectives	Results	Sample size	Randomization	Blinding	Intention to treat
[67]	Hemodialysis patients of both sexes	Acupressure TEAS Control	The purpose of this study was to test the effectiveness of acupressure and TEAS on fatigue, sleep quality, and depression in patients who were receiving routine hemodialysis treatment	The results indicated that patients in the acupressure and TEAS groups had significantly lower levels of fatigue, a better sleep quality, and less depressed moods compared with patients in the control group based upon the adjusted baseline differences. However, there were no differences between acupressure and TEAS groups in outcome measures	106	Y	Unclear	Unclear
[68]	Participants of 60 years old or above and who were suffering from sleep disturbances	Auricular therapy using Junci medulla Using semen vaccariae Using magnetic pearls	The purpose of this study was to examine the effectiveness of auricular therapy on sleep behaviors in the elderly	There were significant differences among the three groups in terms of the NST ($F(2,117)=6.84$, $P<0.05$) and SE ($F(2,117)=7.69$, $P<0.05$). Significant improvement in the sleep behaviors was observed in the experimental group using magnetic pearls. In a backward multiple regression, the effect of auricular therapy on SE after allowing for age in female participants is of high statistical significance ($F(3,106)=9.04$, $P<0.001$)	120		Unclear	Unclear

[73]	Patients aged >18 years with an apnoea-hypopnoea index between 15 and 30 and who complained about snoring	Didgeridoo lessons and daily practice Control	To assess the effects of didgeridoo playing on daytime sleepiness and other outcomes related to sleep by reducing collapsibility of the upper airways in patients with moderate obstructive sleep apnoea syndrome and snoring	Participants in the didgeridoo group practiced an average of 5.9 days a week (SD 0.86) for 25.3 min (SD 3.4). Compared with the control group in the didgeridoo group daytime sleepiness (difference −3.0, 95% confidence interval −5.7 to −0.3, $P=0.03$) and apnoea-hypopnoea index (difference −6.2, −12.3 to −0.1, $P=0.05$) improved significantly and partners reported less sleep disturbance (difference −2.8, −4.7 to −0.9, $P<0.01$). There was no effect on the quality of sleep (difference −0.7, −2.1 to 0.6, $P=0.27$). The combined analysis of sleep related outcomes showed a moderate to large effect of didgeridoo playing (difference between summary z scores −0.78 SD units, −1.27 to −0.28, $P<0.01$). Changes in health-related quality of life did not differ between groups	25	Y	No	Y

PSQI Pittsburgh Sleep Quality Index; *ESS* Epworth sleepiness scale; *ISI* Insomnia Severity Index; *TEAS* transcutaneous electrical acupoint stimulation; *NST* nocturnal sleep time; *SE* sleep efficiency

References

1. UK Ministry of Health. Report on the pandemic of influenza 1918–19. Reports on public health and medical subjects. London: Ministry of Health; 1920.
2. Novel Swine-Origin Influenza A (H1N1) Virus Investigation Team, Dawood FS, Jain S, Finelli L, Shaw MW, Lindstrom S, Garten RJ, Gubareva LV, Xu X, Bridges CB, Uyeki TM. Emergence of a novel swine-origin influenza a (H1N1) virus in humans. N Engl J Med. 2009;360(25):2605–15.
3. Ti H. Nei ching su wen: the yellow emperor's classic of internal medicine [I. Veith, translator]. Berkeley: University of California Press; 1976.
4. Liu L, Gu J. Analysis on ancient asthma acupuncture treatment characteristic. Shanghai J Acupuncture Moxibustion. 2000;19(5):42–3.
5. Qi L, Huang Q, Liu L. Acupuncture treatment of asthma. Shanghai J Acupuncture Moxibustion. 2005;24(4):24.
6. Yang Y. Analysis on curative effect of 174 cough and asthma cases with acupuncture treatment. Shanghai J Acupuncture Moxibustion. 1994;13(4):153.
7. Zhang Y. Acupuncturing Tanzhong (RN17) to treat 61 bronchial asthma cases. Shenzhen J Integr Tradit Chin West Med. 2001;11(2):100–1.
8. Hu L. Treating 50 asthma cases with acupuncture by stage. J Chengdu Univ TCM. 1999;22(2):30–1.
9. Zhao J, Cui H. Observation on effect of treating 36 remission stage asthma cases with mild-warming moxibustion. China's Naturopathy. 2002;14(2):21.
10. Li G, Bian Y, Li G, et al. Retrospective study on treating chronic pulmonary disease with Xiao Chuan Paste which cures winter diseases in summer. Beijing J Tradit Chin Med. 2008;27(11):835.
11. Dong Z, Hua R, Yang R, et al. Observation on effect of treating 223 asthma patients with Xiao Chuan Paste for 10 years. Chin J Integr Med. 1988;8(6):336–7.
12. Xiaoyu Z. Guiding principles for new drug clinical research of Chinese medicine (Trial). 2002;60–6.
13. Li Z. Treating 216 bronchial asthma cases with cupping and acupoint application. China's Naturopathy. 2006;14(11):54–5.
14. Fan X, Liu J. Analysis on curative effect of treating bronchial asthma of different season and different syndrome with Chinese medicine acupoint application. Chin Acupuncture Moxibustion. 2001;21(3):138–40.
15. Zhang J, Yu X, Liu W. Clinical observation on preventing and curing bronchial asthma with Chinese medicine acupoint application in the hottest and coldest days of a year. Liaoning J Tradit Chin Med. 2001;28(4):247–8.
16. Wu W, Tian X, Wang Q, et al. Clinical observation of treating 174 asthma cases with liver-discharging and lung-regulating therapy. J Beijing Univ Tradit Chin Med. 1990;13(4):19.
17. Zhang Y, Chang J, Chi HH, et al. Randomized controlled trial on treatment of bronchial asthma of qi-deficiency. cold syndrome type by Pingchuan Yiqi granule. Chin J Integr Med. 2007;13(1):27–32.
18. Wu Y, Yao Q, Yu S, et al. Analysis on long-term curative effect of treating 120 asthma cases with strengthen spleen and warming kidney oral paste. Zhejiang J Tradit Chin Med. 2000;35(4):27–32.
19. Long X, Tang Y, Huang J, et al. Clinical study on the effect to CD4+, CD8+ and IgE of bronchial asthma patients of Bufei tablet. J New Chin Med. 2007;39(5):27–8.
20. Cai R, Wu W. Clinical discuss on treating 80 asthma cases in remission stage of spleen insufficiency syndrome. J Guiyang Coll of Tradit Chin Med. 2007;29(2):29–30.
21. Zhang J, Shi G. Clinical observation of treating 85 remission stage asthma cases with Huangqi Liujunzi decoction. Shandong J Tradit Chin Med. 2004;23(4):204–5.
22. Cui H, Wu W, Ren C, et al. Effective observation of treating 20 SDA cases with Wumei Wan. Chin J Basic Med Tradit Chin Med. 2004;10(8):609–10.

23. Gong X, Yao J, Liu F, et al. Clinical observation of treating SDA with Chaipo Pingchuan mixture decoction. J Practical Tradit Chin Med. 2000;16(5):6–7.
24. Mi H, Li J. Searching for bioactive components of Chaipo decoction to treat asthma. Tradit Chin Drugs Res Clin Pharmacol. 1994;5(4):51.
25. Zhao X, Guo X. TCM dietary nursing for asthma patients. Chin Med Mod Dist Educ China. 2010;8(18):101–2.
26. Tao K, Zhou X, Mu X, et al. Clinical observation on treating 64 SDA cases with bailing tablet. J Pract Tradit Chin Med. 1998;11(7):589.
27. Wang H. Dietary therapy recipes of asthma patients. J Nanjing Univ Tradit Chi Med. 1994; 10(6):85–6.
28. Chen G. Fujiang chicken decoction—a recipe for treating asthma. Zhonghua Qigong. 2000;(10):48.
29. Lu P. Experience of "treating winter disease in summer" dietary therapy for elder bronchial asthma. Lishizhen Med Materia Medica Res. 2000;11(2):147.
30. Li J. The treatment summary with Chinese medical differentiation of symptoms and signs on chronic obstructive pulmonary disease. J Henan Univ Chin Med. 2009;24(143):9–11.
31. Luo X. The study of the healing efficacy of Bao Fei Ding Chuan medical liquid on 36 COPD patients. J Tradit Chin Med. 2002;43(4):268–70.
32. Fang Y, Deng T. Traditional Chinese internal medicine. Shanghai: Shanghai Scientific and Technical Press; 1966. p. 175–9.
33. Li S, Wu Q. Professor Cao Shihong's experience of therapy of COPD. Study J Tradit Chin Med. 2002;20(1):28.
34. Hong G. Respiratory muscle fatigue, nutritional disorders and chronic obstructive pulmonary disease. Tradit Chin Med J. 2006;5(2):4–6.
35. Wu Z. Overview of the past decade the development of traditional Chinese medicine external treatment. J External Ther Tradit Chin Med. 2003;12(1):32–3.
36. Li Z. Chinese medical external treatment of disease progress and ideas. [J]. 2003;12(6):3–5.
37. Dong Z. Observation on effect of treating 223 asthma patients with Xiaochuangao for 10 years. China Acad TCM. 1988;6:336.
38. Jia J. The report of 66 cases of COPD with the treatment of acupuncture and rehabilitation. Shaanxi J Tradit Chin Med. 2004;25(12):1125–6.
39. Chen Q, Zhong L, Liu H. Massage therapy for chronic obstructive pulmonary disease. Chin J Clin Rehabil. 2006;10(7):10–2.
40. Liu S, Zhou Y, Chen Y. Study on effect of point massage on promoting sputum exclude in treatment of chronic obstructive pulmonary disease (COPD) during acute episode. Mod Prev Med. 2004;31(5):588.
41. Liu F. Observation on effect of treating COPD patients with Qigong and medicine. Tianjin J Tradit Chin Med. 1986;secondary:3–7.
42. Bai C. A study of Qigong rehabilitation in patients with chronic obstructive pulmonary disease. Chin J Rehabil. 7(4):167–74.
43. Wu WP, Ren CY. How to distinguish pulmonary interstitial fibrosis in traditional Chinese medical way. Tradit Chin Mag. 2005;2,46(2).
44. Liu YQ, Liu GY. The discuss of traditional Chinese medical treatment of pulmonary interstitial fibrosis. Tradit Chin Med Res. 2006;12,19(12).
45. Wu YG, Zhang TH. The theory of collateral disease can guide the traditional Chinese medical treatment of pulmonary interstitial fibrosis. Tradit Chin Med J. 2005;1,23(1).
46. Kong XW. Traditional Chinese medical treatment of idiopathic pulmonary interstitial fibrosis. Mod J Integr Tradit Chin West Med. 2003;1,12(1).
47. Peng YH. The method of using traditional Chinese medicine to treat idiopathic pulmonary interstitial fibrosis. Study J Tradit Chin Med. 2003;10,21(10).
48. Guan TY, Yang J, et al. Acquaintance of traditional Chinese medicine about idiopathic pulmonary interstitial fibrosis. Chin Arch Tradit Chin Med. 2007;5,25(5).
49. Qiu SP. Reflect on the cute of pulmonary interstitial fibrosis with activating blood medication. Tradit Chin Med J Fujian Univ. 2007;8,17(4).

50. Cui YH. Discuss about traditional Chinese medical treatment of pulmonary interstitial fibrosis. J Emergen Tradit Chin Med. 2006;8,15(8).
51. Lu XD, Pang LJ, et al. The research of traditional Chinese medicine about the relationship of pulmonary interstitial fibrosis and lung wither. Liaoning J Tradit Chin Med. 2007;34(3).
52. Jiang LD, Zhang XM, et al. The pathogen and treatment of idiopathic pulmonary interstitial fibrosis. Beijing Tradit Chin Med. 2008;4,27(4).
53. Sun SM. Thousand gold prescription. Beijing: Huaxia Publishing House; 1993:254,432.
54. Li R, Yan ZY, Li WJ, et al. The research on the treatment effect of pulmonary interstitial fibrosis with acupuncture. J Clin Acupuncture Moxibustion. 2004;20(2):11.
55. Liu W. Clinical observation on 32 case of idiopathic pulmonary interstitial fibrosis cured by both traditional Chinese medicine and western medicine. J Tradit Chin Med. 2005;46(9): 675–6.
56. Song JP, Li RQ, et al. The experiment research about the treatment and prevent pulmonary interstitial fibrosis with traditional Chinese medicine. Bull Med Res. 2004;33(2).
57. Wu YG, Tang BQ. The research of the treatment on pulmonary interstitial fibrosis with prescription named Fei Xian Jian. J Beijing Univ Tradit Chin Med. 2005;3,19(1).
58. Lu X, Ye WC, et al. The intervene of prescription of strengthening the body on bleomycin make mice got pulmonary inters titial fibrosis. J Tradit Chin Med. 2008;7,47(7).
59. Li R, Li WJ. The experiment research on the effect of moxibustion on 'Feishu', 'gaohuang' of the mice which were made pulmonary interstitial fibrosis with BLMA5. Chin Acupuncture Moxibustion. 2005;11,25(11).
60. Chase JE, Gidal BE. Melatonin: therapeutic use in sleep disorders. Ann Pharmacother. 1997; 31:1218–26.
61. Lee FC. Facts about ginseng, the elixir of life. Elizabeth: Hollyn International Corp; 1992.
62. Punnonen R, Lukola A. Oestrogen-like effectof ginseng. Br Med J. 1980;281:1110.
63. Newall CA, Anderson LA, Phillipson JD. Herbal medicines: a guide for health-care professionals. London: The Pharmaceutical Press; 1996. p. 145–50.
64. Schulz V, Hansel R, Tyler VE. Agents that increase resistance to diseases. In: Schulz V, Hansel R, Tyler VE, editors. Rational Phytotherapy. New York: Springer; 1998. p. 269–72.
65. Soden K, Vincent K, Craske S, Lucas C, Ashley S. A randomized controlled trial of aromatherapy massage in a hospice setting. Palliat Med. 2004;18(2):87–92.
66. Tsay SL, Cho YC, Chen ML. Acupressure and transcutaneous electrical acupoint stimulation in improving fatigue, sleep quality and depression in hemodialysis patients. Am J Chin Med. 2004;32(3):407–16.
67. Suen LK, Wong TK, Leung AW, Ip WC. The long-term effects of auricular therapy using magnetic pearls on elderly with insomnia. Complement Ther Med. 2003;11(2):85–92.
68. Suen LK, Wong TK, Leung AW. Effectiveness of auricular therapy on sleep promotion in the elderly. Am J Chin Med. 2002;30(4):429–49.
69. Sarris J, Byrne GJ. A systematic review of insomnia and complementary medicine. Sleep Med Rev. 2011;15(2):99–106.
70. Sok SR, Erlen JA, Kim KB. Effects of acupuncture therapy on insomnia. J Adv Nurs. 2003;44(4):375–84.
71. Spence DW, Kayumov L, Chen A, et al. Acupuncture increases nocturnal melatonin secretion and reduces insomnia and anxiety: a preliminary report. J Neuropsychia Clin Neurosci. 2004; 16(1):19–28.
72. Montakab H. Acupuncture and insomnia. Forsch Komplementarmed. 1999;6 Suppl 1:29–31.
73. Zhang YF, Ren GF, Zhang XC. Acupuncture plus cupping for treating insomnia in college students. J Trad Chin Med. 2010;30(3):185–9.
74. Gong YL, Zhang YB, Han C, Jiang YY, Li Y, Chen SC, Liu ZY. Clinical observation on therapeutic effect of the pressing plantar reflex area with wooden needle for treatment of patients with insomnia. Zhongguo Zhen Jiu. 2009;29(11):935–7.
75. Zhou MY. The traditional Chinese medicine treatment of neurosis in 75 patients [in Chinese]. Shang Hai Zhong Yi Yao Za Zhi. 1989;7:5.

76. Zhang H, Cao XL, Sun XQ, et al. The treatment of insomnia of Anshen pill in 151 patients [in Chinese]. JTCM. 2000;41:418–9.
77. Li Y, Xu BY, Xiao F. Effect of modified xiaoyao powder for improving sleep in patients with psychological stress insomnia. Zhongguo Zhong Xi Yi Jie He Za Zhi. 2009;29(3):208–11.
78. Xue CC, O'Brien KA. Modalities of Chinese medicine. In: Leung PC, Xue CC, Cheng YC, editors. A comprehensive guide to Chinese medicine. River Edge: World Scientific Publishing; 2003.
79. Tsang HWH, Chan EP, Cheung WM. Effects of mindful and non mindful exercises on people with depression: a systematic review. Br J Clin Psychol. 2008;47(3):303–22.
80. Wang F, Wang WD, Zhang RR, et al. Influence of different qigong practices on sleep quality in patients with type 2 diabetes accompanied by insomnia. J Beijing Univ Tradit Chin Med. 2009;32(9):636–40.
81. Young T, Peppard PE, Gottlieb DJ. Epidemiology of obstructive sleep apnea: a population health perspective. Am J Respir Cir Care Med. 2002;165:1217–39.
82. Li F, Fisher KJ, Harmer P, Irbe D, Tearse RG, Weimer C. Tai chi and self-rated quality of sleep and daytime sleepiness in older adults: a randomized controlled trial. J Am Geriatr Soc. 2004;52(6):892–900.
83. Hanley J, Stirling P, Brown C. Randomised controlled trial of therapeutic massage in the management of stress. Br J Gen Pract. 2003;53(486):20–5.
84. McDowell JA, Mion LC, Lydon TJ, Inouye SK. A nonpharmacologic sleep protocol for hospitalized older patients. J Am Geriatr Soc. 1998;46(6):700–5.

Further Readings

Ancoli-Israel S, Roth T. Characteristics of insomnia in the United States: results of the 1991 National Sleep Foundation Survey. I Sleep. 1999;22 Suppl 2:S347–53.

Attele AS, Wu JA, Yuan CS. Multiple pharmacological effects of ginseng. Biochem Pharmacol. 1999;58:1685–93.

Bent S, Padula A, Moore D, Patterson M, Mehling W. Valerian for sleep: a systematic review and meta-analysis. Am J Med. 2006;119:1005–12.

Bixler EO, Kales A, Soldatos CR, Kalse JD, Healy S. Prevalence of sleep disorders: a survey of the Los Angeles metropolitan area. Am J Psychiatry. 1979;136:1257–62.

Block KI, Gyllenhaal C, Mead MN. Safety and efficacy of herbal sedatives in cancer care. Integr Cancer Ther. 2004;3(2):128–48.

Buscemi N, Vandermeer B, Pandya R, et al. Melatonin for treatment of sleep disorders, evidence report/technology assessment no. 108. Rockville, MD: Agency for Healthcare Research and Quality; Prepared by the University of Alberta Evidence-based Practice Center, under Contract NO. 290–02–0023; November 2004. AHRQ Publication No. 05–E002–2.

Carlson LE, Garland SN. Impact of mindfulness-based stress reduction (MBSR) on sleep, mood, stress and fatigue symptoms in cancer outpatients. Int J Behav Med. 2005;12(4):278–85.

Chen ML, Lin LC, Wu SC, Lin JG. The effectiveness of acupressure in improving the quality of sleep of institutionalized residents. J Gerontol A Biol Sci Med Sci. 1999;54(8):M389–94.

Dawson D, van den Heuvel CJ. Integrating the actions of melatonin on human physiology. Ann Med. 1998;30(1):95–102.

Dietz BM, Mahady GB, Pauli GF, Farnsworth NR. Valerian extract and valerenic acid are partial agonists of the 5-HT5a receptor in vitro. Brain Res Mol Brain Res. 2005;138(2):191–7.

Donath F, Quispe S, Diefenbach K, Maurer A, Fietze I, Roots I. Critical evaluation of the effect of valerian extract on sleep structure and sleep quality. Pharmacopsychiatry. 2000;33:47–53.

Folkard S, Arendt J, Clark M. Can melatonin improve shift workers' tolerance of the night shift: some preliminary findings. Chronobiol Int. 1993;10:315–20.

Ford DE, Kamerow DB. Epidemiologic study of sleep disturbance and psychiatric disorders. An opportunity for prevention. JAMA. 1989;262(11):1479–84.

Foster S, Tyler VE. Valerian. In: Foster S, Tyler VE, editors. Tyler's honest herbal. New York: Haworth Press; 1999. p. 377–8.

Guilleminault C, Cathala JP, Castaigne P. Effects of 5-hydroxytryptophan on sleep of a patient with a brain-stem lesion. Electroencephalogr Clin Neurophysiol. 1973;34:177–84.

Hajak G. Epidemiology of severe insomnia and its consequences in Germany. Eur Arch Psychiatry Clin Neurosci. 2001;251(2):49–56.

Houghton PJ. The scientific basis for the reputed activity of Valerian. J Pharm Pharmacol. 1999;51(5):505–12.

Leger D, Guillrminault C, Delahaye C, Paillard M. Prevalence of insomnia in a survey of 12,778 adults in France. J Sleep Res. 2000;9(1):32–5.

Li F. The study of the effect of point application on pulmonary function of COPD patients. Liaoning J Tradit Chin Med. 2008;8(12):938(2).

Li F, Fisher KJ, Harmer P, Irbe D, Tearse RG, Weimer C. Tai chi and self-rated quality of sleep and daytime sleepiness in older adults: a randomized controlled trial. J Am Geriatr Soc. 2004;52(6):892–900.

Liu P. Clinical efficacy research about traditional Chinese medical treatment of pulmonary interstitial fibrosis. China Pract Med. 2008;7,3(19).

Liu W. Effect of Kechuan plaster on the quality of life of patients with COPD and the mechanism of its action in preventive treatment of disease. Beijing Hospital of TCM Affiliated to Capital Medical University 2008;8(12):938(2).

Lu QZ. Zhang Shi Yi Tong. Beijing: China Press of Traditional Chinese Medicine; 1995. p. 85.

Mason LI, Alexander CN, Travis FT, et al. Electrophysiological correlates of higher states of consciousness during sleep in long-term practitioners of the transcendental meditation program. Sleep. 1997;20(2):102–10.

McCrae CS, Lichstein KL. Secondary insomnia: a heuristic model and behavioral approaches to assessment, treatment and prevention. Appl Prev Psychol. 2001;10:107–23.

Mellinger GD, Balter MB, Uhlenhuth EH. Insomnia and its treatment. Prevalence and correlates. Arch Gen Psychiatry. 1985;42(3):225–32.

Morin CM, Koetter U, Bastien C, Ware JC, Wooten V. Valerian-hops combination and diphenhydramine for treating insomnia: a randomized placebo-controlled clinical trial. Sleep. 2005; 28(11):1465–71.

Muller CE, Schumacher B, Brattstrom A, Abourashed EA, Koetter U. Interactions of valerian extracts and a fixed valerian-hop extract combination with adenosine receptors. Life Sci. 2002;71(16):1939–49.

Murphy PJ, Myers BL, Badia P. Nonsteroidal anti-inflammatory drugs alter body temperature and suppress melatonin in humans. Physiol Behav. 1996;59(1):133–9.

National Academies—Committee on the Framework for Evaluating the Safety of Dietary Supplements. Prototype monograph on melatonin. Dietary supplements: a framework for evaluation safety. Washington: The National Academies Press; 2004. p. D1–71.

Ohayon MM, Hong SC. Prevalence of insomnia and associated factors in South korea. J Psychosom Res. 2002;53(1):593–600.

Ohayon MM. Epidemiology of insomnia: what we still need to learn. Sleep Med Rev. 2002;6(2):97–111.

Ohayon MM, Smirne S. Prevalence and consequences of insomnia disorders in the general population of Italy. Sleep Med. 2002;3(2):115–20.

PDR for herbal remedies. Montvale: Medical Economics; 1998.

Petrie K, Dawson AG, Thompson L, Brook R. A double-blind trial of melatonin as a treatment for jet lag in international cabin crew. Biol Psychiatry. 1993;33:526–30.

Plushner SL. Valerian: valeriana officinalis. Am J Health Syst Pharm. 2000;57(4):328–33.

Qiu SP, Wang YH, et al. The affection of activating blood medication named San Leng, E Zhu to pulmonary interstitial fibrosis mice's lung shape and hydroxyproline. J Fujian Med Univ. 2007;8,41(5).

Reynolds JEF. Martindale: the extra pharmacopea. 31st ed. London: The Royal Pharmaceutical Society of Great Britain; 1996. p. 336–7.
Richards K, Nagel C, Markie M, Elwell J, Barone C. Use of complementary and alternative therapies to promote sleep in critically ill patients. Crit Care Nurs Clin North Am. 2003;15(3):329–40.
Richards KC. Effect of a back massage and relaxation intervention on sleep in critically ill patients. Am J Crit Care. 1998;7(4):288–99.
Salter S, Brownie S. Treating primary insomnia—the efficacy of valerian and hops. Aust Fam Physician. 2010;39(6):433–7.
Santos MS, Ferreira F, Cunha AP, Carvalho AP, Ribeiro CF, Macedo T. Synaptosomal GABA release as influenced by valerian root extract—involvement of the GABA carrier. Arch Int Pharmacodyn Ther. 1994;327(2):220–31.
Sheng L, Yao L, et al. Research on the affection of the resisters of leech and earthworm on pulmonary interstitial fibrosis of experiment mice. Tradit Chin Med Res. 2006;12,19(2).
Simon G, Vonkorff M. prevalence, burden, and treatment of insomnia in primary care. Am J Psychiatry. 1997;154(10):1417–23.
Soulairac A, Lambinet H. Effect of 5-hydroxytryptophan, a serotonin precursor on sleep disorders. Ann Med Psychol. 1977;1:792–8.
Suen LK, Wong TK, Leung AW, Ip WC. The long-term effects of auricular therapy using magnetic pearls on elderly with insomnia. Complement Ther Med. 2003;11(2):85–92.
Suen LK, Wong TK, Leung AW. Effectiveness of auricular therapy on sleep promotion in the elderly. Am J Chin Med. 2002;30(4):429–49.
Surrall K, Smith JA, Bird H, Okala B, Othman H, Padwick DJ. Effect of ibuprofen and indomethacin on human plasma melatonin. J Pharm Pharmacol. 1987;39(10):840–3.
Taibi DM, Bourguignon C, Taylor AG. Valerian use for sleep disturbances related to rheumatoid arthritis. Holist Nurs Pract. 2004;18(3):120–6.
van den Heuvel CJ, Reid KJ, Dawson D. Effect of atenolol on nocturnal sleep and temperature in young men: reversal by pharmacological doses of melatonin. Physiol Behav. 1997;61(6):795–802.
Wang M, Fan L. Classification and dietary therapy of asthma remission stage. J Henan Univ Chin Med. 2004;19(6):85–6.
Weyerer S, Dilling H. Prevalence, burden, and treatment of insomnia in the community: results from the Upper Bavarian Field Study. Sleep. 1991;14(5):392–8.
Wyatt RJ, Zarcone V, Engelman K, et al. Effects of 5-hydroxytryptophan on the sleep of normal human subjects. Electroencephalogr Clin Neurophysiol. 1971;30:505–9.
Xia C. Disease diagnosis and treatment experience of chronic obstructive pulmonary disease. J Emerg Trad Chin Med. 2002;11(6):500.
Zhu Q. Main point of development of Chinese external method of treatment. J External Ther Tradit Chin Med. 2010;19(1):3–5.
Zhu Q. Path of External Therapy of Traditional Chinese Medicine development. J External Ther Tradit Chin Med. 2003;12(2):34–5.

Chapter 16
Counseling Patients with Chronic Lung Disease: Interdisciplinary Strategies for Reducing Distress

Kathleen F. Sarmiento and Linda Berg-Cross

Abstract Patients with chronic lung disease (CLD) experience a progressively debilitating loss of lung function over time. The symptom of breathlessness is commonly cited as the most distressing aspect of living with CLD, whether due to emphysema, asthma, interstitial lung disease, or cystic fibrosis. Current therapies, both allopathic and alternative, target relief of symptoms, but do not reverse loss of lung function. As a result, anxiety and depression are prevalent among patients with CLD. Counseling patients on how to live with their disease and maximize functionality is a critical but often overlooked aspect of patient care. This chapter focuses on the approach to counseling patients with CLD, addressing five pillars of optimum functioning.

Keywords Anxiety • Chronic obstructive pulmonary disease • Counseling • Respiratory disease

Overview and Introduction

The number of people suffering from chronic lung disease (CLD), including chronic obstructive pulmonary disease (COPD), cystic fibrosis (CF), interstitial lung disease (ILD), and asthma, is increasing annually. The majority of this increase is due to an

K.F. Sarmiento, MD, MPH (✉)
Division of Pulmonary and Critical Care Medicine, University of Maryland School of Medicine, 685 West Baltimore St., MSTF 800, Baltimore, MD 21201, USA
e-mail: katiesarmiento@gmail.com

L. Berg-Cross, PhD, ABPP, CBSM
Department of Psychology, Howard University, 525 Bryant St, NW, Washington, DC 20059, USA

L. Chlan and M.I. Hertz (eds.), *Integrative Therapies in Lung Health and Sleep*, Respiratory Medicine 4, DOI 10.1007/978-1-61779-579-4_16,

ever-rising prevalence of asthma and COPD. Advances in medical therapies and improved access to care have contributed to patients with CLD surviving longer. Asthma affected more than 30 million people in the United States in 2004, and more than 300 million people worldwide in 2007. Although COPD is considered the fourth leading cause of death in the United States and fifth leading cause of death worldwide, the World Health Organization projects it will become the third leading cause of death by 2030 [1]. Healthcare utilization by patients with CLD, and the economic burden this imposes through both direct care costs and indirect costs (income loss and work productivity) are significant. Asthma-related costs alone in 2004 were more than $30 billion [2].

Treatment options have remained limited, with most aimed at symptomatic relief rather than disease reversal or prevention of progression. As a result, increasing attention has been given to integrative, complementary, and alternative therapies, and nonpharmacologic strategies of symptom management such as pulmonary rehabilitation, psychotherapy, intensive outpatient outreach programs, mind–body therapy, and manipulation therapies. There are also many sham therapies marketed to patients with CLD, preying on the desperation breathlessness creates. Distinguishing sham treatments, which have no positive effects and often profound negative effects, from reputable complementary and alternative medicines (CAM) is difficult since many popular CAM treatments have not been scientifically evaluated. However, if a patient answers "yes" to any of the five following questions, a sham treatment is almost certain. Are they advising me to ignore or shun traditional medical advice? Are they unwilling to communicate with my medical providers? Is my physician wary about me seeking this CAM? Am I committed to pay for services for a certain period of time or number of sessions? Have there been any complaints about the service or provider to the Better Business Bureau? These simple questions can be used to guide the healthcare provider in determining use of unproven therapies in persons with CLD.

CLDs are often progressively debilitating and create more than their share of desperate people. For example, among COPD patients more than 50% complain about not being able to complete the activities they like to do and over 15% live in fear that their disease will cripple or eventually kill them. This chapter addresses the role of psychological interventions and the approach to counseling patients with CLD. While the focus is on COPD, the issues and treatments are applicable to all types of CLD.

Evidence on Counseling Patients About Lifestyle and on Psychological Interventions

Expanded Provider Roles When Treating CLD

Desperate people search for hope—some magic bullets that will reduce their pain, increase their pleasure, and give meaning to their daily routines. The primary healthcare provider or specialist monitoring a desperate patient with CLD wields enormous psychological power because the patient is dependent on the provider or physician for this hope. There is increasing importance in today's practice of medicine to tailor therapies to the needs of the individual patient. This applies not only to the allopathic medications a patient is prescribed, but also to the non-pharmacologic, integrative approach to symptom relief. Where the practice of medicine may once have been predominantly paternalistic, it is now more of an art of negotiation.

Time spent with patients during office visits is precious and limited. Much of this time is spent obtaining an interval history, including establishing what a patient can and cannot do physically, and devising a plan of care. Often this plan focuses on the addition or subtraction of a medication, or a recommendation for other counseling or rehabilitation programs. Given the variety of support services available to COPD patients, including physical therapists, social workers, psychologists, pharmacists, family members, and friends, physicians often assume patients will utilize these functional and psychological supports when needed. In reality, many patients receive little to no auxiliary support.

It has been shown in other chronic diseases such as heart failure, cancer, and rheumatologic disease that psychological dysfunction can adversely affect medical outcomes [3–8]. Health-related quality of life has consistently been shown to be decreased in patients with CLD. When disease is very advanced, as is often seen in those awaiting lung transplantation, rates of depression and anxiety are particularly high compared to the general population [9–13]. Treating mood disorders, through either or both medication and counseling, improves quality of life and the perception of psychosocial support [13–19].

An Approach to Counseling the CLD Patient: The COPD Quality of Life Wheel

When a patient feels their quality of life is suboptimal despite adhering to recommended therapies, they become desperate for alternative treatments. They are often too embarrassed or unwilling to disclose to their physician any trials with sham therapies, which are often unregulated and not approved by the United States Food and Drug Administration (FDA). The physician with a desperate patient is in the same position as a parent with a restless child—if the parent does not give the child a choice of activity A, B, or C, the child risks getting into trouble by engaging in activities D, E, and F. The following discussion presents data supporting the effectiveness of each spoke of the wheel. It then focuses on what practitioners and their staff can do in the course of a routine office visit to orient and motivate patients to create behavior goals related to each spoke of the wheel.

Although termed "The COPD Quality of Life Wheel," these principles are applicable to all patients with CLD. The wheel (Fig. 16.1), developed by the authors of this chapter, is based on five patient-initiated and patient-maintained strategies that can increase the odds that they will enjoy life for a longer period of time: (1) mood, (2) exercise, (3) sleep, (4) social support, and (5) environmental construct. These are

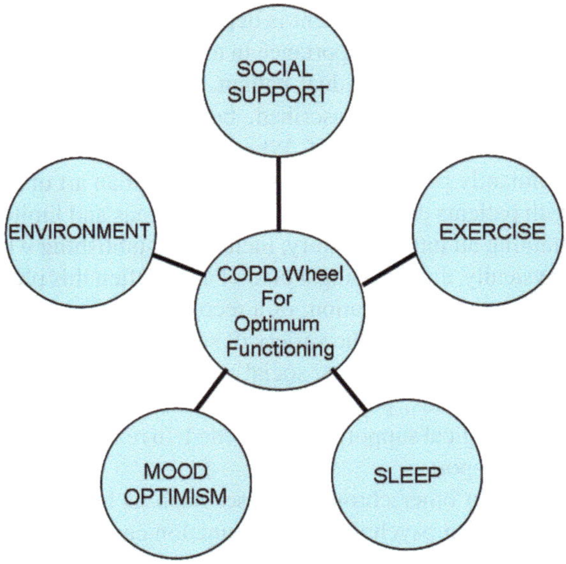

Fig. 16.1 COPD wheel for optimum functioning

the "magic bullets" that evidence-based interdisciplinary medicine keeps in the arsenal. These strategies have active ingredients along with a strong placebo effect that together can help many patients cope more effectively. It is the physician's role to introduce these concepts to the patient and to refer the patient to specialists when needed. Referrals to sleep disorder specialists, mental health providers, physical therapists, occupational therapists, social workers, and support groups (i.e., for smoking cessation) are all appropriate.

Patients should be able to fill in the wheels with all the activities they do each week to help themselves. Self-help groups can employ the COPD wheel to structure their meetings.

Wheel 1: Social Support for the Patient with CLD

This wheel is comprised of healthcare team members as well as members of the patient's social circle, including friends and family, who are often the ones to provide day-to-day patient care. The ability of a caregiver to provide adequate supportive care is one of the key factors in delaying or preventing institutionalization of a person with chronic illness [20]. There have been numerous studies comparing different models of care delivery, including early discharge [21–26] (following hospitalization for acute exacerbations) and home/community-based management [27–35]. Outcomes included hospital length of stay, rates of readmission after discharge from acute hospitalizations, emergency department visits, morbidity, mortality, functional status, and quality of life. In each study, the intervention group received intensive follow up and interaction with a healthcare provider, case manager, or caregiver. Most studies showed no harm to patients in intervention groups, and generally positive outcomes, though the literature is inconsistent at best.

Despite the importance of caregivers in executing a successful discharge home and in delivering ongoing daily care, the needs of the caregiver have received little to no attention [36]. Many end-stage COPD patients in their last year of life are worried about burdening their caregiver [37]. One retrospective review designed to assess the needs of COPD patients in their last year of life included survey information from the caregivers of 209 deceased patients. More than 95% of these patients received help from family and friends in their last year of life [38], with weekly time commitments ranging from 5 h (15%) to more than 40 h (41%). Caregivers helped with household tasks, personal care, and medication administration. The only specific need of the caregiver was to be better informed of the patient's prognosis; 78% did not know that the patient was going to die within a year and would've wanted to have been informed of this. Other studies have shown high rates of depression and loneliness for both patients and their spouses. Addressing the needs of the caregiver should thus also be an important objective of any plan of care formulated by healthcare teams.

For those patients with end-stage lung disease, palliative care and hospice services are an excellent option [39]. Palliative care is interdisciplinary care provided with the goal of relieving suffering and improving quality of life. Hospice care is appropriate for all patients who have a prognosis of less than 6 months if a disease follows its natural course and can be provided on an inpatient and outpatient basis. This service offers care for the patient and support and respite for the caregiver. Patients and families receiving hospice support report better symptom control, emotional and spiritual support, feel more respected, and consistently feel their care is better than those patients who die without hospice care [40]. Hospice care also reduces the cost of providing care in the final year of life. This has significant economic implications given the prediction that COPD will be the third leading cause of death by 2020. Interestingly, COPD patients residing at home with less than a 2-year prognosis who participated in a hospice-based model of care reported better outcomes of self-management of illness, awareness of illness-related community resources, greater vitality, better physical functioning, and higher self-rated health than randomized control subjects [41]. A general guideline for assessing whether a hospice referral is appropriate for a pulmonary patient is outlined in the Medicare Hospice Eligibility Guidelines, but is based on a decrease in functional capacity with breathlessness at rest and poor response to bronchodilator therapy, disease progression as evidenced by emergency room visits and hospitalizations, and the presence of a low oxygen saturation at rest. Dependence in more than two activities of daily living (i.e., eating, bathing, getting dressed, using the bathroom, and mobility) or weight loss of greater than 10% of usual body weight due to poor feeding are also suggestive of a prognosis of less than 6 months [42].

Finally, the value of an involved healthcare team should not be underestimated. For example, something as simple as a daily phone call to review a patient's plans for the day has been shown to significantly increase activities of daily living and quality of life in patients with severe COPD [43]. Routine office visits can also effectively employ interventions that increase self-efficacy. Research has shown that targeting small specific behavior changes leads to more functional improvements and increased self-efficacy [44]. The most important question for the physician to ask the desperate patient to increase their self-efficacy is, "If you woke up tomorrow and were feeling much more in control of your life, how would you know?" If the patient says, "Well, for beginners I wouldn't be so sleepy all day!" then the task of the physician is to help the patient improve the quality of his/her sleep with cognitive behavioral therapy for insomnia (CBT-I) directives. If they say, "I would be able to put on my own slippers without assistance" the task is to figure out how the slippers can be placed at a height accessible to the patient or what assistive devices should be introduced. Not surprisingly, the number of years since diagnosis and the level of impaired activities independently predict self-efficacy, highlighting the bidirectional nature between incapacities and feelings of self-efficacy [45]. However, most patients are motivated to achieve even small improvements and targeting behaviors that are of importance to the patient make the most sense.

Wheel 2: Monitoring and Reinforcing Exercise Routines

Wheel 2 is probably the spoke of the wheel patients most understand and embrace as a key to maintaining functionality. It is also the area in which they are most likely to receive help and encouragement from the interdisciplinary medical team. Pulmonary rehabilitation programs are well accepted and are a part of standard care for pulmonary patients. Built around exercise routines and encouragement, they have repeatedly been shown to increase functioning and survival as well as reduce costs of total medical care. After participation in a rehabilitation program, there are increases in maximum exercise tolerance, aerobic capacity, endurance time during submaximal testing, functional walking distance, and strength of peripheral and respiratory muscles. These benefits are appreciated even in the absence of spirometric improvement on pulmonary function testing. The effect size of pulmonary rehabilitation largely exceeds what can be achieved by the best pharmacological therapy [46–52]. Although increasing in popularity, pulmonary rehabilitation programs may not be readily available or accessible to all patients. Encouraging behavioral lifestyle modifications (taking the stairs instead of elevator, walking, yard work, and participation in recreational sports activities) to increase physical activity may provide as much benefit as a traditional exercise program [53].

However, the physician should also encourage exercise by giving very specific directives. For example, being given a specific task such as "I'd like you to keep a diary of how much you are walking each day with the pedometer, and try to increase it five steps a day until I see you next time" is a far better directive than "Try using a pedometer to make sure you are walking enough." And indeed research has confirmed that physician-prescribed pedometer homework improves functioning more than no such homework [54, 55]. If using a pedometer is the number one self-administered exercise aid, learning and practicing yoga is a close second. Research has repeatedly shown that functionality increases among those who practice yogic breathing. And most importantly, even the most severely ill patients can empower themselves by practicing modified yoga routines or simple, mindful breathing exercises [56, 57]. Breath training has been shown to be an effective tool to reduce breathlessness related to performing activities of daily living and to improve quality of life [58–60].

Wheel 3: Behavioral Sleep Therapy Increases Quantity and Quality of Sleep

Secondary insomnia refers to sleep problems that are primarily associated with an intrusive event such as a primary medical problem (COPD). Since half of all COPD patients have significant sleep disturbances, secondary insomnia is a major comorbid condition that significantly affects daytime functioning [61–63]. Secondary insomnia, much like primary insomnia, has devastating psychological consequences including but not limited to impaired immune function, depressed mood, impaired memory, impulsiveness, fatigue, daytime sleepiness, compromised problem-solving, lowered frustration threshold, and forced expiratory volume. When a respiratory disease co-occurs with insomnia, the impact on functioning and quality of life is significantly greater than the impact of the chronic illness alone [64–66].

Problems with sleep are often multifactorial, and may become magnified with disease progression. There is a diurnal variation in airway muscle tone, with constriction of the airways occurring in the very early hours of the morning. Respiratory muscle tone also decreases during sleep. These physiologic changes increase the likelihood of hypoxemia and sleep-disordered breathing, both of which affect sleep quality and increase morbidity and mortality. Sleep in CLD patients is also affected by medications (bronchodilators increase heart rate, which may lead to feelings of anxiety) and mood disorders, which have a bidirectional relationship with sleep problems. That is, anxiety and depression both provoke sleep problems and are themselves provoked by poor sleep [67–69].

Standard evaluation of secondary insomnia requires asking the following five questions:

1. Are you sleepy during the day?
2. Does it take you more than 30 min to fall asleep?
3. Do you find yourself waking up during the night even if you don't have to go to the bathroom?
4. Is it difficult to fall back asleep when you wake up in the night?
5. Are you groggy and unrefreshed in the morning?

For a diagnosis of secondary insomnia, the patient must endorse item 1 and must answer "yes" to at least one additional question.

Research has indicated that CBT-I is highly effective in treating secondary insomnia, with 60–80% of patients achieving significant clinical benefits from treatment. Sleep parameters such as sleep efficiency, sleep onset latency (SOL), and sleep quality all improve with CBT-I without any additional intervention targeting the chronic illness [61]. Insomnia studies specifically including comorbid respiratory disorders have shown CBT-I to be more effective than stress management and wellness training. CBT-I is also more effective than a home-based audio relaxation treatment, though audio relaxation is more effective than receiving no treatment at all [70]. Home video instruction in CBT-I that was followed up by phone consultations also was able to improve sleep efficiency, SOL, quality, time spent in bed, wake time during the night as well as pain perception, mood, and social functioning [71]. Similarly, half of obstructive sleep apnea (OSA) cases with comorbid insomnia reach nonclinical levels of insomnia according to subjective insomnia, sleep quality, and sleep impairment with CBT-I [72].

While many patients with insomnia will need to be referred to a behavioral sleep specialist for an intense seven-session intervention, there are three "first-line" interventions that can be used by all healthcare professionals, regardless of whether CLD coexists [73].

Sleep Restriction. This technique involves restricting the amount of time that a person spends in bed to the actual hours that they are currently sleeping. Assume a patient indicates that they are only getting 5 h of sleep a night but they are going to bed at 11 and getting up at 8 a.m. They are spending a frustrating 4 h a night, lying there, "trying" to fall asleep and having problems breathing. Besides the nightly frustrations, they are conditioning themselves to stay awake on future nights in the bedroom environment. Sleep restriction requires that the person only go into bed for the amount of time they are actually sleeping. Sleeping only 5 h would dictate that the patient goes to bed at 2 a.m. Sleep onset must occur rapidly in order to obtain a full 5 h of sleep. If this works, one can try to lengthen the sleep period by incrementally going to bed 15 min earlier after a few nights and then continuing this lengthening of sleep, 15 min at a time, until one is awakening well rested. It is critical that, in the early stages of treatment, the patient understands and accepts that they will feel continue to feel sleepy, fatigued, and frustrated.

Stimulus Control. The second technique attempts to refocus all the bedroom stimuli so that they elicit sleep. The patient is not to study in bed, eat in bed, use their laptop in bed, entertain friends on their bed, or use the bed for any other reason than to sleep. In this way, getting in bed is repeatedly paired with falling asleep and can become a strong conditioned cue for sleep. This is particularly challenging for severe COPD patients who spend much of the day at home without activity. When patients refuse to stay out of the bed during the day, they can try to control the stimuli in the bedroom by facing in one direction during the day and turning the direction of their pillow around for sleeping. Other stimulus control possibilities are keeping the pillow that they use for sleep hidden and take it out only when they are ready for sleep. Other sleep onset stimuli include wearing an eye mask or taking out a specific blanket only when it is time to go to bed.

No napping. The no daytime napping directive ensures increased sleepiness at night and this is critical for improving nighttime sleep.

A skilled behavioral sleep therapist is often needed to create the cognitive interventions that will work most effectively for a particular client and are considered part of the "first-line" treatments in CBT-I. Many of the cognitive interventions are focused on inhibiting nighttime ruminations and hyper-focusing on problems. These activities plague many COPD patients, fueling and exacerbating their insomnia. A myriad of psychological interventions can be used to inhibit worrying, including distraction strategies, building new narratives, testing irrational beliefs, visual erasers, verbal and visual metaphors, journaling, gratitude exercises, and dozens of relaxation strategies. When breathing problems provoke panic attacks during the night, a combination of relaxation, visual anchors, and self-talk are often effective in significantly improving sleep quality and coping [74, 75].

Wheel 4: Helping Patients Increase Positive Moods and Optimism

Creating a More Positive Mood

When a patient feels that they are in control of their daily life, regardless of the course of the disease, they live longer and more functional lives [76, 77]. Meta-analyses confirm that solution-oriented psycho-educational interventions can increase feelings of self-control by promoting problem-solving about current and future challenges, thereby having a significant therapeutic effect on patient status [78].

COPD patients with anxiety disorders have more negative thought processes than COPD patients without anxiety, even when adjusted for pulmonary function [79]. Treatment of anxiety with anxiolytics and antidepressants reduces symptoms of distress. Psychosocial interventions are effective in reducing patient stress and increasing perceived support [80–85]. COPD psychosocial researchers have defined the following five areas where patients need to feel empowered to exert self-control: (a) mood control, which involves being able to get themselves out of the inevitable funks or "woe is me" moods; (b) tools to de-escalate bouts of frustration and anger; (c) self-control, particularly of the activities of daily living; (d) adaptability, which involves controlling social and environmental stressors (indoor pollutants, weather, etc.); and (e) lifestyle factors, including controlling diet, exercise, social life, and hobbies. There are several tools available, such as the COPD Self-Efficacy Scale [86] that can help providers identify and review areas patients feel most vulnerable, then target these specific areas for self-empowerment.

The Relationship Between Mood and Sleep

Optimizing sleep is an important target when trying to improve one's mood. Individuals who are predisposed to be depressed, anxious, or angry are most likely to suffer from poor sleep. What all three types of people share in common is high levels of arousal. It is hard for them to relax enough to have restorative sleep. On the other hand, it is generally true that happy-go-lucky, resilient individuals tend to have very few sleep problems. People who trust that despite today's troubles, tomorrow will be a better day, find sleep restorative. Like so many psychological issues, those who are blessed with positive traits keep reaping additional benefits, while those who are sensitive, high strung, temperamental, or otherwise difficult by nature, keep on having additional challenges which they must tackle.

Depression is the most frequent co-occurring disorder with insomnia. There are over 1,500 published articles that have shown a link between depression and sleep [87]. While 20% of patients with insomnia suffer from depression [88, 89], up to 85% of depressed individuals have a sleep problem. For people with OSA, rates of clinical depression can affect up to 45% of patients [90]. Given that patients with COPD have increased levels of both anxiety and depression, the effects on their sleep are particularly damaging and the potential benefits of learning to reduce negative affect are vital.

Many times sleep problems precede and provoke clinical depression. The evidence that insomnia can incite depression comes from many different sources. Longitudinal studies that tracked insomnia patients showed they were four times more likely to develop major depression over the next 3 years compared to patients without insomnia. This pattern of insomnia preceding depression has been found among all age groups, including older adults and younger adults. In fact, in one study elderly insomniacs were six times more likely to experience an initial episode of depression compared to their well-sleeping friends [91]. But the effects are bidirectional. Depression that initially exists without insomnia is often a ticking bomb for the emergence of a sleep problem. Untreated depression breeds insomnia [68, 69].

So if someone with a chronic lung problem has both depression and insomnia, where do you start treatment? It turns out that if you get treated for depression, there is a good chance your sleep problems will disappear, although a significant minority of people will still have insomnia problems even after their depression has lifted. If treated for insomnia, there is a good chance the depression will disappear although in a significant minority of people, the depression will remain and need to be treated [92]. Interestingly, depressed adults who start an antidepressant can ignite a more rapid antidepressant response if they improve their sleep. Thus, improved sleep may potentiate the effects of antidepressant therapy. Thus, working on both the insomnia and the depression seems the best way to get on the road to health.

The bidirectional relationship between insomnia and mood disorders is likely due to the shared pathophysiologic mechanisms that regulate both sleep and mood. Data have shown that both insomnia and depression are related to over-activation of the hypothalamic-pituitary-adrenal (HPA)—the part of the nervous system that controls the turning on and turning off of the fight/flight response.

The major treatment for depression is cognitive behavior therapy (CBT). Referrals for CBT, effective for treating comorbid depression in a wide range of chronic disorders, have been found to have only a positive effect on patients with COPD. One meta-analysis contained a combination of interventions, including

CBT, psychotherapy, and relaxation interventions. They concluded that while psychological interventions can reduce anxiety, it has not yet been demonstrated that they have a strong effect on functioning [93]. Hopefully future studies that focus on CBT interventions adapted for respiratory problems will strengthen the evidence for this approach.

Creating Optimism: Example of a Story from "The Doc"

Hundreds of research studies have linked optimism to better health and a better quality of life when ill [94]. For some, religion or spiritual teachings fuel their optimism. For others, social support from friends and family is the well of optimism. But sometimes, it is a person in authority, like a physician, reframing our situation or giving us some philosophical lifeline that makes us more resilient. Suddenly, instead of a "poor me" narrative, a few well-placed words can help us tune into how our own heroism and grit can let us live successfully, even with the indignities of a chronic disease. Every gifted physician learns how to dispense such conversational "pills" of hope. For example, one clever colleague found coins to give her patients. She told them to keep the coin near their bed and first thing, each morning, to flip the coin: if it came up "heads," it meant they would find the inner resources to have a good day; if it was "tails," it meant a day of frustration and despair. Since all the coins had "heads" on both sides, patients were reminded of the potential for coping each morning!

Another colleague tells patients that she wants to share the wisdom of the Cherokees. The Cherokees believe that there are two battling wolves inside every one of us. One wolf is Despair. He is filled with anger, self-pity, and resentment. The other wolf is Optimism. He is filled with joy, love, and hope. Patients with COPD can feel the struggle between the two wolves battling inside of them. The doctor then asks the patient if they want to know which wolf will win in their case. When they say "yes," he says, "the wolf that wins is always the one you choose to feed."

A favorite parable to nurture optimism is *The Carrot, the Egg and the Coffee Bean*. It can be photocopied and given to patients who in their desperation have lost both hope and optimism. The story is as follows: A young woman went to her mother and told her about her life and how things were so hard for her. She did not know how she was going to make it and wanted to give up. She was tired of fighting and struggling. Her mother took her to the kitchen. She filled three pots with water and placed each on a high fire. Soon the pots came to a boil. In the first, she placed carrots, in the second she placed eggs, and in the last she placed ground coffee beans. She let them sit and boil, without saying a word. In about 20 min she turned off the burners. She fished the carrots out and placed them in a bowl. She pulled the eggs out and placed them in a bowl. Then she ladled the coffee out and placed it in a bowl. Turning to her daughter, she asked, "Tell me, what do you see?" "Carrots, eggs, and coffee," she replied. She brought her closer and asked her to feel the carrots. She did and noted that they were soft. She then asked her to take an egg and break it. After pulling off the shell, she observed the hard-boiled egg. Finally, she asked her to sip the coffee. The daughter smiled as she tasted its rich flavor. The daughter then asked, "What does it mean, Mother?" Her mother explained that each of these objects had faced the same adversity—boiling water—but each reacted differently. The carrot went in strong, hard, and unrelenting. However after being subjected to the boiling water, it softened and became weak. The egg had been fragile. Its thin outer shell had protected its liquid interior. But, after sitting through the boiling water, its inside became hardened. The ground coffee beans were unique, however. After they were in the boiling water, the beans had actually changed the water. The water that could have proved lethal, became something new, meaningful, and nurturing. It brought out the best in the coffee bean. "Which are you?" she asked her daughter. "When adversity knocks on your door, how do you respond? Are you a carrot, an egg, or a coffee bean?"

Think of this: Which am I? Am I the carrot that seems strong, but with pain and adversity, do I wilt and become soft and lose my strength? Am I the egg that starts with a malleable heart, but changes with the heat? Did I have a fluid spirit, but with hard times, have I become hardened and stiff? Or am I like the coffee bean? The bean actually changes the hot water, the very circumstance that brings the pain. If you are like the bean, when things are at their worst, you will discover and release the unknown, miraculous parts of yourself. You will be able to change the bleakest situation into a meaningful and growth-enhancing occasion for yourself and your loved ones. How do you handle adversity? When adversity strikes, ask yourself … Are you a carrot, an egg, or a coffee bean? [95]

Wheel 5: Environmental Modifications and Technology to Facilitate Optimum Functioning

Patients with chronic lung problems have to expend more energy to do the same activities as someone without a chronic lung problem. COPD patients have an accelerated loss of aerobic capacity, which correlates with mortality [96]. Because independent living relies on being able to do the basic activities of daily living, decreased capacity to perform these tasks is existentially frightening and frustrating. The only way individuals with advanced chronic lung problems can get the same amount done as a non-ill person is to learn more efficient ways of performing everyday tasks. One way of achieving this energy savings is by design changes to one's home and environment. When funds are not available for the modifications, creative no-cost solutions can be found (e.g., taking doors away and becoming barrier free rather than retrofitting doors with levers). Some of the top modifications in the home that conserve a patient's energy are as follows: rollators (walkers), lever handles, adjustable height kitchen tops, remove carpeting to expose wood floors, using HEPA filters, extra low rise steps outside (to accommodate rollators), ultralight pots and pans, shower seats, house carts, and controlling indoor humidity levels. Patients often benefit from physicians "normalizing" the use of these modifications, by stressing how they can increase functioning, independence, and life satisfaction.

Environmental modifications for chronic illness will rely more and more heavily on social media for peer sharing about easy modifications as well as high-tech experts creating robots to individualize accommodations. Right now, an internet-based dyspnea self-management program (DSMP) has demonstrated that on-line patients showed increased self-efficacy for managing dyspnea symptoms and for maintaining more activities in daily living compared to a similar group without access to the social/educational media [97]. On a far more sophisticated and personalized scale, the KSERA project (Knowledgeable Service Robots for Aging) in the Netherlands is building three prototype houses to demonstrate how resident robots can help COPD patients in their daily lives by following the patient through the house, making helpful suggestions, offering advice, and learning their habits. The robot will be able to open doors, take food items in and out of the refrigerator, turn devices on and off, and encourage a patient to increase their activity. The robots can also monitor the owner's physical condition and environmental air quality. They can warn, advise, and support them in hazardous situations, enabling improved self-management and decreased hospitalization [98].

Summary and Conclusions

Current guidelines for allopathic practitioners are based on evidence-based reviews for each therapy. Medications and pulmonary rehabilitation are the mainstays of most treatment plans for patients with CLD. Pulmonary rehabilitation did not gain wide acceptance for several years due to the lack of effect on improving spirometric lung function. Broadening outcomes to include quality of life measurements made benefits of therapy more recognizable and valuable. As such, the physician educated on the importance of identifying patients' values and goals of therapy will be more likely to be successful in holistically treating his or her patients. Tangible and targeted goals of therapy, such as being able to walk a flight of stairs without stopping or being able to put on one's shoes, will bring more pleasure to a patient when accomplished than when goals are ill-defined or, worse-yet, meaningful only to the physician (change in spirometry but no subjective change in symptoms).

The role of the provider must thus extend beyond the prescription pad. Many allopathic physicians are not trained to counsel their patients about anxieties and fears related to their illness, nor do they feel they have enough time to undertake such an important task during a typical clinic visit. Many health-related quality of life questionnaires do not include room for free-text responses about what a patient may value. Thus, even if such tools are utilized to gauge a patient's functional status, a patient's goals and opinions about their treatment plan will be overlooked without an ensuing dialogue. There is a need to educate physicians and other healthcare providers on how to converse effectively and efficiently with patients to establish a plan of care together.

While evidence supporting the effectiveness of counseling patients with CLD on the five aspects of the COPD wheel is lacking, it is an area of clinical practice that should be further explored. There is strong evidence demonstrating the effectiveness of each spoke of the wheel on improving overall self-efficacy and perception of disease. Initiating a dialogue with patients allows other goals of treatment to present themselves. After all, it is not only the patient who is desperate for treatment but also the physician who feels desperate when no further treatments can be offered.

Directions for Future Research

There are many opportunities for research that arise from the discussion above. There is a clear need for increased education of physicians on how to effectively counsel patients with CLD in an efficient and effective manner. Ample opportunities exist for educational research on curriculum development to meet this goal, including determining which specialties should be included and at what level of training should this occur (medical school, residency, fellowship, attending). Development of screening tools to guide practitioners through the process of identifying patients' needs, and a protocol for using them, is also needed. For example, a short questionnaire could be created addressing not only health-related quality of life but also individual goals and values. A directory of resources should be made available not only to providers but also to patients and caregivers. This directory may include links to reputable CAM and integrative medicine websites, educational resources, and provider directories. Research potential exists for each spoke of the wheel as well: how active counseling impacts sleep, mood, optimism, and willingness and ability to exercise. Finally, there is an urgent need to further explore the needs of the caregiver, as they are the backbone of the support system for patients with CLD.

References

1. Murray CJ, Lopez AD. Mortality by cause for eight regions of the world: global burden of disease study. Lancet. 1997;349:1269–76.
2. Kamble S, Bharma M. Incremental direct expenditure of treating asthma in the United States. J Asthma. 2004;46:73–80.
3. Karajgi B, Rifkin A, Doddi S, et al. The prevalence of anxiety disorders in patients with chronic obstructive pulmonary disease. Am J Psychiatry. 1990;147:200–1.
4. Kim HF, Kunik ME, Molinari VA, et al. Functional impairment in COPD patients: the impact of anxiety and depression. Psychosomatics. 2000;41:465–71.
5. Grady KL, Jalowiec A, White-Williams C, et al. Predictors of quality of life in patients with advanced heart failure awaiting transplantation. J Heart Lung Transplant. 1995;14:2–10.
6. Woodman CL, Geist LJ, Vance S, et al. Psychiatric disorders and survival after lung transplantation. Psychosomatics. 1999;40:293–7.
7. Squier HC, Ries AL, Kaplan RM, et al. Quality of well-being predicts survival in lung transplantation candidates. Am J Respir Crit Care Med. 1995;152:2032–6.
8. Berkman LF, Leo-Summers L, Horwitz RI. Emotional support and survival after myocardial infarction. A prospective, population based study of the elderly. Ann Intern Med. 1992; 117:1003–9.

9. Viramontes JL, O'Brien B. Relationship between symptoms and health-related quality of life in chronic lung disease. J Gen Intern Med. 1994;9:46–8.
10. Singer HK, Ruchinskas RA, Riley KC, et al. The psychological impact of end-stage lung disease. Chest. 2001;120:1246–52.
11. Anderson KL. The effect of chronic obstructive pulmonary disease on quality of life. Res Nurs Health. 1995;18:547–56.
12. Craven J. Psychiatric aspects of lung transplantation: The Toronto Lung Transplant Group. Can J Psychiatry. 1990;35:759–64.
13. Brenes GA. Anxiety and chronic obstructive pulmonary disease: prevalence, impact, and treatment. Psychosom Med. 2003;65:963–70.
14. Argyropoulou P, Patakas D, Koukou A, et al. Buspirone effect on breathlessness and exercise performance in patients with chronic obstructive pulmonary disease. Respiration. 1993;60: 216–20.
15. Papp LA, Weiss JR, Greenberg HE, et al. Sertraline for chronic obstructive pulmonary disease and comorbid anxiety and mood disorders. Am J Psychiatry. 1995;152:1531.
16. Smoller JW, Pollack MH, Systrom D, et al. Sertraline effects on dyspnea in patients with obstructive airways disease. Psychosomatics. 1998;39:24–9.
17. Borson S, McDonald GJ, Gayle T, et al. Improvement in mood, physical symptoms, and function with nortriptyline for depression in patients with chronic obstructive pulmonary disease. Psychosomatics. 1992;33:190–201.
18. Eiser N, West C, Evans S, et al. Effects of psychotherapy in moderately severe COPD: a pilot study. Eur Respir J. 1997;10:1581–4.
19. Kunik ME, Braun U, Stanley MA, et al. One session cognitive behavioural therapy for elderly patients with chronic obstructive pulmonary disease. Psychol Med. 2001;31:717–23.
20. Cain JC, Wicks MN. Caregivers attributes as correlates of burden in family caregivers coping with chronic obstructive pulmonary disease. J Fam Nurs. 2000;6:46–8.
21. Taylor S, Eldridge S, Chang YM, et al. Evaluating hospital at home and early discharge schemes for patients with an acute exacerbation of COPD. Chron Respir Dis. 2007;4:33–43.
22. Murphy N, Byrne C, Costello R. An early supported discharge programme for patients with exacerbations of chronic obstructive pulmonary disease (COPD) in Ireland. All Ireland J Nurs Midwifery. 2002;22:815–20.
23. Davison AG, Monaghan M, Brown D, et al. Hospital at home for chronic obstructive pulmonary disease: an integrated hospital and community based generic intermediate care service for prevention and early discharge. Chron Respir Dis. 2006;3:181–5.
24. Cotton MM, Bucknall CE, Dagg KD, et al. Early discharge for patients with exacerbations of chronic obstructive pulmonary disease: a randomized controlled trial. Thorax. 2000;55: 902–6.
25. Davies L, Wilkinson M, Bonner S, et al. "Hospital at home" versus hospital care in patients with exacerbations of chronic obstructive pulmonary disease: prospective randomized controlled trial. BMJ. 2000;32:1265–8.
26. Hernandez C, Casas A, Escarrabill J, et al. Home hospitalization of exacerbated chronic obstructive pulmonary disease patients. Eur Respir J. 2003;21:58–67.
27. Watson PB, Town GI, Holbrook N, et al. Evaluation of a self-management plan for chronic obstructive pulmonary disease. Eur Respir J. 1997;10:1267–71.
28. Poole PJ, Chase B, Frankel A, et al. Case management may reduce length of stay in patients with recurrent admissions for chronic obstructive pulmonary disease. Respirology. 2001;6:37–42.
29. Bourbeau J, Collet JP, Schwartzman K, et al. Economic benefits of self-management education COPD. Chest. 2006;130:1704–11.
30. Bourbeau J, Julien M, Maltais F, et al. Reduction of hospital use in patients with chronic obstructive pulmonary disease. Arch Intern Med. 2003;163:585–91.
31. Smith BJ, Adams R, Appleton SL, et al. The effect of a respiratory home nurse intervention in patients with chronic obstructive pulmonary disease (COPD). Aust N Z J Med. 1999; 29:718–25.

32. Hermiz O, Comino E, Marks G, et al. Randomized controlled trial of home based care of patients with chronic obstructive pulmonary disease. BMJ. 2002;325:938–40.
33. Monninkhof EM, van der Valk P, van der Palen J, et al. Effects of a comprehensive self-management programme in patients with chronic obstructive pulmonary disease. Eur Respir J. 2003;22:815–20.
34. Egan E, Clavarino A, Burridge L, et al. A randomized control trial of nursing-based case management for patients with chronic obstructive pulmonary disease. Lippincotts Case Manag. 2002;7:170–9.
35. Rabow MW, Dibble SL, Pantilat SZ, et al. The comprehensive care team: a controlled trial of outpatient palliative medicine consultation. Arch Intern Med. 2004;164:83–91.
36. Caress AL, Luker KA, Chalmers KI, et al. A review of the information and support needs of family carers of patients with chronic obstructive pulmonary disease. J Clin Nurs. 2009;18:479–91.
37. Jones JI, Kirby A, Ormiston P, et al. The needs of patients dying of chronic obstructive pulmonary disease in the community. Fam Pract. 2004;21:310–3.
38. Elkington H, White P, Addington-Hall J, et al. The health care needs of chronic obstructive pulmonary disease patients in their last year of life. Palliat Med. 2005;19:485–91.
39. von Gunten CF. Palliative care for pulmonary patients. Am J Respir Crit Care Med. 2010;182:725–31.
40. Teno JM, Clarridge BR, Casey V, et al. Family perspectives oon end-of-life care at the last place of care. JAMA. 2004;291:88–93.
41. Aiken LS, Butner J, Lockhart CA, et al. Outcome evaluation of a randomized trial of Phoenix-Care Intervention: program of case management and coordinated care for the seriously chronically ill. J Palliat Med. 2006;9:111–25.
42. Gazelle G. Understanding hospice-an underutilized option for life's final chapter. N Engl J Med. 2007;357:321–4.
43. Wewel AR, Gellermann I, Schwertfeger I, et al. Intervention by phone calls raises domiciliary activity and exercise capacity in patients with severe COPD. Respir Med. 2008;102:20–6.
44. Davis AH, Carrieri-Kohlman V, Janson SL, et al. Effects of treatment on two types of self-efficacy in people with chronic obstructive pulmonary disease. J Pain Symptom Manage. 2006;32:60–70.
45. Inal-Ince D, Savci S, Coplu L, et al. Factors determining self-efficacy in chronic obstructive pulmonary disease. Saudi Med J. 2005;26:542–7.
46. LaCasse Y, Wong E, Guyatt GH, et al. Meta-analysis of respiratory rehabilitation in chronic obstructive pulmonary disease. Lancet. 1996;348:1115–9.
47. Stewart AL, Hays RD, Wells KB, et al. Long-term functioning and well-being outcomes associated with physical activity and exercise in patients with chronic conditions in the Medical Outcomes Study. J Clin Epidemiol. 1994;47:719–30.
48. Bourjeily G, Rochester CL. Exercise training in chronic obstructive pulmonary disease. Clin Chest Med. 2000;21:763–81.
49. Sevick MA, Dunn AL, Morrow MS, et al. Cost-effectiveness of lifestyle and structured exercise interventions in sedentary adults: results of project ACTIVE. Am J Prev Med. 2000;19:1–8.
50. Troosters T, Gosselink R, Decramer M. Short- and long-term effects of outpatient rehabilitation in patients with chronic obstructive pulmonary disease: a randomized trial. Am J Med. 2007;109:207–12.
51. Dermon E, Marchand E, et al. Pulmonary rehabilitation in chronic obstructive pulmonary disease. Ann Readapt Med Phys. 2000;50:602–26.
52. Steele BG, Belza B, Cain KC, et al. A randomized clinical trial of an activity and exercise adherence intervention in chronic pulmonary disease. Arch Phys Med Rehabil. 2008;89:404–12.
53. Berry MJ, Rejeski WJ, Miller ME, et al. A lifestyle activity intervention in patients with chronic obstructive pulmonary disease. Respir Med. 2010;104:829–39.
54. de Blok BM, de Greef MH, ten Hacken NH, et al. The effects of a lifestyle physical activity counseling program with feedback of a pedometer during pulmonary rehabilitation in patients with COPD: a pilot study. Patient Educ Couns. 2006;61:48–55.

55. Hospes G, Bossenbroek L, ten Hacken NH, et al. Enhancement of daily physical activity increases physical fitness of outclinic COPD patients: results of an exercise counseling program. Patient Educ Couns. 2009;75:274–8.
56. Donesky-Cuenco D, Nguyen HQ, Paul S, et al. Yoga therapy decreases dyspnea-related distress and improves functional performance in people with chronic obstructive pulmonary disease: a pilot study. J Altern Complement Med. 2009;15:225–34.
57. Pomidori L, Campigotto F, Amatya TM, et al. Efficacy and tolerability of yoga breathing in patients with chronic obstructive pulmonary disease: a pilot study. J Cardiopulm Rehabil Prev. 2009;29:133–7.
58. Hochstetter JK, Lewis J, Soares-Smith L. An investigation into the immediate impact of breathlessness management on teh breathless patient: randomised controlled trial. Physiotherapy. 2005;91:178–85.
59. Wu X, Hou L, Bai W. Effects of breathing training on quality of life and activities of daily living in elderly patients with stable severe chronic obstructive pulmonary disease. Chinese J Rehabil Med. 2006;21:307–10.
60. Garrod R, Dallimore K, Cook J, et al. An evaluation of the acute impact of pursed lips breathing on walking distance in nonspontaneous pursed lips breathing chronic obstructive pulmonary disease patients. Chron Respir Dis. 2005;2:67–72.
61. Lichstein KL. Secondary insomnia: a myth dismissed. Sleep Med Rev. 2006;10:3–5.
62. Klink M, Quan SF. Prevalence of reported sleep disturbances in a general adult population and their relationship to obstructive airways diseases. Chest. 1987;91:540–6.
63. Cormick W, Olson LG, Hensley MJ, et al. Nocturnal hypoxaemia and quality of sleep in patients with chronic obstructive lung disease. Thorax. 1986;41:846–54.
64. Gooneratne NS, Gehrman PR, Nkwuo JE, et al. Consequences of comorbid insomnia symptoms and sleep-related breathing disorder in elderly subjects. Arch Intern Med. 2006;166:1732–8.
65. Katz DA, McHorney CA. Clinical correlates of insomnia in patients with chronic illness. Arch Intern Med. 1998;158:1099–107.
66. Milross MA, Piper AJ, Norman M, et al. Subjective sleep quality in cystic fibrosis. Sleep Med. 2002;3:205–12.
67. Chang PP, Ford DE, Mead LA, et al. Insomnia in young men and subsequent depression. The Johns Hopkins Precursors Study. Am J Epidemiol. 1997;146:105–14.
68. Jansson-Frojmark M, Lindblom K. A bidirectional relationship between anxiety and depression, and insomnia? A prospective study in the general population. J Psychosom Res. 2008;64:443–9.
69. Johnson EO, Roth T, Breslau N. The association of insomnia with anxiety disorders and depression: exploration of the direction of risk. J Psychiatr Res. 2006;40:700–8.
70. Rybarczyk B, Lopez M, Benson R, et al. Efficacy of two behavioral treatment programs for comorbid geriatric insomnia. Psychol Aging. 2002;17:288–98.
71. Rybarczyk B, Lopez M, Schelble K, et al. Home-based video CBT for comorbid geriatric insomnia: a pilot study using secondary data analyses. Behav Sleep Med. 2005;3:158–75.
72. Krakow B, Ulibarri V, Melendrez D, et al. A daytime, abbreviated cardio-respiratory sleep study (CPT 95807–52) to acclimate insomnia patients with sleep disordered breathing to positive airway pressure (PAP-NAP). J Clin Sleep Med. 2008;4:212–22.
73. Perlis ML, Jungquist C, Smith MT, Posner D, editors. Cognitive behavioral treatment of insomnia: a session-by-session guide. 1st ed. New York: Springer; 2005.
74. Rose C, Wallace L, Dickson R, et al. The most effective psychologically-based treatments to reduce anxiety and panic in patients with chronic obstructive pulmonary disease (COPD): a systematic review. Patient Educ Couns. 2002;47:311–8.
75. Livermore N, Sharpe L, McKenzie D. Panic attacks and panic disorder in chronic obstructive pulmonary disease: a cognitive behavioral perspective. Respir Med. 2010;104:1246–53.
76. Surtees PG, Wainwright NW, Luben R, et al. Mastery, sense of coherence, and mortality: evidence of independent associations from the EPIC-Norfolk Prospective Cohort Study. Health Psychol. 2006;25:102–10.
77. Nguyen HQ, Donesky-Cuenco D, Carrieri-kohlman V. Associations between symptoms, functioning, and perceptions of mastery with global self-rated health in patients with COPD: a cross-sectional study. Int J Nurs Stud. 2008;45:1355–65.

78. Devine EC, Pearcy J. Meta-analysis of the effects of psychoeducational care in adults with chronic obstructive pulmonary disease. Patient Educ Couns. 1996;29:167–78.
79. Porzelius J, Vest M, Nochomovitz M. Respiratory function, cognitions, and panic in chronic obstructive pulmonary patients. Behav Res Ther. 1992;30:75–7.
80. Antoni MH, Baggett L, Ironson G, et al. Cognitive-behavioral stress management intervention buffers distress responses and immunologic changes following notification of HIV-1 seropositivity. J Consult Clin Psychol. 1991;59:906–15.
81. Lutgendorf SK, Antoni MH, Ironson G, et al. Changes in cognitive coping skills and social support during cognitive behavioral stress management intervention and distress outcomes in symptomatic human immunodeficiency virus (HIV)-seropositive gay men. Psychosom Med. 1998;60:204–14.
82. Spiegel D, Bloom JR, Yalom I. Group support for patients with metastatic cancer. Arch Gen Psychiatry. 1981;38:527–33.
83. Blumenthal JA, Jiang W, Babyak MA, et al. Stress management and exercise treatment in cardiac patients with myocardial ischemia: effects on prognosis and mechanisms. Arch Intern Med. 1997;157:2213–23.
84. Frasure-Smith N, Prince R. The ischemic heart disease life stress monitoring program: impact on mortality. Psychosom Med. 1985;47:431–45.
85. Napolitano MA. Development of a pulmonary-specific quality of life scale (PQLS). Ann Behav Med. 1999;21:S168.
86. Wigal JK, Creer TL, Kotses H. The COPD self-efficacy scale. Chest. 1991;99:1193–6.
87. Armitage R. Sleep and circadian rhythms in mood disorders. Acta Psychiatr Scand Suppl. 2007;433:104–15.
88. Mellinger GD, Blater MB, Uhlenhuth EH. Insomnia and its treatment: prevalence and correlates. Arch Gen Psychiatry. 1985;42:225–32.
89. Overland S, Glozier N, Sivertsen B, et al. A comparison of insomnia and depression as predictors of disability pension: the HUNT Study. Sleep. 2008;31:875–80.
90. Millman RP, Fogel BS, McNamara ME, et al. Depression as a manifestation of obstructive sleep apnea: reversal with nasal continuous positive airway pressure. J Clin Psychiatry. 1989;50:348–51.
91. Perlis ML, Smith LJ, Lyness JM, et al. Insomnia as a risk factor for onset of depression in the elderly. Behav Sleep Med. 2006;4:104–13.
92. Morawetz D. Depression and insomnia. Aust Fam Physician. 2000;29:1016.
93. Baraniak A, Sheffield D. The efficacy of psychologically based interventions to improve anxiety, depression and quality of life in COPD: a systematic review and meta-analysis. Patient Educ Couns. 2010;doi: 10.1016/j.pec.2010.04.010
94. Carver CS, Scheier MF, Segerstrom SC. Optimism. Clin Psychol Rev. 2010; doi: 10.1016/j.cpr.2010.01.006
95. The Carrot, the Egg, and the Coffee Bean. http://www.bored.com/parablesite/index.html
96. Cooper CB. Airflow obstruction and exercise. Respir Med. 2009;103:325–34.
97. Nguyen HQ, Carrieri-Kohlman V, Rankin S, et al. Is internet-based support for dyspnea self-management in patients with chronic obstructive pulmonary disease possible? Results of a pilot study. Heart Lung. 2005;34:51–62.
98. KSERA Project. http://ksera.ieis.tue.nl/

Afterword

Marshall I. Hertz and Linda Chlan

Dramatic changes have occurred during the past 30 years in regard to complementary, alternative, and integrative therapeutic approaches—for acute illness, for chronic medical conditions, and for disease prevention and health maintenance. Clearly, the public has become increasingly aware and accepting of their utility: In fact, it estimated that more than one-third of adults in the United States use at least one of these therapies [1]. At least in part due to pressure from patients, healthcare providers have gradually adopted a more open-minded attitude to these therapies. Health insurers and major healthcare organizations have also added many of these approaches to their benefit plans and services, and many have developed formal integrative therapy programs and clinics. Despite all of this there is lively debate, both in scientific journals and in the lay press [2], regarding the value, efficacy, and clinical applicability of integrative therapies.

In this volume, we have tried to put into perspective the current state of science and practice related to selected integrative therapies for lung diseases, critical illness, and sleep disorders. We have learned that a wide variety of nontraditional therapies are being employed for a diverse group of disorders, ranging from asthma to lung cancer to critical illness. We have also learned that the extent to which these therapies are used for individual disorders is highly variable. For example, asthma has been treated using many nontraditional means for hundreds or thousands of years (as detailed by Li et al. in Chap. 15 and by Fine and Blumenthal in Chap. 3); while there are few, if any, descriptions of their use for pulmonary fibrosis and pulmonary hypertension (refer to Chap. 5).

The major question to be answered about any therapy is, "Does it work?" This simple question often defies a simple answer, as discussed in detail by Halm and Katseres in Chap. 2. Although the randomized clinical trial has become the "gold standard" for evaluating the efficacy of medical treatments, there are few examples of large, randomized, blinded clinical trials of integrative therapies for lung disease—and the vast majority of the published literature reports case series and small clinical trials. This may appear to be a deficiency at first glance; however, other methods of evaluation may, in fact, be more useful for more complicated interventions and for those involving more subjective endpoints. In addition, many integrative therapies

L. Chlan and M.I. Hertz (eds.), *Integrative Therapies in Lung Health and Sleep*, Respiratory Medicine 4, DOI 10.1007/978-1-61779-579-4

(e.g., massage and yoga) are not amenable to blinding; in these cases, qualitative research methods and evaluation of "therapy bundles" may be more useful than a randomized clinical trial. In addition, the mechanism by which integrative therapies provide benefit to patients may be indirect. For example, the use of massage therapy during medical illness may result in improved clinical outcomes—not due to a direct effect of the massage on the mechanism of illness but because the massage improved the patients' ability to complete the medical therapy. In this case, a randomized clinical trial of massage vs. no massage might incorrectly conclude that there was no difference between the groups, particularly when the results are corrected for the amount of medical therapy they received.

Another important theme is that there are major interindividual differences in response to most therapies, which can be lost when attention is only paid to the average response. This is no different for integrative or alternative therapies than for allopathic therapies. The plethora of medications that are available for hypertension, constipation, and allergic disorders is powerful testimony that different people respond differently to medications. Likewise, it should not be a surprise that the benefit of yoga for COPD patients, for example, is quite variable from patient to patient (as discussed in Chap. 4).

Partly as a result of the large spectrum of available integrative therapies, major deficiencies remain in our evidence base regarding their efficacy for patients with lung disease and other major medical illness. Specifically, there are still major gaps in our understanding of which nontraditional medical therapies are effective; by which mechanisms they are effective; and for which patients and conditions they are effective. This has led the National Institutes of Health to create the National Center for Complementary and Alternative Medicine (NCCAM), whose mission is "to define, through rigorous scientific investigation, the usefulness and safety of complementary and alternative medicine interventions and their roles in improving health and health care" [3]. In addition, at least 47 academic medical centers have formed the Consortium of Academic Health Centers for Integrative Medicine, whose mission is to advance the principles and practices of integrative healthcare within academic institutions [4]. These and other organizations and funding sources will further the basic, preclinical, and clinical research that is needed to answer the many remaining questions regarding the most effective ways complementary and integrative therapies can be employed to treat disease and improve human health.

References

1. Complementary and alternative medicine use among adults and children: United States, 2007. National Health Statistics Reports. No. 12. 10 Dec 2008.
2. Freedman DH. The triumph of new-age medicine. The Atlantic. July/Aug 2011.
3. http://nccam.nih.gov/
4. http://www.imconsortium.org.

Index

MIX
Papier aus verantwortungsvollen Quellen
Paper from responsible sources
FSC® C105338

If you have any concerns about our products,
you can contact us on
ProductSafety@springernature.com

In case Publisher is established outside the EU,
the EU authorized representative is:
Springer Nature Customer Service Center GmbH
Europaplatz 3, 69115 Heidelberg, Germany

Printed by Libri Plureos GmbH
in Hamburg, Germany